THIRD, REVISED EDITION

with 492 illustrations, of which 308 are
color photomicrographs
and 78 electron photomicrographs

Color Atlas & Textbook of Tissue and Cellular Pathology

by Professor WALTER SANDRITTER
Director of the Pathological Institute,
Freiburg University

with the assistance of
Dr. G. BENEKE, Professor W. KNOTH, Dr. H. LÖFFLER, Dr. K. NOESKE,
Professor K. H. SALFELDER and Professor J. SCHORN†

Translated and edited by
WILLIAM B. WARTMAN, M.D.
Morrison Professor of Pathology,
Northwestern University, Chicago

YEAR BOOK MEDICAL PUBLISHERS · INC.
35 EAST WACKER DRIVE · CHICAGO

Year Book Medical Publishers, Inc. 1969.

What is hardest of all to do?
What seems to you the easiest:
To see with your own eyes,
What your eyes lay before you.

GOETHE

To the memory of

ARNOLD LAUCHE

September 14, 1890 – September 29, 1959

Director of the Pathological Institute of the University of Frankfort on the Main

1943 – 1959

GEORG HERZOG

November 4, 1884 – April 2, 1962

Director of the Pathological Institute of the University of Giessen

1926 – 1954

Preface to the Third German Edition

Not quite four years after the appearance of the first edition of this book, a third edition has become necessary. Seemingly the terse text and schematic diagrams of this atlas have proved a useful guide to students in their study of the complexities of abnormal histological structures. Thus the basic premise of the book has been given new support.

The text has been carefully gone over and in certain places has been revised or expanded. Some of the illustrations have either been replaced or the old ones improved (Figs. 6, 78, 92, 116, 123, 128, 134, 187, 223, 259, 314, 319, 356a, 389, 437, 474, 492).

I wish to thank Dr. STEPHANI for help with the index and Miss BARNERFOR for assistance with the photographs and drawings.

Freiburg, Summer 1968

W. SANDRITTER

Preface to the Second German Edition

The first edition of *Histopathologie* was sold out in a surprisingly short time. This favorable reception of the book may be traced chiefly to the previous lack of a student textbook on histopathology. The translation of the second edition of the book into several other languages as well as co-editions (English, Italian, Japanese, Spanish) makes clear that pathological anatomy is still a common world language.

In the second edition, some of the chapters have been enlarged (lymph nodes, bones, endocrine glands) and several new have ones been added: *Skin*, by Professor W. KNOTH, Department of Dermatology, University of Giessen; *Blood and bone marrow*, by Dr. H. LÖFFLER, Department of Medicine, University of Giessen, and *Fungi and parasites*, by Professor K. SALFELDER, Director of the Institute of Pathology, Merida University, Venezuela. Dr. G. BENEKE, chief physician at the Pathological Institute, has written the chapter on *Bones* and Dr. K. NOESKE has expanded the chapter on *Lymph nodes*.

I have to thank many colleagues for much constructive criticism and many helpful suggestions. My particular thanks go also to the many students who have taken the trouble to call attention to various mistakes.

I am indebted for histological preparations to the following to whom I extend my thanks: Professor KAHLAU, Frankfurt, Professor KRACHT, Hamburg, Dr. HÜBNER, Frankfurt. I have received much valuable aid from lengthy discussions with Dr. MÖLBERT, Freiburg, Professor HEDINGER, Lausanne, Professor BOHLE, Tübingen, Professor GUSEK, Hamburg, Dr. THOENES and Dr. BANNASCH, Würzburg, Dr. GIESEKING, Münster, Dr. KORB and Dr. TOTOVIĆ, Marburg. Professor ALTMANN, Würzburg, has kindly allowed me to use Figure 223.

Several American colleagues have generously provided electron photomicrographs for use in several of the chapters. This expanding dimension of morphology is now responsible for so much of our newer knowledge that a textbook lacking this bridge between histology and biochemistry is no longer conceivable.

My fellow workers at the Institute have generously given much help in the preparation of the second edition. I am especially indebted to Dr. B. LEDERER and to our photographer, Mr. M. HESSE.

Senator SCHATTAUER and Professor MATIS have always encouraged me with understanding and energetic support. For this I express to them my heart-felt thanks as well as for their success in increasing greatly the number of illustrations and the contents of the book without increasing the price, for which I know the purchasers of this book will also be thankful.

Giessen, May 1966

W. SANDRITTER

Preface to the First German Edition

In considering the functions of a textbook of pathology intended for students of medicine, particularly in the context of current knowledge of pathology, one comes to the conclusion that *teaching can profitably stem from the optical aspect, that is, from the microscopic and submicroscopic picture.* The "typical" microscopic structure should be the constant companion of the student in his clinical studies and serve as a firm foundation for his evaluation of the diseases he sees. From this point of view, pathological histology and cytology are more than a propos for examinations – more importantly, they are a supplement to the textbooks of clinical medicine and pathology and can be used simultaneously with them. Needless to say, however, this book can never replace the study of actual histological sections.

In order to accomplish the purposes of the book, the material has been organized around the *principles of special pathology,* the correlation to clinical cases being thus facilitated and the student's knowledge of general pathology enlarged. The comments on general pathology in the Introduction and the corresponding illustrations may be used to review this subject. It was included for the special benefit of the beginner in order to guide him in his interpretation of the photomicrographs in the latter part of the book. The technical comments explaining the proper use of the microscope are intended similarly.

This book is oriented toward the student and the beginner in pathology. However, in view of the great amount of material, choices had to be made. We have made an effort to give preference to the typical and the representative – in view of the multiplicity of choices, this was a most difficult task. Illustrative schematic drawings have been included for clarification and, as far as is practical within the scope of the book, depict simplified didactic versions of functional aspects of pathological processes.

The illustrations are a paramount feature of the book. The explanations of the pictures have been kept as brief as possible and have been placed on the page opposite so that picture and text may be easily compared. The organization of the book into a sort of atlas has brought about many difficulties – the brevity of the explanations being among them – yet, in the end, it seemed to us that the benefits of this plan far outweighed its shortcomings. The text is arranged in such a fashion that an introductory sentence gives a short definition which is followed by a description explaining not only the particular picture under discussion, but also taking into account the common variations. Short references to the macroscopic appearances and pathogenesis are added where they are deemed to help in understanding the microscopic features. A short *literature index,* arranged according to special fields, includes both original papers and review articles and should make possible intensive study when this is desired.

The authors of this book hope for attentive observers and readers. Should the book, in addition to being instructive, arouse critical discussion, then it will have fulfilled its purpose.

The most beautiful part of this book, the illustrations, is the work of JULIUS SCHORN, M.D. A tragic mishap in the United States has removed him from his most productive work, but my memory of him acted as an incentive for me to finish this book.

Particular thanks are due to the following assistants: Mr. K. WEIL in Frankfort, to whom we owe the schematic drawings, Mr. M. HESSE, photographer at the Institute, and Miss H. NITSCHKE, technical assistant.

Drs. G. BENEKE, K. NOESKE, and B. LEDERER assisted me with valuable advice and energetic support.

We owe Senator F. K. SCHATTAUER a debt of gratitude for his generous patronage; without his indefatigable urging and his understanding this book would never have come to life.

Giessen, Christmas 1964   W. SANDRITTER
                                                                Institute of Pathology,
                                                                Justus-Liebig University, Giessen

"A man is like a bit of Labrador spar, which has no lustre as you turn it in your hand until you come to a particular angle; then it shows deep and beautiful colors."

RALPH WALDO EMERSON

"In learning we have developed the requisite processes of thinking, and this training is not lost as long as we are possessed of our full mental vigor."

THEODOR BILLROTH

Preface to the English Edition

The ways of writing about pathology are infinitely varied and are naturally influenced by the author's background. In the present book, Professor SANDRITTER and associates approach the subject with the experience and techniques of trained observers of form and function and skilled experimentalists, quick at characterization and accurate description of the structural features of disease revealed by the microscope, always on the scent of new approaches, inclined to apply the historical method on occasion, more intent on using the facts of pathology to further the understanding of disease processes than on the acquisition of the facts for their own sake and alert to the impact of the results of animal experiments and of cellular biology on traditional opinions. This makes for easy, agreeable reading and a lively presentation of a subject that has made important additions to knowledge in the past and is now making new and even more exciting contributions.

Although the book is explicitly written for medical students and for young men and women who are beginning their careers as professional pathologists, nevertheless physicians in many special areas of medicine as well as experienced pathologists will find the point of view presented in the book provocative and informative. In essence, the point of view is the study of pathology and, in particular, of special or systematic pathology, taking as a starting point the evidence provided by the light and electron microscopes. This evidence is supplemented by pertinent information obtained from the macroscopic appearances of diseased organs and tissues, the clinical features of disease and the results of experiments on animals. The method used to make clear the authors' viewpoint is a simple one – the study of an atlas of remarkable photomicrographs of type lesions illustrating the principles of general pathology and the characteristic diseases of the different organ systems of the body. Not only are the illustrations fully described and the important features carefully marked, but many of the disease processes are concisely summarized in a series of unusually lucid diagrams. Thus, the student is carefully guided through the complexities of the microscopic appearances of diseased cells and tissues.

The authors have at all times kept clearly in mind that the chief value of pathology for most students is to improve their understanding of disease and to help them in their practical work at the bedside. For example, the results of recent studies with the electron microscope are so carefully woven into the fabric of the book that the reader easily perceives how they join the facts of traditional morphology with those of biochemistry and cellular biology to produce a coherent pattern. Indeed, it may truthfully be said that the book looks at pathology from the fundamental angle of molecular biology. In this respect, the authors have pointed out the path we shall all tread in the years to come.

The beauty of the illustrations, apparent even at a glance, stands forth as an exceptional feature of the book. Study of them will make clear the care with which the material for illustration has been selected, the skill with which it has been photographed and labeled and the excellence of the reproduction and printing. These things speak for themselves, and of themselves are valuable additions to the literature of pathology.

The task of translating the book has been a pleasant one. I have tried faithfully to convey the authors' ideas as I understand them and to preserve something of the flavor of their style, while at the same time putting the book into English which will not be foreign to the ear. I have edited the book, for the most part, only to the extent of bringing terminology into accordance with commonly used American and English practice. In certain parts of the book the German points of view are somewhat different from those given in most books in English. I have not attempted to modify these sections, believing that, for the student and teacher alike, it is valuable to know that there are different ways of looking at many angles of medicine. Too often, the student is unaware that different viewpoints are not only possible but actually exist.

The first German edition of this book carried the title *Histopathologie*, and this title has also been used for the second German edition although the scope of the book has been greatly expanded. With the permission of Professor Sandritter, we have changed the title for the English edition, which is a translation of the second German edition, to *Color Atlas and Textbook of Tissue and Cellular Pathology*, since it gives a better idea of the contents of the book.

I have been fortunate during the preparation of the translation to have the advice and help of my colleagues and students. PETER HERDSON, M.D., has reviewed the parts dealing with electron microscopy, and HERBERT M. SOMMERS, M.D., the chapter on Fungi and Parasites. ROBERT B. JENNINGS, M.D., and JOSEPH C. SHERRICK, M.D., have given advice on portions of the chapter on General Pathology and the chapter on the Spleen and Lymph Nodes. Two of my medical students, L. D. VOEGELE and M. STEWART, have helped with the translation of the latter part of the book. To all of them and to my secretaries, particularly to Mrs. LOWELLA RIVERO, and to the publishers, go my sincere thanks for all their help and to Dr. PETER HERDSON for assistance with proofreading.

Chicago, August 1966   W. B. WARTMAN

Contents

List of the Electron Photomicrographs

I wish to express my sincere thanks to the many colleagues who have so generously loaned electron photomicrographs and to the publishers who have kindly consented to their publication. Unfortunately it was not possible to cite the literature and publisher in the legends for the illustrations.

Professor W. BERNHARD, Institut de Recherches Scientifiques sur le Cancer, Villejuif, Seine
Figs. 384, 386, 387

Dr. P. BANNASCH, Pathologisches Institut der Universität Würzburg
Figs. 214, 217, 218

Dr. C. BIAVA, Loyola University, School of Medicine, Department of Pathology, Chicago, Illinois
Figs. 215 and 216 from: Labor. Invest. *13*: 1099 (1964), The Williams and Wilkins Company, Baltimore, Maryland; Fig. 219: American Journal Path. *46*: 775 (1965), Harper & Row Publishers; Fig. 221: Labor. Invest. *13*: 301 (1964), The Williams and Wilkins Company, Baltimore; Fig. 222: Labor. Invest. *13*: 301 (1964)

Dozent Dr. CAESAR and Dr. SCHIRASAWA, Pathologisches Institut der Universität Kiel
Fig. 24

Dozent Dr. CAESAR, Pathologisches Institut der Universität Kiel
Figs. 253, 267, 268

Professor W. GUSEK, Pathologisches Institut der Universität Hamburg
Figs. 33, 34, 35, 36, 37, 385, 388

Dozent Dr. GIESEKING, Pathologisches Institut der Universität Münster
Figs. 14, 25, 26, 27, 29, 107, 108, 109, 110, 111
From the monograph: Mesenchymale Gewebe und ihre Reaktionsformen im elektronenmikroskopischen Bild. G. Fischer, Stuttgart 1966

Professor H. HAGER, Neuropathologisches Institut der Universität Gießen
Figs. 17, 18, 367, 368, 369, 370
Fig. 362 from: Beitr. Path. *130*: 422 (1964), Fig. 3 – G. Fischer-Verlag, Stuttgart

Dr. G. HÜBNER, Pathologisches Institut der Universität Köln
Fig. 213

Prof. KLEINSCHMIDT, Hygiene-Institut der Universität Frankfurt
Fig. 98

Dr. G. KÖPPEL, Elektronenmikroskopische Abteilung des Pathologischen Instituts in Gießen
Fig. 99

Dozent Dr. KORB, Pathologisches Institut der Universität Marburg
Figs. 53, 54, 55, 56, 57

Professor H. LAPP and Dr. NIKULIN, Pathologisches Institut der Universität Frankfurt
Fig. 97
from: Frankfurter Zschr. für Path. *74* (1965)

Dr. G. MAJNO and Dr. G. E. PALADE, Department of Pathology, Harvard Medical School, Boston, Mass.
Fig. 22 from: J. Biophys. Biochem. Cytol. *11*: 571 (1961)

Professor F. MILLER, Elektronenmikroskopische Abteilung des Pathologischen Institutes der Universität München
Figs. 30, 31, 211, 212, 235

Dr. MOVAT and Dr. N. V. P. FERNANDO, University of Toronto, Department of Pathology, Canada
Fig. 23 from: Labor. Invest. *12*: 895 (1963).

Professor H. POPPER and Professor F. SCHAFFNER, Mount Sinai Hospital, New York
Fig. 220

Dr. H. PROSE, Dr. L. LEE and Dr. S. BALG, New York University, School of Medicine, Department of Pathology
Fig. 16: Amer. J. Path. *47:* 493 (1965).

Dr. N. F. RODMAN, Dr. R. G. MASON and Dr. K. E. BRINKHOUS
Fig. 96 from: Federation Proceedings *22:* 1356 (1963)

Dr. SCHÄFER, Medizinische Universitätsklinik Würzburg
Fig. 254

Dr. H. E. SCHROEDER, Zahnärztliches Institut der Universität Zürich, Schweiz
Figures produced at: Dental Institute, University of Aarhus, Abt. f. Elektronenmikroskopie, Dänemark
Fig. 11 and Fig. in Table 4

Dozent Dr. W. THOENES, Pathologisches Institut der Universität Würzburg
Figs. 236, 252, 254 – in Verh. Dtsch. Ges. Path. (1965), S. 14, G. Fischer-Verlag, Stuttgart

Dozent Dr. TOTOVIĆ, Pathologisches Institut der Universität Marburg, Laboratorium für Elektronenmikroskopie
Figs. 15, 19, 28, 231, 232, 233, 234, 237
Fig. 15 and Fig. 19 in Virch. Arch. *340:* 251 (1966), Springer-Verlag

Dozent Dr. WESSEL, Pathologisches Institut der Universität Bonn
Fig. 13

Dr. J. WIENER, D. SPIRO and R. G. LATTES, Columbia University, New York, Department of Pathology
Fig. 32 from Amer. J. Path. *47:* 457 (1965).

Introduction – General Pathology

A certain amount of practical knowledge and skill, particularly with respect to use of the light microscope, is desirable on the part of the reader if he is to get the most good from reading a textbook of histopathology. Profitable use of the microscope requires knowledge of its construction and of the interrelations of its individual parts. Furthermore, it is only possible to interpret a histological slide after one is informed as to how the tissue has been prepared for cutting and how it has been stained. A solid foundation in normal Histology and General Pathology goes without saying, for the principles of General Pathology are used constantly in Special Pathology.

Preliminary Technical Remarks

Use of Microscope

The light source, the lens system with its diaphragms and the eye must all be correctly aligned with one another in order to obtain optimal information from a histological section. Artificial light, which consists predominantly of yellowish red light rays, can be corrected by a blue filter so that it will approximate daylight. Köhler's principle is commonly used to adjust the light source, since by using this principle it is possible to illuminate only the object area that is to be examined and that entirely uniformly. With a microscope with a built-in light source, swing in the front lens of the condenser. Focus the microscope on the specimen and stop down the *field diaphragm*. Rack up the condenser as far as possible and then lower it slowly, thus focusing the field diaphragm within the specimen area.

Center the condenser with the two centering screws, if necessary (the condensers of many student microscopes are permanently centered so that this step may be omitted). Open the field diaphragm until its shadow disappears from the field of view. The field diaphragm should always be adjusted so that its image just disappears behind the edge of the eyepiece stop. Adjust image contrast and, if necessary, sharpness – but not image brightness – with the *condenser (aperture) diaphragm* by opening it entirely and then closing it down just far enough to remove glare from the specimen. Unstained objects can be seen best when the condenser diaphragm is closed as far as possible or with a phase contrast microscope. With blurred images, reducing the condenser diaphragm will increase the contrast.

The microscopic image is produced by diffraction of the light by the structures in the histological preparation in the focal plane at the back of the objective (primary image). The secondary image, which is the one observed in the ocular, arises from magnification of the primary image.

Objective and ocular must be properly matched. In usual histological practice, an ocular with a 10× magnification is used with the following objectives, in which the first number gives the magnification and the second the numerical aperture of the objective, which is a measure of its resolving power:

1. *Scanning lens:* objective 2.5 to 5.0 – magnification 25–50×.
2. *Low magnification:* objective 10/0.25 – magnification 100×.
3. *High dry magnification:* objective 40/0.65 – magnification 400×.

For still higher magnification, especially for examination of smears of cells (blood, lymph node), oil immersion objectives (100/1.25) are available with a magnification up to 1,000×.

When using the microscope, the following suggestions will prove helpful. With a monocular microscope, always keep both eyes open, since the adjustment for distance obtained in this way prevents rapid eye fatigue due to constant accommodation.

The lowest magnification should always be used before going to the other objectives because it is easier to orient the various structures under low magnification.

If the image is blurred, you should think of the possibility of the slide being upside down with the cover-slip resting on the stage of the microscope.

Preparation and Staining of Histological Sections

Sections are prepared from blocks of tissue measuring about 1×1 cm. The selected tissue is usually hardened and fixed in formol (ordinary 40% commercial formalin diluted with water $1:9$ so that the resulting solution is about 4%). The *hardening* results from coagulation and denaturation of protein, while the *fixation* arrests autolysis and bacterial decomposition. In order to prepare sections 5–10 micra thick, the tissue must have a consistency suitable for cutting. To obtain this, the tissue may either be frozen (at $-20°$ C.) with carbon dioxide snow and cut on the frozen-section microtome (this method is used particularly for demonstrating fat or for rapid diagnosis of biopsy specimens at the time of surgery) or the tissue can be processed through a series of alcohols (from 70 to 100%), methyl-benzoate, and benzol into paraffin with a melting point of 56° C. Liquid paraffin at 60° C. penetrates the finest tissue spaces and produces a good cutting consistency. After cutting on a microtome, the sections are mounted on microscopic slides and stained, after first being deparaffinized with xylol.

Note: Frozen sections permit demonstration of neutral fat – in paraffin sections, the fat is dissolved by alcohol and the droplets of fat appear as optically empty spaces in the tissue.

The methods used for *histological staining* have been developed empirically and the physical-chemical basis for them is not exactly known except in a few cases. Electrostatic binding, among other factors, plays a principal role. Negatively charged groups, for example, nucleic acids (phosphate groups) or proteins (-COOH groups) or the mucopolysaccharides (-COOH.SO$_4$), bind with the basic dye groups, which behave as cations. Acid dyes (e. g., eosin) with electron negative charges bind predominantly with positively charged protein groups (NH$_2$-groups). Excess and easily soluble dye in the tissue is removed after staining by differentiation in water, alcohol or weak acid. Finally, the water is removed with 70 and 96% alcohol, the section immersed in a clearing agent (xylol), mounted in Permount or Canada balsam and covered with a cover-slip.

For further details on histological techniques, see Davenport, Lilly, Humason, etc.

Histochemistry deals with specific and sometimes quantitative identification of chemical substances in tissues, such as nucleic acids, certain proteins, carbohydrates, enzymes, etc. (see Pearse, 1960).

Artifacts in histological sections are caused chiefly by improper fixation, embedding (cracks or tears) or staining (transparent, unstained flaws).

Table 1 reviews the features of some commonly used stains. *Fluorescence microscopy,* in which tissues are stained with fluorescing dyes and examined under ultraviolet light, allows detection of certain substances, e. g., immunologically active proteins, because the ultraviolet light rays (e. g., 350 Mμ) liberate secondary rays in the visible range (compare Figs. 358 and 361 on p. 218). Some substances show self fluorescence, e. g., lipids, porphyrins and elastic fibers.

Table 1. **Staining Methods**

Method	Results		Remarks
Hematoxylin-eosin (H & E)	**Blue** *Hematoxylin* Basophilic cytoplasm, nuclei, bacteria, calcium	**Red** *Eosin* Cytoplasm, connective & all other tissues	Fig. 47
van Gieson (v. G.)	**Yellow** *Picric Acid* Cytoplasm, muscle, amyloid, fibrin, fibrinoid	**Red** *Fuchsin* Connective tissue, hyalin	**Black** *Iron Hematoxylin* Nuclei Fig. 52
Elastic stain	**Black** *Resorcin-fuchsin* Elastic fibers	**Red** *Nuclear fast red* Nuclei	Figs. 90, 91
Elastic-van Gieson (E.v.G.)	used in combination with above		Fig. 95
Azan	**Red** *Azocarmine* Nuclei, erythrocytes, fibrin, fibrinoid, acidophilic cytoplasm	**Blue** *Aniline blue, Orange G* Collagen fibers, basophilic cytoplasm mucus	Fig. 225
Silver stain	**Black** *Ammoniacal AgNO$_3$* Reticulum fibers, nerve fibers		Collagen fibers brown Fig. 276
Fat stain	**Red** *Sudan III, Scarlet Red* Neutral fat	**Blue** *Hematoxylin* Nuclei, cytoplasm	Fig. 45
Congo red	**Red** *Congo red* Amyloid	**Blue** *Hematoxylin* Nuclei	Fig. 265
Weigert's fibrin stain	**Blue** *Lugol's solution, Crystal violet* Fibrin, bacteria	**Red** *Nuclear fast red* Nuclei	Not specific for fibrin Fig. 131
Berlin-blue reaction	**Blue** *Calcium ferrocyanide* Hemosiderin, Fe^3	**Red** *Nuclear fast red* Nuclei	Fig. 104
Giemsa (May-Grünwald-Giemsa)	**Blue** *Methyl violet* Nuclei, all basophilic substances	**Red** *Azur-eosin* Eosinophils, cytoplasm & its granules, collagen fibers	Metachromatic: Mast cells violet Melanin green Fig. 278

Table 1. **Staining Methods** (cont'd)[1]

Method	Results		Remarks
Spielmeyer's myelin stain	**Blue-black** *Iron-alum hematoxylin* Myelin, erythrocytes		Fig. 383
Ziehl-Neelsen	**Red** *Carbofuchsin* Acid-fast rods, Tb bacilli, lepra bacilli	**Blue** *Hemalum* Nuclei	Fig. 139
Periodic Acid–Schiff Reaction (PAS)	**Red** *Schiff Reagent* Adjacent hydroxyl groups and amino-alcohols		Neutral and acid polysaccharides Fig. 466
Levaditi	**Black** *AgNO₃-Reduced* *Pyrogallic acid* Spirocheta pallida Listerella mono-cytogenes		Fig. 194
Thionine, Toluidine Blue	**Blue** Basophilic cytoplasm	**Blue** Nuclei	Mucus, mucin, lipids are metachromatic, Fig. 359

1 See Table 3, p. 10 and Table 10, p. 270, for other special stains.

Histological Interpretation and Diagnosis

A famous physician (FRANZ VOLHARD) once said: "*The Gods have put diagnosis before therapy – man must put careful observation and interpretation before diagnosis.*" *Analysis must precede synthesis* as it does in all other branches of knowledge. Analysis begins with the examination of the subject with a clear-cut objective in mind. *Careful observation* of similarities and dissimilarities, the separation of the typical and the atypical, the general from the special, all contribute to the desired knowledge of the subject. The arrangement, color, size and form of the tissue elements and their relations to one another all help to determine the essential characteristics of the various structures under consideration. As such observations cannot be obtained without adequate preparation, a thorough theoretical grounding and a certain amount of experience become essential.

The beginning student will find it helpful in getting exact histological details either to make drawings or to set down his observations in abbreviated, outline form. The student is thus forced to emphasize the essential features and to de-emphasize unessential ones.

After first carefully making the necessary observations, it is then possible to take the second step, that is, to synthesize the observations and make a diagnosis. On the other hand, hasty, careless examination will often lead to an incorrect opinion. In order to arrive at a *diagnosis*, the histological observations need to be classified in some logical manner, usually one which has been reached through a compromise of experience and hypothesis. But, by its very nature, no diagnosis can be considered final, since it can change with the progress of scientific knowledge. Thus, it is understandable that an exact description retains its validity indefinitely, even when the interpretation and diagnosis of a section have already been revised.

The student will therefore be well advised to put his chief effort into a careful description of a microscopic section. In examinations, this is always graded higher than a diagnosis unsupported by accurate description.

In practice, the first step in examining a histological preparation is to look at the section with the *unaided eye*. The shape and the various components of the tissue structures – easily recognized by differences in staining – often provide essential topographical information and have an important influence on the next step in the analysis of the section. An inverted ocular used as a scanning lens will provide an over-all view of the tissue at very low magnification. Ordinary *low-power magnification* can then be used to examine in greater detail the structures already seen with the inverted ocular. In this way, a rough over-all picture of the essential elements of the lesion is formed. Further details can also be distinguished with *low magnification*, such as the size and position of the nuclei and the structure of the cytoplasm. This magnification is probably the most useful of all, for at a magnification of about one hundred-fold, all the essential structures are well seen without losing the over-all architectural relationships. A drawing at this stage of the examination will fix the typical findings firmly in mind. Practically all histological preparations can be diagnosed with low magnification. *Higher magnification* is used only to clarify individual details, such as the shape and division of nuclear chromatin, mitoses, and so forth.

Such a methodical approach is an essential prerequisite for profitable observation and correct diagnosis.

Notes on General Pathology[1])

These brief, almost stenographic, introductory remarks about general pathology are intended only as a means of making it easier to understand the complexities of special pathology. Reference to the appropriate illustrations of the book permits its use as a guide to the principles of general pathology.

A knowledge of general pathology is an excellent foundation for the study of disease. The knowledge so obtained can be applied in nearly all special situations, since *the host in reacting to the many different pathological stimuli that may affect it has only a limited number of possible responses available*. These originate essentially from either transient or permanent increase *(anabolism)* or decrease of metabolism *(catabolism)* or from *work failure*. In addition, complex tissue responses occur in *circulatory disturbances*, the various forms of *inflammation* and in *tumors*.

---

1 For a more detailed treatment of the subject see the textbooks of ANDERSON, BOYD, FLOREY, MONTGOMERY, MUIR-CAPPELL, PEREZ-TAMAYO and ROBBINS as well as HENKE-LUBARSCH.

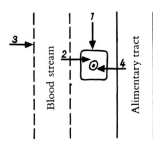

Fig. 1. See text for explanation.

In theory, pathological stimuli can reach the cells and tissues in various ways (Fig. 1):

1) *directly* (e. g., trauma, radiant energy). 2) by way of the *blood stream* or the *lymphatics* with resultant direct cell injury (e. g., toxins, alterations of the vascular contents as in thrombosis). 3) *indirectly*, when the stimulus acts on the *vessel walls*, a secondary circulatory disturbance then causing the cell injury (e. g., nervous derangement of permeability). 4) the pathological stimulus can come from the *alimentary tract*. Finally, primary (e. g., inborn) defects of metabolism may cause secondary cellular reactions.

The following diagram sets out the possible reactions of the organism to pathological stimuli in simple fashion (Fig. 2).

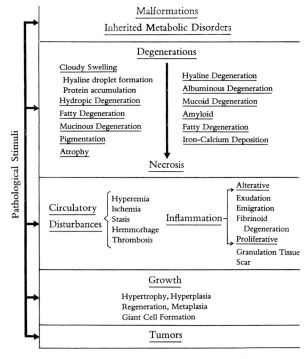

Fig. 2. Schematic survey of possible host reactions to pathological stimuli.

Malformations : Inherited Metabolic Disorders

Malformations or *metabolic disorders* can develop in the embryonal (up to the third month of pregnancy) and fetal periods (after the third month) either because of inborn errors in the genetic material or of the action of pathological stimuli (e. g., teratogens). These manifest themselves, for example, either in *agenesis* (absence of enzymes, e. g., galactosemia; defective organ formation) or *aplasia* or *hypoplasia* (absence or faulty development of existing organs). A great number of different manifestations can be produced in this way.

Degenerations

The different sorts of *degeneration* are morphological manifestations of metabolic disturbances either of cells (left-hand column of Fig. 2) or of intercellular substances (right-hand column of Fig. 2).

Cloudy swelling and hydropic degeneration (Fig. 3) result from disturbance of the metabolic systems that maintain the ionic environment of cells (so-called ion pumps). When these regulatory mechanisms fail, then sodium and water flow into the cells and potassium leaves them. As a result, the mitochondria swell and the cytoplasm appears to be filled with fine "protein granules" *(cloudy swelling)*. The resulting cloudiness is due to increased scattering of light *(Tyndall effect)*. The mitochondria may also be transformed into water-filled vesicles *(hydropic transformation* of mitochondria). The water may accumulate in the ground substance or cause widening of the cisternae of the endoplasmic reticulum (hydropic degeneration). Compare Figure 224 (light photomicrograph) with Figures 53, 56, 217 and 213 ff. (electron photomicrographs). Also see pp. 14 and 147.

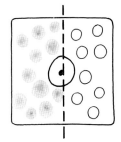

Fig. 3. Cloudy swelling (left), hydropic degeneration (right).

Nuclei may also show swelling *(degenerative nuclear swelling)*. This must be distinguished, however, from physiological or *functional nuclear swelling*, which is often accompanied by enlargement of the nucleolus and is a reflection of increased metabolic work.

Hyalin droplet degeneration (protein accumulation) should be distinguished from cloudy swelling (Fig. 4). The microscopical appearances of the two conditions can be similar, but in hyalin droplet degeneration active work is performed by the cell (anabolism) with accumulation of protein (cytoplasmic coacervation), for example, the reabsorption of protein in the renal tubules. Such reabsorption of material is accomplished by pinocytosis, in which small vesicles are formed by constriction of the cell membrane (see Table 4 and Fig. 33). Phagocytosis, on the other hand, is the process by which the cytoplasm takes up large, formed materials, such as bacteria (see Table 4 and Figs. 17, 18, 35, 36).

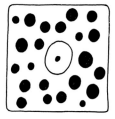

Fig. 4. Hyalin droplet degeneration (protein reabsorption).

See Figure 225 (light photomicrograph) and Figures 235–237 (electron photomicrographs).

The term *fatty degeneration* (perhaps better called fatty change or fatty metamorphosis) describes the appearance of microscopically visible fat, either in the form of fine (Fig. 5, right) or large (Fig. 5, left) droplets. The size of the droplets depends upon the proportion of neutral fat (large droplets contain little phospholipid). Normally, fat is taken up in the form of fatty acids, which is accomplished through pinocytosis. The fatty acids are synthesized to triglycerides, bound to phospholipids and proteins, and delivered to the blood as lipoproteins. Any disproportion between the amounts of triglycerides (e. g., increased alimentary supply) or of phospholipids (e. g., choline deficiency) or failure of energy coupling (oxygen or enzyme deficiencies) leads to accumulation of fat, i. e., to fatty degeneration.

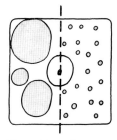

Fig. 5. Fatty degeneration.

See Figures 45 and 184 (light photomicrograph) and Figures 55, 213 and 233 (electron photomicrographs).

Fat phanerosis may develop in *necrobiosis* (perceptible, slow cell death) in which structurally intact fat tissue is broken down into microscopically visible droplets.

In disordered carbohydrate metabolism, glycogen droplets may appear (e. g., in the kidney in diabetes), or mucinous degeneration develop (production of mucopolysaccharides but without secretion) as, for example, in mucinous carcinoma (signet-ring cells, Fig. 6).

See Figure 421, p. 249.

Alteration of the character of mucin secretion may also result in obstruction of excretory ducts (e. g., cystic fibrosis of the pancreas).

Fig. 6. Signet ring cell.

See Figure 179, p. 114.

Glycogen storage disease is caused by an *inborn error* of carbohydrate metabolism.

Pigments are naturally colored materials that are laid down in either diffuse or granular fashion. They usually have as the chief component either *protein* (e. g., melanin), *lipid* (lipopigments, e. g., lipofuscin) or derivatives of *hemoglobin* (hemosiderin or siderin, hematoidin, bile pigment). In addition, a number of *exogenous pigments* may be seen.

See the following Figures:

Lipofuscin, pp. 17, 35, 116	Bile pigment, p. 116, 136
Melanin, p. 266	Malaria pigment, p. 116
Hemosiderin or siderin, pp. 16, 76	Exogenous pigments, pp. 94, 168
Hematoidin, pp. 16, 168	

Table 2 gives the most important differential characteristics of the different pigments.

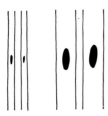

Atrophy of cells (Fig. 7) results from inactivity or chronic metabolic deficiency, is manifested by reduction in cell size *(simple atrophy)* and eventually results in reduction of cell number *(numerical atrophy)*.

See Figures 34, 116, 186, 200.

Degeneration of the connective and supporting tissues affects chiefly the *ground substance*. It may result in unsheathing of the fibers, infiltration of fat and mucin and deposition of foreign substances.

Fig. 7. Atrophy, hypertrophy.

The word *"hyalin"* describes tissue structures that have the following macroscopic and microscopic appearances: homogeneous, glassy, translucent material that stains with eosin (see Table 3 and pp. 140, 152, 256). **Epithelial hyalin,** e. g., the colloid of the thyroid gland differs from **connective tissue hyalin.** In the latter, recent studies with the electron microscope (GIESEKING, 1966) show one form of hyalin characterized by *swelling* (splitting of collagen fibers, loss of cross-striations, changes in protoplasmic fibrils, Fig. 25 a) and another by *reconstitution*. In the latter, instead of parallel arranged bundles of collagen fibers, there is a disarrayed network of elementary fibrils, which have been reconstituted from lysis of the collagen (fibrolysis) in acute inflammation (Fig. 31). *Precipitated hyalin* is another form, of which examples are fibrinoid degeneration e. g. in necrosis (Fig. 24 and p. 154) and amyloid. In hyalinization of arterioles (*arteriolar hyalin*, Fig. 32), electron microscopy discloses between the muscle fibers of the media a structureless, finely granular material having the structural characteristics of basement membrane protein. In all likelihood, this material comes from the blood plasma (Wiener *et al.*, 1965). Hyalin in the glomeruli also

Table 2. Pigments

Substance	Components	Location	Iron Reaction	Fat Stain	H_2O_2	Acid	Base	PAS[1]	Ag NO$_3$[2]	Fluorescence[3]	Gmelin Test
Lipofuscin Figs. 15, 43	unsaturated oxidized fatty acids	Parenchymal cells	–	(+)	(+)	–	–	+	+[4]	+	–
Ceroid	unsaturated oxidized fatty acids	intracellular (mesenchymal)	–	+	–	–	–	+	±	+	–
Melanin Fig. 456	tyrosine derivatives	intracellular	–	–	+	–	(+)	–	+[5]	–	–
Siderin Hemosiderin Figs. 13, 104, 206, 260, 369	iron glycoprotein	intracellular	+	–	–	+	–	+	+	–	–
Hematoidin Figs. 14, 261	bilirubin	extracellular	–	–	–	+	+	–	–		+
Bile Pigment Fig. 183	bilirubin biliverdin	intra– and extracellular	–	–	–	+	+	–			+
Malarial Pigment Fig. 182	hemoglobin derivative	intracellular	(+)	–	+	+	+	–		+	
Formalin Pigment Fig. 262	protoporphyrin	extracellular	–	–	–	–	+	–		–	
Exogenous Pigments Fig. 263	e. g., carbon, silver, etc.	intra– and extracellular	–	–	–	–	–	–	–	–	–

1 Periodic acid–Schiff reaction for demonstration of polysaccharides (α glycol).
2 Reduced silver.
3 Primary fluorescence without staining.

4 Brown.
5 Black.
(+) Indicates a weak reaction.

shows similar electron-microscopic characteristics. Such investigations indicate that the word hyalin includes several alterations of the tissues, each with a distinctive structure, origin and chemical structure. Hyalin is therefore merely a working hypothesis employed in the context of light microscopy and must be analyzed differently in each individual case.

Amyloid is a "hyalin" substance that stains specifically and shows a fibrous structure without periodicity (this is debated) when examined with the electron microscope (Figs. on pp. 162, 170). It is formed chiefly in the cells of the reticuloendothelial system and deposited extracellularly. Preferred sites are spleen, liver, kidney, adrenals and intestines. For additional details, see p. 170.

See the photomicrographs on pp. 118, 144, 162, 170, 184.

Table 3. Distinguishing Characteristics of Hyalin, Amyloid, Fibrinoid and Fibrin

Stain	Hyalin	Amyloid	Fibrinoid	Fibrin	Remarks
Hematoxylin Eosin	red homo-geneous	red homo-geneous	red homo-geneous	red fine fibers or homo-geneous	
van Gieson	red	yellow	yellow	yellow	
Congo Red	–	red	–	–	
Methyl Violet	–	red	–	–	metachromatic red
Azan	blue	red	red	red	
Weigert's Fibrin Stain	–	–	±	±	depending on the fixative used and on the age of the fibrin
Digested by Trypsin Pepsin	–	–	+	+	
	–	–	–	–	
Tissue Reaction	–	occasional giant cells	slight acute in-flammation, granulation tissue, histiocytes	granula-tion tissue	

Note: Hyalin – no tissue reaction. *Fibrinoid* – almost always a tissue reaction: granuloma, e.g. Aschoff nodules (p. 46), or granulation tissue (panarteritis, p. 64).

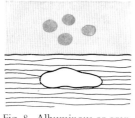

Fig. 8. Albuminous or granular protein degeneration (above), muco-cystic degeneration (below).

Albuminous or granular protein degeneration and mucoid degeneration of the connective tissues (Fig. 8) result from disintegration of the ground substance with precipitation of protein in cartilage or other tissues having a low metabolic rate. Protein complexes appear in the ground substance, or there is an increase in mucopolysaccharides. The collagen fibers are exposed in the process and finally destroyed, with the result that cysts are formed (*muco-cystic degeneration*, e.g., in a meniscus). *See p. 218.*

Necrosis

Necrosis (focal death of tissue) is recognized morphologically by destruction of cell nuclei (pyknosis = nuclear shrinkage, karyolysis = nuclear dissolution, karyorrhexis = fragmentation of nuclei, Figs. 9, 19), homogenization of the cytoplasm and distinctly increased eosinophilia. (See also pp. 38, 43, 144, 222.)

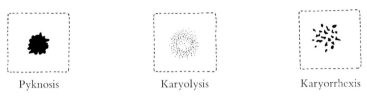

| Pyknosis | Karyolysis | Karyorrhexis |

Fig. 9. Diagram of the different manifestations of nuclear destruction.

In the early or acute stages, denaturation of proteins occurs and evokes a leukocytic reaction. Later, the necrotic tissue is resorbed by granulation tissue and finally a scar is formed. There are, however, various other paths that differ from this ordinary sequence of events, as shown in Figure 10. In occasional cases, regeneration occurs with complete restitution of tissue integrity (e. g., liver, especially in young persons).

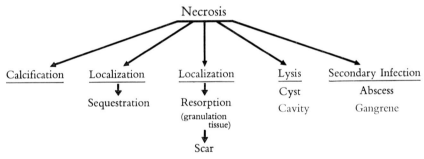

Fig. 10. Sequelae of necrosis. *(See pp. 38, 40, 100, 120, 126, 128.)*

Electron Microscopy

The advances in the field of electron microscopy have added a new dimension, that of ultrastructure, and it is essential to consider the significance of this fact with respect to general pathology. The advancing edge of this new dimension is closing the large gap between light microscopy and biochemistry. Electron microscopy, and in particular histochemical electron microscopy, is making visible for the first time those cellular structures that are the morphological bases of metabolic processes. This new knowledge has greatly increased our understanding of disease. Structure and function are no longer to be conceived of as antagonists, but rather as parts of a whole (see D. W. KING, 1966).

The electron micrographs that follow on the next pages have to do with certain angles of general pathology. Those illustrating special pathology are placed under the sections on the respective organs.

In attempting to present the electron microscopic basis of general pathology in tabular form (pp. 14, 15), it is realized that the brevity of the tabular form imposes severe restrictions. Only the barest outline of the alterations of cell organelles can be indicated. However, the juxtaposition achieved in the table makes it clear that at the level of ultrastructure, as well as at the level of light microscopy, there are no *specific* cellular lesions and the most widely different injurious agents may call forth quite similar reactions.

---

1 The rule shown in the electron micrographs is one micron in length unless otherwise indicated.

Normal Liver Cell

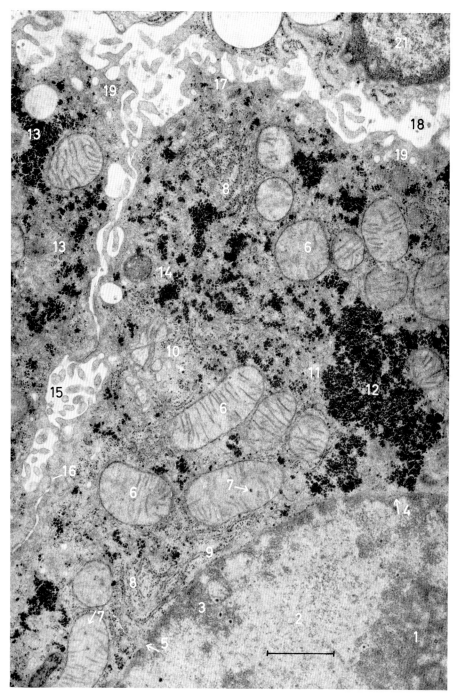

Fig. 11. Normal liver cell of the mouse. Electron photomicrograph (Dr. SCHROEDER). 20,600 ×.

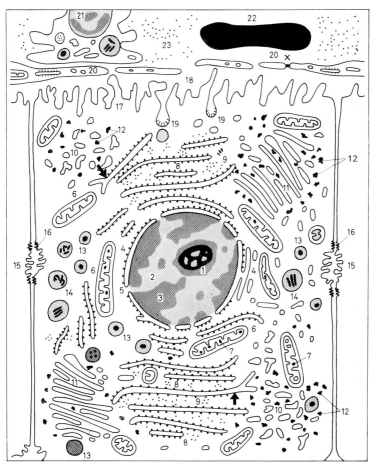

Fig. 12. Diagram of the electron microscopic appearance of a normal liver cell (the same legend numbers are used in Fig. 11). 1. *nucleolus* (forms ribosomes and transfer – RNA). 2. *loose chromatin* (euchromatin: synthesis of messenger RNA). 3. *dense chromatin* (heterochromatin: genetic building block). 4. *double membrane* of the nucleus with a partial outer border of ribosomes. 5. *pores in the nuclear membrane*. 6. *mitochondria* with cristae (citric acid cycle, respiratory enzymes, part of fatty acid synthesis). 7. *matrix granules* of the mitochondria (lipoprotein with cations. Ion transport?). 8. *rough endoplasmic reticulum* (RER) with outer border of *ribosomes*. In Figure 12 transformation of rough endoplasmic reticulum (RER) into smooth endoplasmic reticulum (SER). Protein is synthesized on the ribosomes and *polysomes* (aggregates of ribosomes, 9; see Fig. 30) with the help of messenger – RNA. In the cisternae of the RER protein transport occurs. The *Golgi zone* (10) serves as a condensation and packaging station. II. *smooth endoplasmic reticulum* (SER). Cisternae without ribosomes. The RER and SER together form a membrane system [the *endoplasmic reticulum* (ER) is the same as the biochemist's microsome fraction] with organ specific enzymes (STAUDINGER, 1962): hydrolases (with a detoxifying function), glucose-6-phosphatase (glycogen metabolism). Steroid synthesis, etc. 12. *glycogen* (particles uniformly measuring 150–400 Å in diameter and having a rosette arrangement). 13. *cytosomes* ("microbodies") with thick inner bodies (precursors of lysosomes?). 14. *lysosomes* with enclosing membrane (see Table 4). Hydrolytic enzymes: acid phosphatase, β-glucuronidase, cathepsin, peroxydase, etc. 15. *bile canaliculi* with microvilli. 16. *desmosomes* (tight cell junctions close to the bile canaliculi). 17. *microvilli* on the surfaces of cells extending into the space of Disse (18) (a basement membrane is lacking in liver sinusoids). 19. *pinocytotic vacuoles* and vesicles (uptake of colloid particles, fat, etc.). 20. endothelial cell process with wide pores; x, endothelial cell pore with diaphragm. 21. stellate Kupffer cell. 22. erythrocyte. 23. denatured blood plasma (redrawn from JEZEQUEL, 1962; PORTER and BONNEVILLE, 1965).

Table 4. **Pathological Alterations of Cell Organelles**

Normal	Pathological	Remarks
	Mitochondria a) swelling matrix type cristal type mixed type THOENES, 1964	*Microscopic:* the picture of cloudy swelling arises from marked mitochondrial swelling involving the matrix (matrix type of swelling). The cristal type of swelling is unremarkable by light microscopy. *Cause:* O_2 deficiency, toxins, substrate deficiency. *Metabolic effect:* decrease in ATP, DPN, oxidative phosphorylation; also conversion to vacuoles (so-called vacuolar transformation or hydropic degeneration. See also RER below and Figures 56, 213, 217, 231, 232.
	disappearance of matrix granules	In O_2 deficiency, necrosis. See Figure 56.
 15,000 ×	b) structural changes 	*Microscopic:* no equivalent. *Cause/precursor:* Vitamin E deficiency, cirrhosis of liver, tumors, chronic alcoholism. *Metabolic effect:* great increase in enzymes of the citric acid cycle, ATP increased. See Figure 386.
	c) membrane changes 	Increase or decrease of the mitochondrial membrane, lengthening or shortening of the cristae, formation of gaps in the lamellae, myelin figure degeneration, lysis of membranes. *Cause:* e. g., high CO_2 tension (lung), toxins, tumors, icterus, etc. See Figures 218, 386.
	d) matrix changes clearing condensation aggregation 	Clearing and condensation of the matrix in different sorts of injuries. Matrix aggregates (mitochondrial bodies) in methyl-cholanthrene application, alcoholism, necrosis. Often contain calcium (e. g., in nephrocalcinosis). See Figures 57, 213, 214, 234.
	Rough Endoplasmic Reticulum a) changes in form and size H_2O H_2O	*Microscopic:* Vacuolar or hydropic degeneration. *Cause:* O_2 deficiency, toxins. *Metabolic effect:* decreased protein synthesis. The vacuoles form from the cisternae of the RER and SER, mostly with loss of ribosomes attached to the membranes of the RER. See Figures 53, 214, 217, 231.
	b) fragmentation, vesiculation 	Appearance at the onset of necrosis. Loss of ribosomes. See Figures 57, 211, 231.
	c) "finger print" degeneration concentric layering of membranes (so-called myelin figures) 	Regeneration in chronic intoxication; increased cellular activity. See Figure 218.
29,000 ×	d) changes in ribosome distribution loss of ribosomes 	Toxins, carcinogenesis, vitamin C deficiency, necrosis. See Figures 214, 217.

Table 4 is based in large part upon the excellent papers of MILLER, 1958, and TRUMP et al., 1965.

Table 4 (cont.)

Normal	Pathological	Remarks
 50,000×	e) Alterations of ribosomes and polysomes: disappearance of aggregates of 80 S ribosomes (= polysomes), appearance of 50 S and 30 S ribosomes (biochemical) See Figs. 211, 235.	*Microscopic:* the granular basophilia of the cytoplasm disappears, diffuse basophilia appears. Decreased protein synthesis, e. g., in carbon tetrachloride, thioacetamid intoxication.
 29,000×	Smooth Endoplasmic Reticulum a) focal or diffuse increase b) associated with storage fault (e. g. glycogen in Gaucher's disease) 	*Microscopic:* hyalin cytoplasm. *Cause:* starvation, alcohol, toxins, carcinogenic agents, detoxification, steroid synthesis, fatty degeneration. e. g. accumulation of kerasin. *Microscopic:* PAS-positive material (SCHÄFER et al., 1966). See Figures 218, 221.
 15,000×	*Golgi apparatus* swelling of cisternae, hypertrophy 	In oxygen deficiency, secretion, hibernation.
Cytosome 29,000× Lysosome 20,000× acid phosphatase 20,000×	Cytosomes, Lysosomes a) *Cytosomes:* disappear with onset of necrosis, simultaneous increase in acid phosphatase activity (see adjoining figures for electron-microscopic evidence) and decrease of succinic dehydrogenase. b) *Autolysosomes:* absorption and digestion of the cell's own substance (seen in the middle picture to the left and in Fig. 212). The remainder of the debris = lipofuscin granules. c) *Phagolysosomes:* destruction and digestion of foreign substances by pinocytosis or phagocytosis. membrane-bound vesicles fibrin in Schwartzman phenomenon (Fig. 16) siderin (siderosomes) (Figs. 13, 369) lysosome protein or hemoglobin storage (Figs. 235, 236) microvilli phagocytosis of bacteria (Figs. 18, 35)	*Cytosomes: Microscopic:* necrobiosis with marked cytoplasmic eosinophilia. *Autolysosomes:* The contents consist of membrane fragments (RER, SER, mitochondria, glycogen, etc.) which are found in limited injury of all cells with high metabolic activity (e. g., starvation, hepatitis, vitamin E deficiency). In calcification, so-called Schaumann bodies in giant cells (Boeck's disease). *Phagolysosomes:* Ingestion of foreign materials or foreign bodies always leads to membrane formation through invagination of the cell membrane. Microscopically, iron for example can be demonstrated by the Berlin-blue reaction. Protein accumulation manifests itself as hyalin droplet inclusions. Bacteria are demonstrated by special staining (Fig. 139). Common also are accumulations of nuclear fragment (Fig. 171). (Literature: De DUVE, WEISSMANN.)
fatty degeneration	diffuse increase of SER (see Figs. 55, 213, 233)	*Microscopic:* Cytoplasmic fat droplets.
structureless ground substance	*Condensation* of matrix (increased electron density): toxins, O$_2$ deficiency. *Clearing* of matrix (decreased electron density, hydration): with various injurious agents (diffuse, vacuolar) (e. g., Figs. 19, 231).	

Electron photomicrographs by Dr. SCHROEDER, Zürich. Picture of acid phosphatase by Dr. HAGER, Giessen.

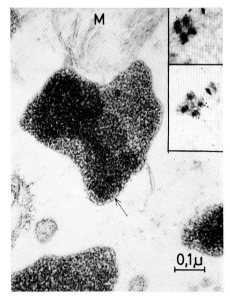

Fig. 13. Macrophage resulting from injection of iron and showing siderosomes (membrane →) with both large particles (siderin) and finely granular ones (ferritin, 55 Å, see inset B). 75,000 ×. M = mitochondrion. 450,000 × (Dr. WESSEL)[1].

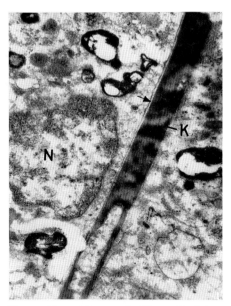

Fig. 14. Hematoidin crystal (K) contained in a macrophage and surrounded by invaginated cell membrane (→). N = nucleus (see Fig. 261). 25,000 × (Dr. GIESEKING).

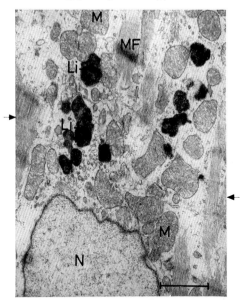

Fig. 15. Perinuclear lipofuscin (Li) in heart muscle (cat). N = nucleus. MF and arrow = myofilaments with Z bands. M = mitochondria. 12,000 × (Dr. TOTOVIC)[2].

1 WESSEL and GEDIGK, 1959.
2 SOMORAJSKI et al., 1965.
3 PROSE, et al., 1965.

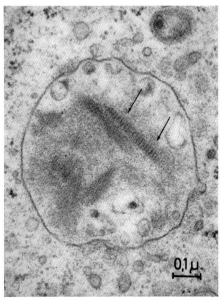

Fig. 16. Fibrin showing cross bands (typical periodicity →) lying in a cytoplasmic vacuole in a Kupffer cell following administration of endotoxin ("fibrin-clearing" mechanism in the Shwartzman phenomenon). 71,000 × (Dr. PROSE)[3]. See Fig. 107.

16

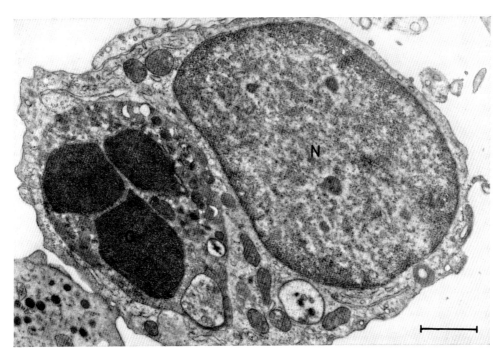

Fig. 17. Phagocytosis of a necrotic leukocyte by a macrophage (G = granulocyte). N = nucleus of the macrophage. 16,000× (Dr. Hager), see Nelson *et al.*, 1962.

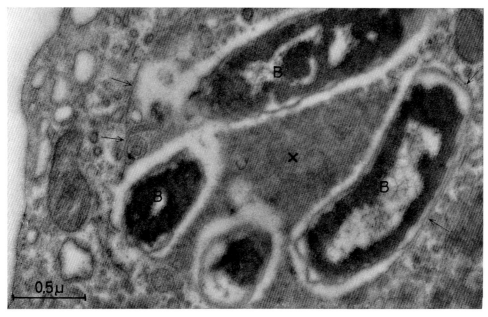

Fig. 18. Phagocytosis of colon bacilli by a macrophage. The large phagocyte is filled with dense, homogeneous substance (x) and four intact bacteria (B). The membrane of the phagosome can be identified (→). 40,000× (Dr. Hager).

17

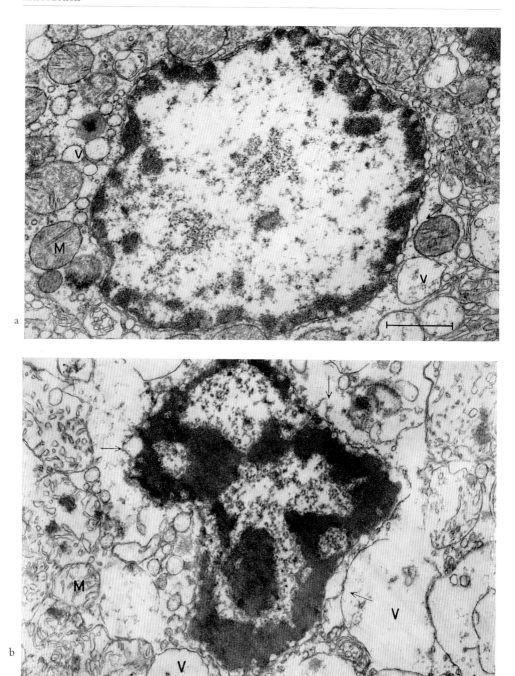

Fig. 19, a, b, c, d: different stages of cell destruction leading to pyknosis. Distal renal tubule of a rat with an experimentally produced infarct of the kidney.

a) hyperchromatic nuclear wall, i. e., increased margination of chromatin on the nuclear membrane plus pallor of the interior. → lifting of the outer lamella of the nuclear membrane. M = mitochondria, V = vacuole in ER (vacuolar degeneration).

Nuclear Pyknosis

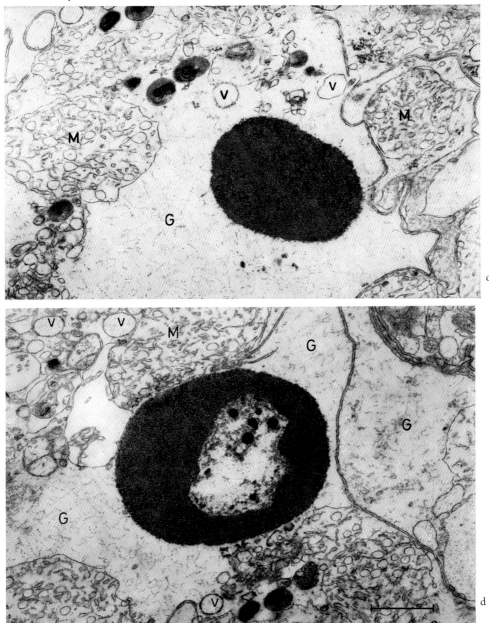

b) shrinkage of the nucleus with beginning thickening and clumping of the chromatin. → lifting of the outer lamella of the nuclear membrane. V = large cytoplasmic vacuole.

c) and d) far-advanced pyknosis with pronounced condensation of nuclear chromatin. The nuclear membrane is no longer distinguishable. Mitochondria (M) markedly swollen, edema and pallor of the ground substance (G), vacuoles (V) in the ER. Cytosomes (C) still partially preserved. Magnification for Figs. 19 a-d 17,000× (Dr. TOTOVIC). See TOTOVIC, 1966; ALTMANN et al., 1966.

19

Circulatory Disturbances

The *circulatory disturbances*, like inflammation, involve complex processes in a variety of tissues. These processes take place in the terminal circulatory channels, the arterioles, meta-arterioles, capillaries and venules. Even under normal conditions, there is a changing interplay of hyperemia (in activity) and anemia (at rest), which, under pathological conditions, change to *passive* (stasis of blood) or *active hyperemia* or to *ischemia*. *Stasis* indicates stagnation of the blood current with hemoconcentration. If the stasis persists, necrosis will result. Depending upon local factors, there will develop either an *anemic infarct* (coagulation necrosis: in organs supplied with end-arteries, e. g., heart, kidney, spleen, etc.) or a *hemorrhagic infarct* (necrosis and hemorrhage, e. g., in lung, intestine).

Hemorrhage may occur for various reasons (e. g., injury of capillary walls, deficiency of platelets, deficiency of fibrinogen). Derangement of the coagulation mechanism together with slowing of the blood stream and endothelial injury results in formation of a thrombus which either breaks off *(embolus)*, becomes organized, calcified or softened interiorly *(putrid softening)* or is dissolved *(fibrinolysis)*.

See the following Figures:

Congestion, p. 76, 120	Hemorrhagic infarct, p. 80, 104
Stasis, p. 76, 120	Hemorrhage, p. 224
Anemic infarct, p. 38, 150, 154	Thrombosis, p. 68

Inflammation

Inflammation consists of a series of complex reactions by vascular and connective tissue elements to a tissue injury. In the acute phase, there is *hyperemia, fluid exudation* (if chiefly blood serum = *serous inflammation*; if chiefly fibrinogen = *fibrinous inflammation*; if accompanied by hemorrhage = *hemorrhagic inflammation)* and *emigration* of leukocytes *(purulent inflammation)*.

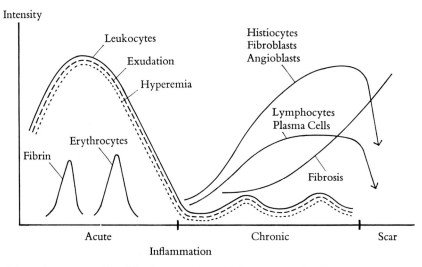

Fig. 20. Schematic representation of the tissue reactions to inflammatory stimuli.

See the following Figures:

Serous inflammation, pp. 22, 48, 90, 106	Hemorrhagic inflammation, p. 88
Fibrinous inflammation, pp. 50, 83, 107	Purulent inflammation, p. 44, 54, 92, 112, 122, 164, 225

In the *chronic stages*, proliferation of connective tissue cells, histiocytes and capillaries predominate *(granulation tissue)*. Different morphological appearances and functional disturbances are produced, depending upon the duration of the injury, the amount of denatured protein (necrotic tissue, fibrin) deposited or the presence of foreign bodies in the tissue. Essentially, there is proliferation of *fibroblasts*, young connective tissue (fibrosis → scar), *histiocytes* (phagocytic function) [now thought to come from blood monocytes! (LEDER, 1967)] and *new capillaries* (nutritional function). There are also varying numbers of lymphocytes, plasma cells, mast cells and polymorphonuclear leukocytes.

On the basis of the cell type, some authors separate a *cellular form of proliferating granulation tissue*, which is rich in lymphocytes and histiocytes, from *granulation tissue in a narrow sense* (only capillary twigs and fibroblasts), and from an *infiltrating form of granulation tissue* which appears between the local tissue elements and may be transformed into them.

Among the chief functions of granulation tissue the following may be mentioned:

1. *resorption*, e. g., the resorption of necrotic tissue, thrombi or fibrin (Fig. 49);
2. *tissue replacement*, e. g., replacement of defects in the skin or mucous membranes (Fig. 322);
3. *localization*, e. g., walling off of an abscess (Fig. 471).

The result is always the formation of a *scar* to replace the defect caused by loss of local parenchymatous tissue.

See p. 40, 46, 53, 64, 92, 105, 130, 184, 198, 200, 202.

Macroscopic: Immature granulation tissue: red. Scar tissue: white, glistening, fibrous and tough.

Fibrinoid degeneration or necrosis (Fig. 21) develops after severe acute disturbance of vascular permeability with subsequent sudden leakage of blood plasma into the vessel wall and the surrounding connective tissue. Because of this, the vascular tissues are either obscured or destroyed (see Table 3 and p. 23). The blood plasma proteins combine chemically with collagen or the tissue mucopolysaccharides (BENEKE, 1963). Fibrin is often demonstrable with both the light and electron microscopes (Fig. 24). A slight, fleeting leukocytic reaction or secondary proliferation of histiocytes (e. g., Aschoff nodules in rheumatic fever) or granulation tissue (e. g., in periarteritis nodosa) may follow, with consequent resorption of the fibrinoid (see pp. 23, 46, 64, 154).

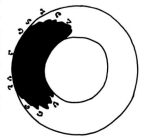

Fig. 21. Fibrinoid necrosis in an artery.

Circumscribed nodules of granulation tissue are seen in granulomatous inflammation (histiocytic granuloma, e. g., Aschoff nodules; foreign body granuloma; epithelioid granuloma of tuberculosis, etc.).

See pp. 46, 98, 198.

By the term "specific inflammation" is meant a tissue reaction distinguished by a characteristic (specific) morphological appearance that suggests the etiologic agent, e. g. tuberculosis which shows a typical arrangement of cells and tissues (often with necrosis). It should be noted, however that such lesions are specific only in a limited sense, since epithelioid cell granulomas, for example, may occur in diseases of different causes (tuberculosis, syphilis, brucellosis, histoplasmosis, sarcoid, etc.).

See the following Figures: Tuberculosis, pp. 54, 98, 100; Syphilis, p. 122.

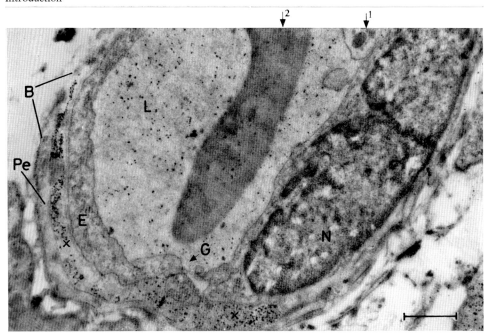

Fig. 22. Serous inflammation: acute, serous exudation of blood plasma from a venule 3 minutes after administration of serotonin and intravenous injection of HgS (black particles), cremaster muscle of rat. L = lumen, G = opening between two endothelial cells, XX = plasma with HgS in a cleavage space between endothelial cells (E) and pericytes (Pe) or basement membrane (B), N = nucleus of an endothelial cell, → 1 thrombocyte, → 2 erythrocyte. 14,000 × (MAJNO et al., 1961).

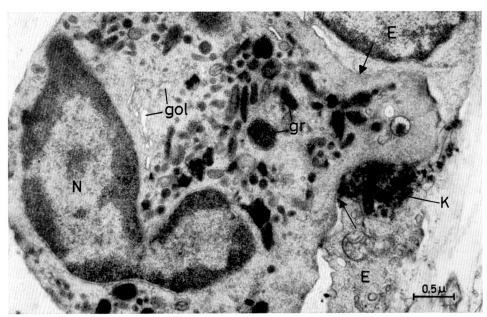

Fig. 23. Early stage of leukocyte emigration, 5 minutes after heat injury (54–56° C. for 10–15 sec.; rat omentum). A polymorphonuclear leukocyte (N = nucleus, gr = granule, gol = golgi zone) has pushed a cytoplasmic process between two endothelial cells (E). In the picture → indicates the borders of the endothelial cells. In between there is carbon, previously given intravenously. 23,500 × (MOVAT et al., 1963).

Acute Inflammation

In *serous inflammation*, fluid leaks from the blood vessels. Figures 22 and 23 show what happens. The tight junctions between the endothelial cells (normally desmosomes, Fig. 12) are lost. Through these pores (0.1 to 0.8 μ) blood serum escapes and collects under the basement membrane or the pericytes (Figs. 22 and 23). *Leukocytes* also pass through these pores (Fig. 23). Exudation of *fibrinogen* is thought to take place in a similar fashion. Once outside the vessels, it polymerizes to fibrin. Because a thick layer of fibrin may be deposited on and be bound to the collagen fibers, a homogeneous, eosinophilic microscopic appearance results that is referred to as *fibrinoid swelling* or *degeneration*. The acid pH of the inflamed area causes the collagen fibers to loosen (tuft-like splintering, Fig. 25a). In addition, fibrin may be deposited between the protofibrils *(fibrinoid necrosis)*. Leukocytic proteolytic enzymes often cause tissue liquefaction (abscess), during which process the collagen fibers are re-formed into monomeric tropocollagen (Fig. 25b, *reconstituted hyalin*, GIESEKING, 1966).

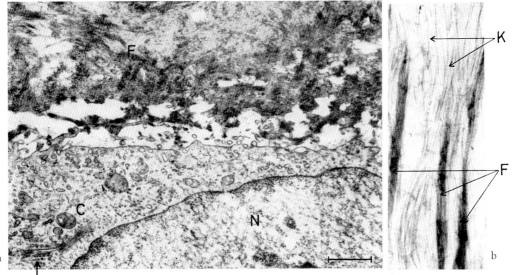

a
b

Fig. 24a and b. Fibrinoid swelling (degeneration) in the Arthus phenomenon. a) Intestinal serosa (i. v. injection of human albumin followed in 12 days by a local application of human albumin). Mesothelial cell (N = nucleus, → = SER, C = cytosome). Layer of fibrinoid (F) in which the periodicity of fibrin is not visible. 12,000 ×. b) Cornea of the eye (produced experimentally as in 24a). K = collagen fibers showing distinct periodicity, F = coating of the collagen by fibrin deposits lacking cross-striations. 16,250 × (Dr. CAESAR, Dr. SCHIRASAWA).

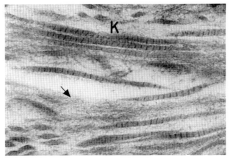

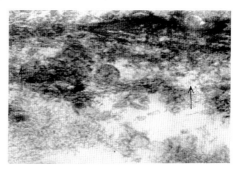

Fig. 25a and b. Fibrolysis: a) loosening of the collagen fibers by the tissue acidity of inflammation (K shows distinct periodicity) and splintering into protofibrils (→) without cross striations (hyaline swelling) 30,000 ×.

b) Disintegration of collagen fibers (→) into fine micellar particles through the action of the proteolytic enzymes of leukocytes. Liquefaction of tissues. 50,000 × (Dr. GIESEKING).

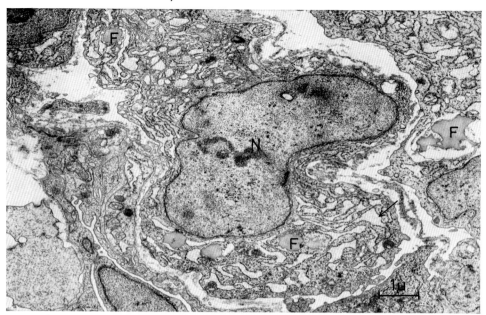

Fig. 26. Fibroblast from a 5-day-old myocardial infarct. N = nucleus. The cytoplasm contains an abundance of rough endoplasmic reticulum (e. g., at →), showing partially dilated cisternae. F = cytoplasmic fat droplet. 10,000× (Dr. KORB). Synthesis of collagen fibers follows with formation of tropocollagen and deposition of it on the intracellular protofibrils in the region of the RER (Fig. 27). The protofibrils aggregate extracellularly to form elemental collagen fibrils (GIESEKING, 1966).

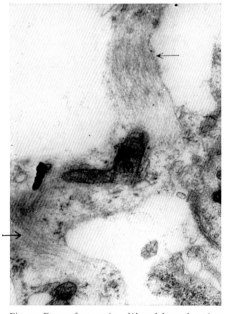

Fig. 27. Parts of an active fibroblast showing intracellular (→ lower left) and extracellular (→ upper right) protofibrils. 22,000× (Dr. GIESEKING).

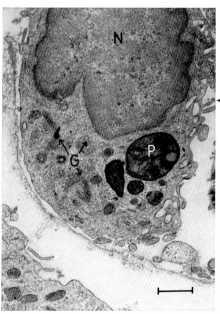

Fig. 28. Histiocyte showing phagolysosomes (P) and a distinct cytoplasmic process → (resorption!). G = Golgi apparatus. N = nucleus. 9,000× (Dr. TOTOVIC).

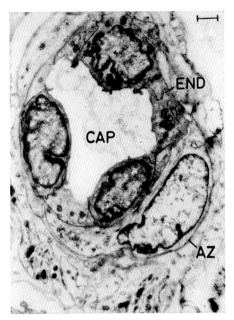

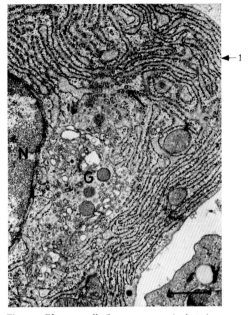

Fig. 29. Granulation tissue showing newly formed capillary (CAP = capillary lumen) with endothelial cells (End) and adventitial cells (AZ). 6,500× (Dr. GIESEKING).

Fig. 30. Plasma cell (bone marrow) showing closely packed cisternae of RER (→ 1), rosette-like arrangement of the ribosomes (polysomes →), G = Golgi zone. 12,000× (Dr. MILLER).

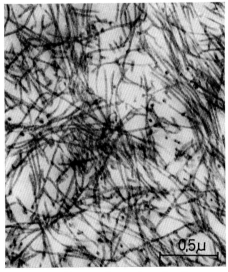

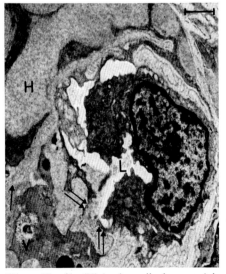

Fig. 31. Hyalin transformation of collagenous tissue (pleural plaque) showing cross-striations (reconstituted hyalin). 30,000× (Dr. GIESEKING).

Fig. 32. Hyalin (H) in the wall of an arteriole (experimental hypertension in a rat) presenting in the form of finely granular material. L = narrowed lumen, → transition of the thickened basement membrane to hyalin, ⇒ gap in the endothelium, V = vacuole. 8,000× (WIENER et al., 1965).

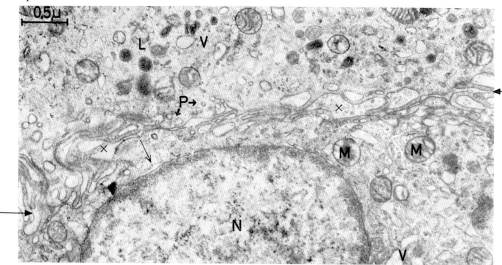

Fig.33. Epithelioid cell in lupus vulgaris (epithelioid cell tuberculosis of the skin, see Fig.320). N = oval nucleus showing reticular karyoplasm, → widening of the perinuclear space (gap in the nuclear double membrane). M = mitochondria, V = vacuoles in ER, X microvilli on the surface of the cell which are closely interdigitated with those of the neighboring cell (above, → indicates the outer border of both cells), P = micropinocytotic vacuoles (uptake of materials). L = lysosomes. 24,000 × (GUSEK)[1].

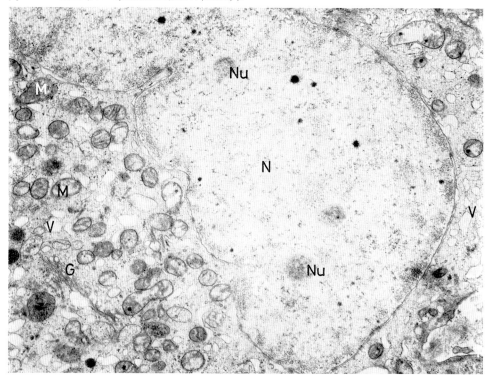

Fig. 34. Epithelioid cell in Boeck's disease (see Fig. 273). Indented nucleus (N) with loose chromatin and many nucleoli (Nu), numerous cytoplasmic mitochondria (M) and vacuoles (V) in the ER, G=Golgi apparatus. 18,000 × (Dr. GUSEK).

1 See GUSEK, 1962; DUMONT, 1965.

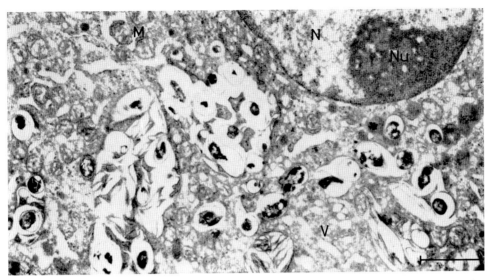

Fig. 35. Epithelioid cell in a BCG-granuloma (injection of attenuated tubercle bacilli, 14 days after inoculation). N = nucleus with marginally situated nucleolus (Nu). In the cytoplasm there are clumps of bacteria in different stages of destruction and enclosed in phagocytic vacuoles. V = vacuoles in ER, M = mitochondria. All membranes (mitochondrial, ER) are fuzzy from the action of the infectious agent. 17,000× (Dr. GUSEK).

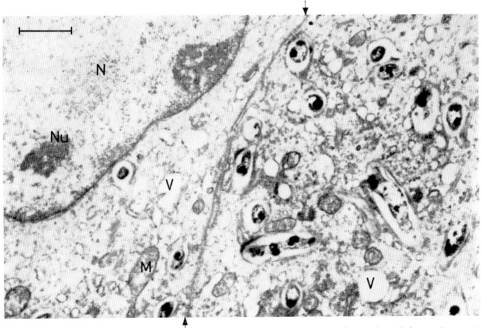

Fig. 36. Epithelioid cells in leprosy. The left-hand cell shows a nucleus (N) with loose chromatin and nucleoli (Nx). Right-hand cell (→ edge of cell). The cytoplasm contains numerous lepra bacilli (seen in longitudinal and cross sections) in different stages of disintegration. M = mitochondria, V = ER vacuoles. Both the mitochondria and the membranes are preserved better than in Figure 35. 15,000× (Dr. GUSEK).

Growth

The term *regeneration* describes an increase in the parenchymal cells of an organ or tissue. An increase in metabolism is manifested morphologically by enlargement of cells and cell nuclei (hypertrophy, see Fig. 7). Later, there may be an increase in the number of cells *(numerical hypertrophy* or *hyperplasia)*. (See p.34). This can develop into metaplasia, for example, the transformation of ciliated epithelium into squamous epithelium. In this instance, the basal cells of the tissue have differentiated into epithelium foreign to the particular situation.

See pp.44, 82, 200.

Giant cells appear under various conditions and in a variety of forms (Fig. 38). Frequently, they are the result of the increased work of resorption (e. g., Langhans giant cells, foreign body giant cells, osteoclasts). They can also result from fusion of cells or from nuclear division without cytoplasmic division (amitotic division). In many cases, giant cells develop from capillary twigs (e. g., giant cells in an epulis). Touton giant cells are found in chronic resorbing inflammation in fat tissue.

See the following Figures: foreign body giant cell, p.198; Langhans giant cell, p.98; giant cells in an epulis or brown tumor, p.214; giant cells in an Aschoff nodule, p.46; Touton giant cells, p.197; Hodgkin and Reed–Sternberg giant cells, p.176; osteoclasts, p.204; placental giant cell, p.188; tumor giant cell, p.262.

Tumors

Benign and malignant *tumors* are *autonomous*, that is, they are distinguished by their independence from the regulatory mechanism of the total organism, so that the host tissues are either displaced *(benign tumors)* or *destroyed*. *Invasive growth* and seeding of cell colonies in distant parts of the body *(metastases)* are the hallmarks of *malignant tumors*. See p.230 ff.

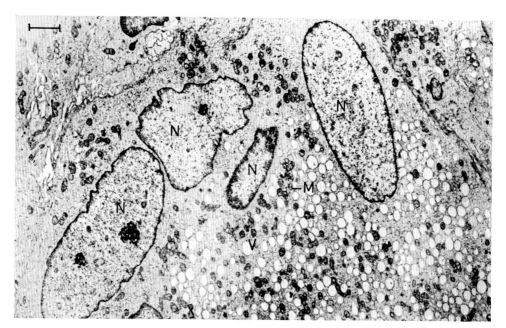

Fig. 37. Langhans giant cell in skin tuberculosis. Many nuclei (N) with loose chromatin and nucleoli. Numerous mitochondria (M) and ER vacuoles (V). 8,000× (Dr. GUSEK).

Giant Cells

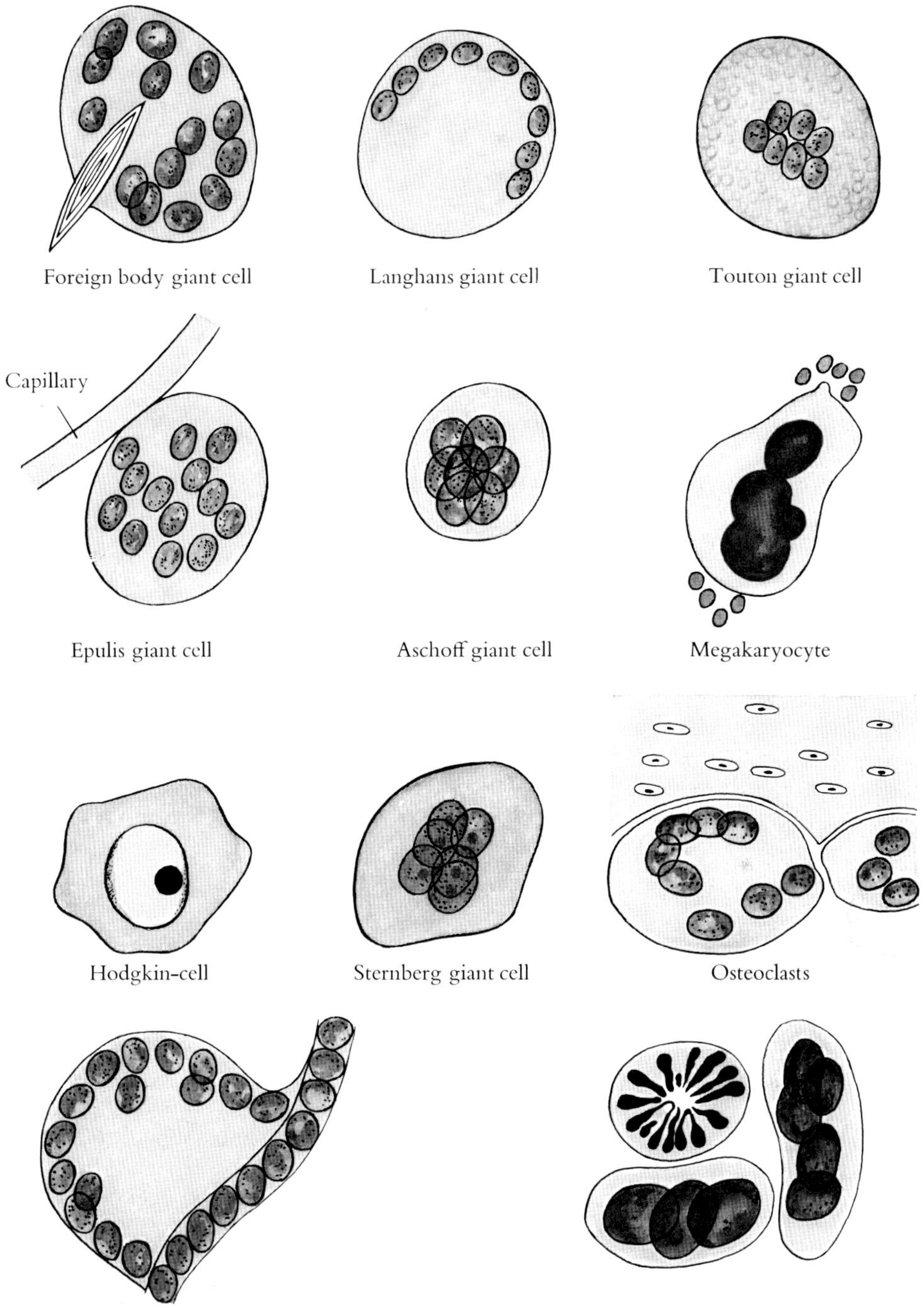

Foreign body giant cell   Langhans giant cell   Touton giant cell

Capillary

Epulis giant cell   Aschoff giant cell   Megakaryocyte

Hodgkin-cell   Sternberg giant cell   Osteoclasts

Placental giant cell   Tumor giant cells

Fig. 38. Comparison of various giant cells seen under normal and pathological circumstances.

Addendum

The student and young physician can easily forget that the pathologist has an important function to play in the preservation and care of the state of health. In practice, this function is often manifestly concerned with the examination of *biopsy material*, since frequently the decision between life and death for the patient depends upon the pathologist's diagnosis. An *unequivocable histological opinion* can lead the clinician to a single, simple diagnosis. In many cases, the correct interpretation of the histological appearance is suggested by the clinical findings, being dependent upon such things as the site from which the biopsy specimen was taken and the age and sex of the patient. This information is often essential for pathological diagnosis. For this reason, it is important that the form accompanying the request for examination of an important biopsy specimen be completely filled out by the person submitting it. Likewise, the fixation of the biopsy specimen must be just right (aqueous 40% formalin diluted 1:9, the ratio of specimen to volume of fixative at least 1:20, thickness of tissue block not more than 1 cm.). As to the biopsy itself, it is essential that *both normal and diseased tissue be removed*, so that the two can be compared in the histological preparation. In the case of polyps and papillomas, the tissue in the deepest part of the biopsy should be most carefully examined in order to discover possible invasion.

Every piece of tissue removed from a patient should be examined histologically – a requirement that the physician in his own best interests should never neglect, even when the macroscopic appearances seem ever so plain.

If a physician takes to heart these simple rules, he cannot fail to help his patients.

Systemic Pathology

Heart

The brief introductory remarks about the normal microscopic anatomy of each of the organs discussed in the rest of the book are based on standard textbooks, such as MAXIMOFF and DEMPSEY and PORTER.

Heart muscle shows cross-striations, centrally placed nuclei and a syncytial arrangement of the fibers with slender anastomoses. By comparison, *skeletal muscle* shows no such anastomoses between fibers, and the nuclei lie at the periphery of the cells, whereas *smooth muscle*, although showing centrally located nuclei, lacks cross-striations. The cross-striations depend upon the presence of myofilaments with isotropic and anisotropic bands. The intercalated disks are bright, narrow bands that demarcate the longitudinal limits of individual heart muscle cells (see Fig. 43). Between the muscle fibers there is a small amount of connective tissue containing capillaries and larger vessels. Segmentation of the fibers is a frequent postmortem finding in which irregular fractures of the muscle fibers appear, often with a step-like arrangement (see Fig. 45). Between the muscle fibers there is loose connective tissue containing large vessels and capillaries.

The *endocardium* is made up of a single layer of endothelium lying on a bed of loosely arranged elastic and collagen fibers.

The *leaflets of the heart valves* are avascular, covered with endothelium and contain collagen and elastic fibers.

Epicardium and pericardium are both covered with flattened cells and in the epicardium fat tissue is abundant.

In evaluating *pathological changes* in heart muscle, attention should be paid to the width of the fibers, foreign materials in the sarcoplasm (fat, glycogen, etc.), the cell nuclei, and the cellular constituents of the interstitial tissue. In looking at the valves, pay particular attention to vascularization and, of course, to thickening of the valve substance and to surface deposits. The epicardium and pericardium frequently show a coating of fibrin in pathological conditions.

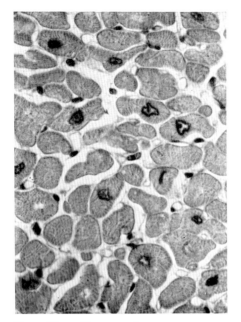

Fig. 39. Normal heart muscle.
H & E, 600×.

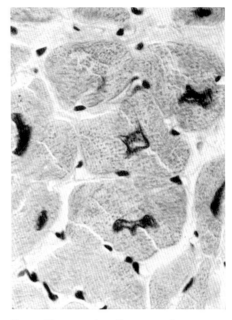

Fig. 40. Hypertrophy of heart muscle.
H & E, 600×.

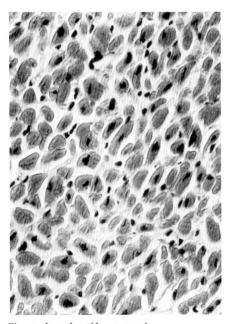

Fig. 41. Atrophy of heart muscle.
H & E, 600×.

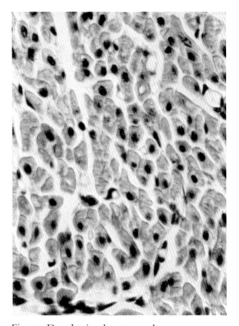

Fig. 42. Developing heart muscle.
H & E, 600×.

Hypertrophy and atrophy of the heart

The four accompanying photomicrographs have been taken at the same magnification in order to permit comparison of the changes in diseased heart muscle with the normal. The changes can be easily appreciated by comparing the *width of the muscle fibers*, the *size and shape of their nuclei* and the *number of nuclei* per section. Compared with **normal heart muscle** (Fig. 39), the myocardial fibers in **cardiac hypertrophy** (Fig. 40, heart weight 650 Gm.) are about three times as thick (in the photograph, normal fibers measure 0.8 cm., and hypertrophied fibers 2–3 cm.). Because of this, the number of nuclei per unit area of the section appears to be decreased. Likewise, the nuclei are nearly double the normal size; their DNA content corresponds to an octoploid value (normal is tetraploid). The nuclei also show bizarre changes in configuration. Some observations suggest that at times hyperplasia, an increase in the number of fibers, can also occur. In the sarcoplasm the thickening of transversely cut myofilaments can be clearly seen and, in comparison to normal myocardium, they are increased both in number and transverse measurement. Notice that normal or even atrophic fibers may appear next to hypertrophied ones.

In **atrophy of heart muscle** (Fig. 41, heart weight 200 Gm.), a relative increase in number of nuclei occurs; that is, a greater number of cell nuclei are seen in a unit area of the section. The fibers are clearly smaller (0.5 cm.) than in normal or hypertrophied hearts and often are also decreased in number *(numerical atrophy)*. In **developing heart muscle** (Fig. 42, 6-year-old child), we likewise find an apparent nuclear increase. The fibers are even smaller than in atrophy (0.4 cm.) and, by comparison, the nuclei are round and deeply stained.

Atrophy of heart muscle frequently is accompanied by an increase of lipofuscin *(brown atrophy)*.

The natural brown color of **lipofuscin pigment** is best brought out by using hematoxylin alone, since it stains only the cell nuclei (Figs. 15, 43). The brown pigment lies at the poles of nuclei in the form of granules of different sizes. This zone is without myofilaments. The pigment is made up chiefly of unsaturated fatty acids (brown color of rancid fat) and may occur normally in heart muscle.

The differentiation of lipofuscin from other pigments is given in Table 2, page 9.

Macroscopically, the organs in brown atrophy are shrunken and brown.

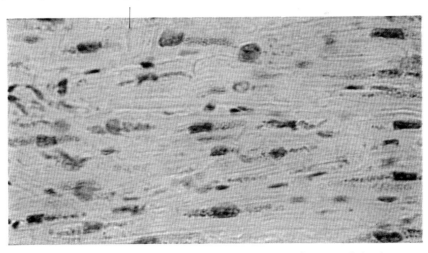

Fig. 43. Lipofuscin in brown atrophy of heart muscle. Hematoxylin, 600×. (→) points to an intercalated disk.

Fatty degeneration – fatty heart

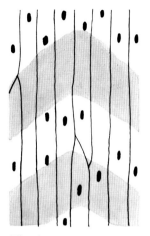 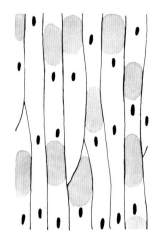

Tigering
of Heart Muscle

Toxic Fatty
Degeneration

Fat Infiltration
of Heart
→ F = Fat tissue
→ M = Muscle

Fig. 44. Fatty degeneration – fat infiltration of heart.

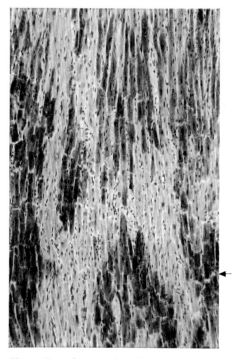 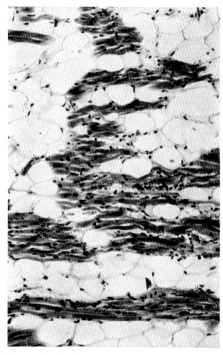

Fig. 45. Fatty degeneration of heart muscle
(tigering); Sudan – hematoxylin, 82×.

Fig. 46. Fat infiltration of heart;
H & E, 148×.

36

Fatty degeneration – Fat infiltration

Fatty degeneration (fatty metamorphosis) of heart muscle must be clearly separated from *fat infiltration* or fatty heart (Fig. 44).

Fatty degeneration appears in two forms:

1. A *band or streak-like form* in which segments of myocardial fibers containing fat alternate regularly with unchanged fibers so that an appearance like that of a tiger's skin results. The fatty streaks lie next to the venous limbs of capillaries. The cause of this form of fatty degeneration is generalized, deficient oxygenation of the heart muscle.

It is seen frequently in aplastic or pernicious anemia, in massive blood loss or so-called *anemic anoxia* and less frequently in leukemia. This sort of fatty degeneration can likewise be caused by generalized oxygen-lack due to disturbances of lung ventilation *(asphyxic anoxia)*.

2. A *disseminated focal form*, affecting irregular areas of the heart, in which there is fatty degeneration of single fibers or portions of fibers, usually in association with other degenerative changes of heart muscle such as clumping of sarcoplasm (see Fig. 59). These changes appear at the edges of myocardial infarcts, after toxic injuries of heart muscle, such as diphtheria or interstitial myocarditis, and after poisoning, for example, with phosphorus, chloroform, ether and lead (see also the electron photomicrographs, pp. 42, 43).

Macroscopically, the heart is dilated and shows small, speck-like, grayish yellow spots.

In fatty degeneration of the myocardium (tigering), the essential changes can be seen at a glance (Fig. 45). In sections stained with Sudan or scarlet-red, the striped pattern of the fatty myocardial fibers clearly contrasts with the unaltered fibers which are stained faintly blue by the hematoxylin. The resemblance to the skin of a tiger is very striking, since the stripes vary in width and often do not run exactly parallel through the entire section of tissue, but branch frequently. High magnification shows that the fat is in the form of fine droplets laid down between the myofilaments (see also Fig. 55). Notice the segmentation of the heart muscle fibers in both the right-hand (→) and left-hand parts of the picture (Fig. 45).

Macroscopically, the heart likewise shows a pattern resembling a tiger's skin with parallel yellow lines alternating with reddish brown muscle. It is especially well seen in the papillary muscles of the left ventricle.

In fat infiltration or fatty heart (Figs. 44, 46) there is both *infiltration of heart muscle with fat, such as occurs elsewhere in obesity, and transformation of connective tissue cells into fat cells.* Even with the unaided eye, one can see that the muscle bundles have been separated by finely distributed fat tissue, which extends into the musculature in tongue-like processes. The amount of subepicardial fat is also increased and, microscopically (Fig. 46, medium magnification), fat can be seen replacing interstitial tissue. The cell nuclei are pressed to the periphery by the fat droplets and the cytoplasm is reduced to a thin membrane. Since the fat content of the cells is dissolved by the process of paraffin embedding, in which alcohol and xylol are used, only optically empty spaces are seen in the section.

Macroscopically, fat infiltration is most pronounced in the right ventricle. The cut surface shows yellow, streak-like infiltration of the myocardium. Frequently, there are also islands of fat beneath the endocardium. In estimating the weight of the heart, especially in cardiac hypertrophy, allowance must be made for the amount of fat tissue. *Clinically*, marked obesity may cause the so-called Pickwick syndrome with elevated diaphragm, hypoventilation, cyanosis polycythemia and cor pulmonale.

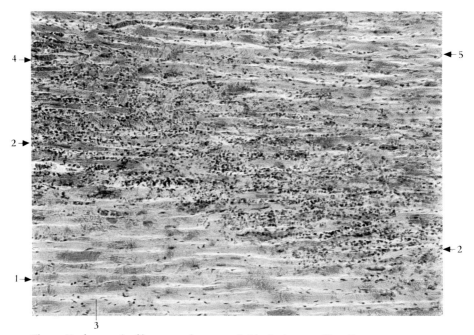

Fig. 47. Fresh necrosis of heart muscle surrounded by leukocytes. H & E, 70×.

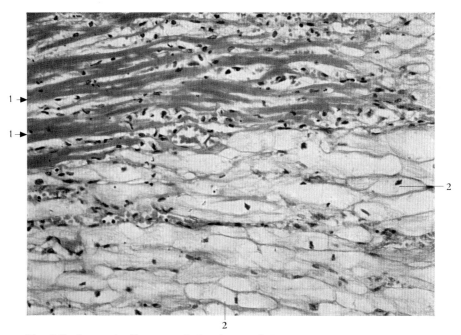

Fig. 48. Fresh necrosis of heart muscle showing sarcolysis. H & E, 225×.

Infarct of the Heart

Infarcts of the heart show ischemic coagulation necrosis resulting from lack of oxygen due to obstruction of the coronary arteries (arteriosclerosis, thrombosis, which are common, or embolism, which is rare).

Table 5 shows the *time sequences* of the macroscopic and microscopic changes and of some of the clinical events.

Table 5. **Time Sequences of Events in Heart Infarcts**

Time	Macroscopic	Microscopic	Other Changes
15 sec.	—	—	ECG changes
30–60 min.	—	Edema of fibers	Electron microscopic changes (Figs. 53, 56) H_2O uptake
2 hrs.	—	Hyalinization of fibers (homogeneous, eosino-philic)	Calcium loss up to 24 hours
3 hrs.	—	Clumping of sarcoplasm Fatty degeneration	Increased sodium content. Decreased enzymes of the citric acid cycle in infarct
4 hrs.	TTC-reaction negative	Necrosis	
6 hrs.	Slight pallor	Leukocytic reaction	
9 hrs.	Yellow, dry, firm	Fully developed necrosis	
18–24 hrs.	Yellow, dry, firm	Fully developed necrosis	Increased enzymes in serum
2–3 wks.	Red granulation tissue	Granulation tissue	
5 wks. 2 mos.	Scar White, firm, fibrous	Scar tissue	

Legend: TTC-Reaction = triphenyltetrazolium chloride reaction (for detection of succinic dehydrogenase).

Figure 47 shows a **new infarct** with fresh muscle necrosis that is about 8 hours old (→ 1) and bordered by a broad zone of leukocytic infiltration (→ 2). At the edge of the infarct, in adjacent myocardium, there is a zone of recent hemorrhage (→ 4), beyond which the myocardium is normal (→ 5). Muscle fibers in the necrotic area lack nuclei and have homogeneous cytoplasm. Notice that the nuclei of the interstitial connective tissue are preserved (→ 3).
Fresh Myocardial Necrosis Showing Sarcolysis. Microscopic examination of the necrotic myocardium with high magnification shows very clearly the homogenization of the sarcoplasm (Fig. 48 and Fig. 57) and the absence of cross-striations (→ 1). The depth of staining with eosin is also noteworthy. Myocardial nuclei have disappeared, although nuclei of the interstitial connective tissue cells are still present. The illustration also shows advanced sarcolysis, or dissolution of necrotic sarcoplasm, leaving only the empty shells of the sarcolemma (→ 2). Essentially the same process, but with clumping of the sarcoplasm, is seen in Figure 59. Capillaries, some collapsed and others dilated, can be recognized in the interstitial tissue. Remnants of the sarcolemma may persist in the scar of an infarct for long periods.

Macroscopic appearance: a circumscribed, lemon yellow, dry, firm area.

Complications of Myocardial Infarcts: rupture of the ventricle with pericardial tamponade, rupture of a papillary muscle (mitral insufficiency may develop), mural thrombosis with arterial embolism, fibrinous pericarditis, acute or chronic ventricular aneurysms, cardiac shock.

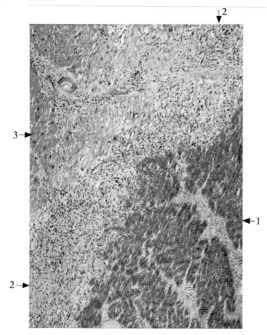

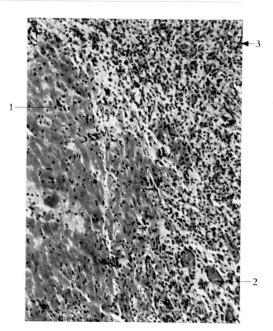

Fig. 49. Organization taking place in a somewhat older myocardial infarct;
H & E, 41 × .

Fig. 50. Organization taking place in a somewhat older myocardial infarct (detail);
H & E, 120 × .

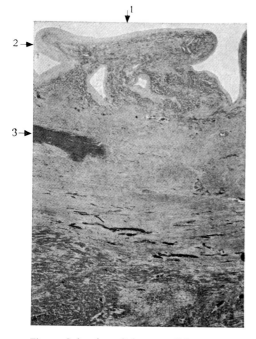

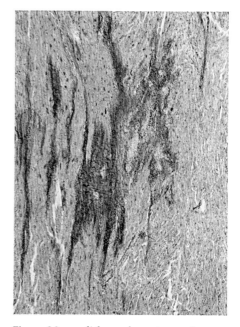

Fig. 51. Subendocardial myocardial scar;
H & E, 15 × .

Fig. 52. Myocardial scars due to incomplete
coronary artery insufficiency;
van Gieson, 39 × .

Necrotic heart muscle will largely be reabsorbed by granulation tissue during the course of 2–3 weeks, depending upon the size of the infarct. In such an **organizing infarct** (Fig. 49), examination of a microscopic section with the unaided eye or at low magnification shows an irregularly shaped, intensely red area which is the *necrotic zone* (→ 1), a richly cellular layer (blue appearing) bordering the necrotic zone (*granulation tissue* → 2), bordered in turn by the less deeply eosin-stained *normal heart muscle* (→ 3). Medium magnification reveals the essential alteration, namely necrotic muscle fibers that have lost their nuclei. Higher magnification shows the loss of cross-striations. The cytoplasm of the myocardial fibers is homogeneous and eosinophilic. In addition, the nuclei of the interstitial tissue have nearly completely disappeared. In adjacent granulation tissue, capillaries can be seen with medium magnification as small, empty, round or ovoid spaces between which there are round cells (lymphocytes, histiocytes, see Fig. 28), fibroblasts and connective tissue fibers having a distinctive smooth, straight shape. The cellular infiltration seen in the granulation tissue extends only slightly into the uninjured myocardium in which well-preserved nuclei can be clearly seen.

Macroscopic: Red granulation tissue intermixed with remnants of yellow necrotic tissue.

Figure 50 is a detail under higher magnification of another somewhat **older infarct in the process of organization** showing the line of division between necrosis and granulation tissue. In the necrotic zone on the left-hand side of the picture are seen once again anuclear muscle fibers with homogeneous, intensely red eosinophilic sarcoplasm. The nuclei of the interstitial connective tissue are partially preserved, and in some places wandering histiocytes can already be seen (→ 1). The granulation tissue is richly cellular and contains dilated capillaries (→ 2). The earliest wandering cells to infiltrate the granulation tissue (→ in picture) are histiocytes (see Fig. 28) with large round to oval nuclei and basophilic cytoplasm. In the upper right-hand part of the figure (→ 3) the granulation tissue is less cellular. A delicate background of fine collagen fibers has appeared between the small rod-shaped nuclei of the fibroblasts (see also Fig. 26).

Compare this picture with the granulation tissue shown on page 52. Notice the similar structure: *wandering histiocytes* – the highly cellular *middle zone* with capillaries, angioblasts, histiocytes, lymphocytes and fibroblasts – and an *outer zone* in which fibrous tissue is being formed.

The final outcome of a myocardial infarct is a **scar of the heart muscle.** Figure 51 is from a section of myocardium taken perpendicular to the endocardium, so that the trabeculae (→ 1) of the inner ventricular surface can be seen. The endocardium is thickened by connective tissue (→ 2) and beneath it the muscle fibers are for the most part preserved, since they are nourished from inside the heart chambers. Next to the myocardium there is a broad layer of practically acellular collagenous tissue: the scar. At the lower margin of the picture, normal myocardium can be seen interspersed with small islands of scar tissue. Within the large scarred area there is a red area (→ 3): fresh necrosis of a surviving remnant of myocardium (recurrent infarct).

Macroscopic: White scar tissue, sometimes intermixed with yellow areas of necrosis.

Myocardial Scars in Coronary Insufficiency (Fig. 52.) *Coronary insufficiency* (BÜCHNER) *develops because of a disproportion between the amount of oxygen needed by the myocardium and the amount of oxygen available to it* (for example, in cardiac hypertrophy or coronary arteriosclerosis with obstruction insufficient to cause massive infarction but sufficient to cause an oxygen deficiency). The essential difference from a myocardial infarct can be seen on naked-eye examination. Instead of a large necrotic area or a large scar in the heart muscle, there are small disseminated, fleck-like scars which in sections stained by van Gieson's method are colored bright red. Heart muscle stains yellow.

Macroscopic: Firm, fibrous, glistening, white scar tissue.

Fine Structure of the Heart Muscle in O_2 Deficiency

In O_2 deficiency, the electron microscope reveals first of all *loss of glycogen*, followed by *edema of the ground substance* and *vacuolation of the endoplasmic reticulum* (vacuolar degeneration) as may be seen in Figure 53. The *mitochondria swell*, and pale, fleck-like patches appear (Fig. 56), the matrix becomes clear (edema) and later the membranes disintegrate. Finally, the *myofilaments* come loose from their attachments at the Z-bands and the cross-striations disappear (Fig. 57).

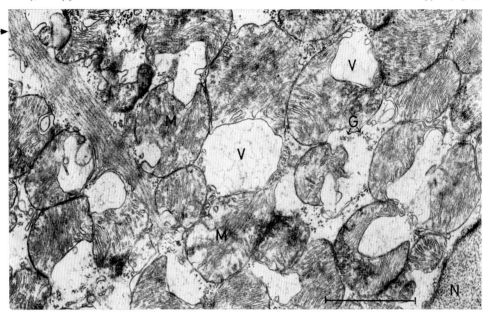

Fig. 53. *Vacuolar (hydropic) degeneration* of myocardium (rat, coronary insufficiency, 15 hours after subcutaneous injection of 75 mg./kg. of isoproterenol sulphate). Many vacuoles (V), partly in the ground substance and partly in the ER, contain finely granular and thready material (protein rich fluid). N = nucleus, M = mitochondria (slightly swollen), G = glycogen, → myofibrils. 24,500 × (Dr. KORB, 1965).

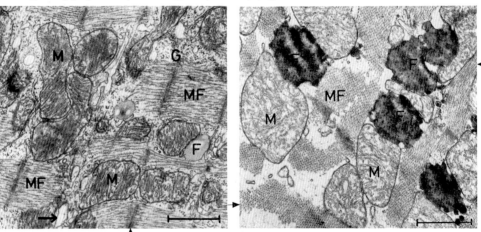

Fig. 54. *Normal rat heart muscle.* There are myofilaments and distinct Z-bands (→). Mitochondria thickly packed with cristae (M) lie between. Scattered throughout are isolated fat droplets (F), as well as glycogen granules (G) and parts of ER (→ inside picture). 14,000 × (Dr. KORB).

Fig. 55. Fatty degeneration (rat myocardium, periphery of an infarct 1 hour old). Fat droplets (F) lie between bundles of myofibrils (MF and →) and are in close contact with swollen mitochondria (M). 15,500 × (Dr. KORB).

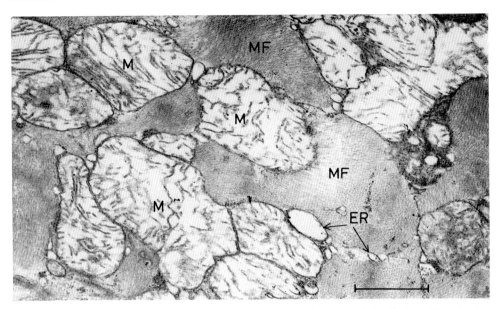

Fig. 56. *Cloudy swelling of heart muscle* (rat: treated as in Fig. 53, after 3 hours). Marked swelling of mitochondria (M), clearing of the matrix and reduction in the number of cristae. MF = myofibrils; the ER shows focal vacuolar dilatation. 19,500× (Dr. KORB).

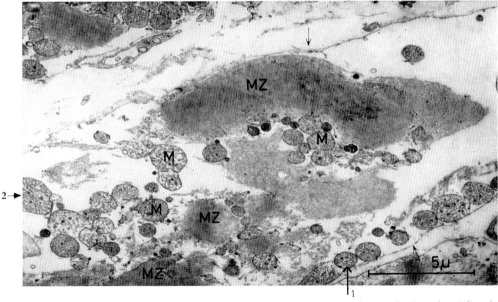

Fig. 57. *Clump-like disintegration and sarcolysis* (heart muscle, cat, 3 hours after production of an infarct by ligation of a coronary artery). There are connected fragments of muscle cells (MZ) showing thickened and clumped myofilaments with disrupted fine structure. In the neighborhood are partly preserved and partly condensed mitochondria (M). → marks the remnants of the sarcolemma. There are so-called matrix aggregates (intramitochondrial granules) in some mitochondria (→ 1, → 2). These, in all likelihood, contain calcium (see Table 4). 6,000× (Dr. KORB).

43

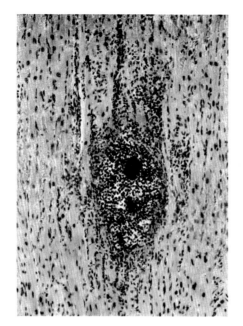

Fig. 58. Metastatic (embolic) abscess of heart muscle;
H & E, 141 × .

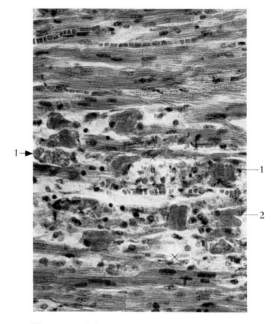

Fig. 59. Diphtheritic myocarditis;
H & E, 315 × .

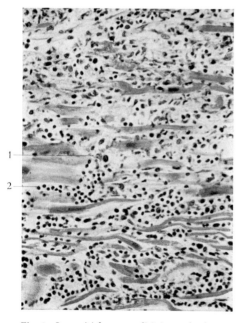

Fig. 60. Interstitial myocarditis in scarlet fever;
H & E, 255 × .

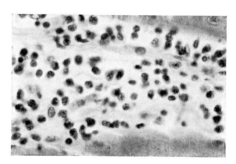

Fig. 61. Idiopathic myocarditis with eosinophils;
H & E, 592 × .

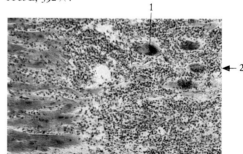

Fig. 62. Idiopathic myocarditis with giant cells;
H & E, 110 × .

Myocarditis

Inflammations of the heart muscle may be grouped as follows:

1. *serous myocarditis,*

2. *purulent myocarditis,*

3. *non-purulent interstitial myocarditis:*

   a) degenerative or parenchymatous inflammation (example: *diphtheria*);

   b) lympho-histiocytic form (example: *scarlet fever*);

   c) granulomatous myocarditis (example: *idiopathic myocarditis* of Fiedler; active *rheumatic fever* with Aschoff nodules).

Serous myocarditis is manifested by inflammatory edema of interstitial tissues (e. g., in thyrotoxicosis and burn injury among others, see the electron micrographs of serous inflammation, Fig. 22).

Purulent myocarditis originates mostly from metastatic colonies of bacteria or from septic arterial emboli (pyemic abscesses, for example, in thrombo-ulcerative endocarditis; they also occur in kidney). Figure 58 shows a **metastatic abscess of the heart muscle** with centrally situated bacterial colonies (globular, dusky heart), destruction of tissue and great infiltration of polymorphonuclear leukocytes. Neighboring tissues are sparsely infiltrated with polymorphs.

Non-purulent, diphtheritic myocarditis (Fig. 59) always shows *degenerative changes of the parenchymatous cells,* and the ordinary features of inflammation are not pronounced (parenchymatous or alterative inflammation). In Figure 59, different stages of myocardial injury can be recognized: homogenization and clumping of sarcoplasm ($\rightarrow$ 1) progressing to sarcolysis (X), so-called toxic myolysis. See also Figure 57. At higher magnification, the injured fibers stain intensely red and have irregular shapes. In addition, some myocardial fibers show focal fatty change (see Fig.44). Histiocytes have mobilized around degenerated fibers ($\rightarrow$ 2), to remove dead and dying debris. In addition, there are occasional polymorphonuclear leukocytes. Healing results in the formation of many small focal scars.

Macroscopic: Dilation of the heart with either small, poorly defined, grayish yellow foci or small scattered scars.

Interstitial myocarditis may occur during the course of scarlet fever. There is *infiltration of lymphocytes and histiocytes* (Fig. 60) and a less conspicuous degenerative component. Between the widely separated muscle fibers there is a sparse infiltration of histiocytes ($\rightarrow$ 1), lymphocytes ($\rightarrow$ 2), fibroblasts and occasional plasma cells and considerable interstitial edema. Some muscle fibers are intact, others are degenerated and some are necrotic.

In some cases of myocarditis of unknown cause **(idiopathic myocarditis with eosinophils),** the myocardium is either diffusely or focally infiltrated with eosinophils (Fig. 61). In addition, granulomatous inflammation **(idiopathic giant cell myocarditis)** (Fig. 62) may occur with a richly cellular infiltration of lymphocytes, fibrocytes and plasma cells and complete destruction of foci of heart muscle. In such cases, the inflammatory exudate contains giant cells having clumped nuclei, the so-called muscle giant cells ($\rightarrow$ 1 and 2).

Macroscopic: Dilatation of the heart. The cut surface shows numerous small, poorly circumscribed, grayish red or grayish yellow fleck-like foci.

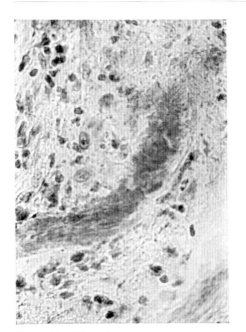

Fig. 63. Fresh fibrinoid necrosis.
H & E, 480×.

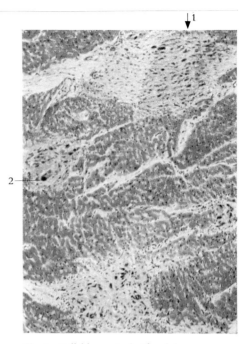

Fig. 64. Full-blown Aschoff nodules.
H & E, 120×.

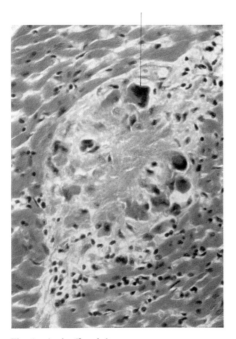

Fig. 65. Aschoff nodule.
H & E, 330×.

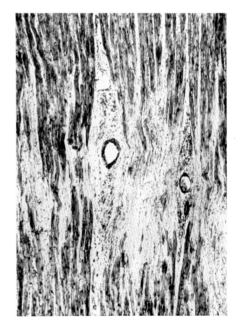

Fig. 66. Rheumatic scar.
H & E, 56×.

Rheumatic Myocarditis

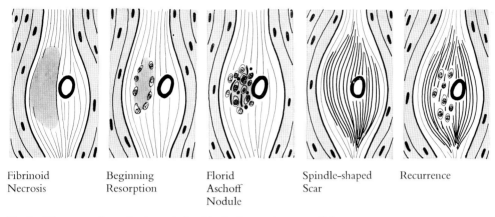

Fibrinoid Necrosis	Beginning Resorption	Florid Aschoff Nodule	Spindle-shaped Scar	Recurrence

Fig. 67. Diagram to show the time relationships in rheumatic myocarditis.

Figure 67 shows the *course of rheumatic myocarditis* in active rheumatic fever. Similar changes take place in the aorta, peritonsilar tissues, heart valves and joints. *The illness begins with fibrinoid swelling (necrosis) of the perivascular connective tissue* (see also Fig. 25a). *The body reacts by producing a histiocytic granuloma containing giant cells which is called an Aschoff nodule* (ASCHOFF, 1904). The histiocytes remove the fibrinoid material (phagocytic function of the histiocytes). *The end stage is a perivascular scar of connective tissue* in which histiocytes have been transformed into fibroblasts and have formed collagen fibers (Fig. 27). *Recurrences* localize preferentially in old scars.

In examining the tissue microscopically, attention should be directed to the large interstitial spaces. Figure 64 was taken at medium magnification and shows many **full-blown Aschoff nodules** (→ 1) with compact accumulations of histiocytes and giant cells (→ 2). High magnification shows the earlier change of **fresh fibrinoid necrosis** (Fig. 63) consisting of bright red, homogeneous material which completely obscures the connective tissues. The host reaction commences immediately with mobilization of histiocytes, which can be recognized by their large, chromatic nuclei, large nucleoli and poorly demarcated, faintly basophilic cytoplasm. A few lymphocytes are also present. Figure 65 shows an **Aschoff nodule** at a somewhat more advanced stage. In the center of this nodule there is fibrinoid material. At the margins there are histiocytes as well as giant cells derived in part from muscle cells (→), since in this case the inflammation has involved the myocardium.

At the termination of the acute inflammatory phase, the histiocytes become oblong in shape and form collagen fibers. As a result, perivascular **rheumatic scars** develop (Fig. 66). These scars appear as elongated and pointed bright red areas. In the illustration, a few solitary histiocytes are still embedded in the scar tissue.

Macroscopic: Dilatation of the heart; small, white focal scars in the healed stage. Almost always accompanied by active or subsiding rheumatic valvulitis.

Endocarditis

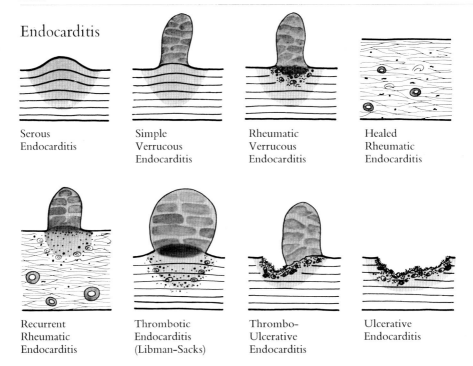

Serous
Endocarditis

Simple
Verrucous
Endocarditis

Rheumatic
Verrucous
Endocarditis

Healed
Rheumatic
Endocarditis

Recurrent
Rheumatic
Endocarditis

Thrombotic
Endocarditis
(Libman-Sacks)

Thrombo–
Ulcerative
Endocarditis

Ulcerative
Endocarditis

Fig. 68. Diagrammatic representations of different sorts of endocarditis.

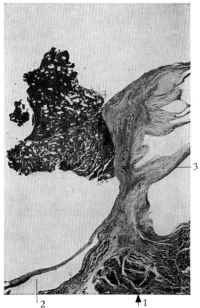

Fig. 69. Recurrent rheumatic verrucous
endocarditis;
H & E, 10×.

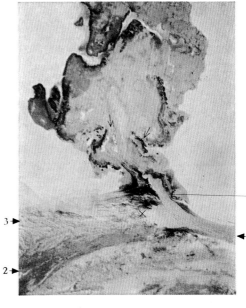

Fig. 70. Thrombo-ulcerative endocarditis;
H & E, 11×.

Endocarditis

Endocarditis is an inflammation of the heart valves and is characterized not only by conspicuous fluid and cellular exudation in the connective tissues of the leaflets or cusps, but also by superimposed thrombosis. The aortic cusps and mitral leaflets are preferentially affected.

There are 5 different sorts of endocarditis. 1. The mildest and most fleeting sort, and perhaps also the precursor of all other forms of endocarditis, is **serous endocarditis** (Fig. 68), in which blood serum proteins exude into the connective tissue of the valves and cause swelling of the fibers and interstitial edema (macroscopic: slight, glistening swelling). 2. **Simple verrucous endocarditis** (Fig. 68) is distinguished from rheumatic endocarditis only by the intensity of the edema and cellular reaction. A break develops in the valvular endothelium which is then overlaid by a thrombus consisting almost exclusively of blood platelets, although a small amount of fibrin is also usually present. The valvular connective tissue shows moderately marked fibrinoid degeneration and a sparse inflammatory reaction (leukocytes and histiocytes). 3. **Rheumatic endocarditis** (Fig. 68) has almost the same microscopic appearance. However, fibrinoid swelling is more marked, and correspondingly there is a more pronounced inflammatory reaction of polymorphonuclear leukocytes and histiocytes. Healing **(burned-out rheumatic endocarditis,** Fig. 68) is accompanied by vascularization and scarification with deformity of the valve. Recurrent attacks of rheumatic endocarditis are frequent **(recurrent rheumatic endocarditis,** Fig. 69).

Macroscopic examination reveals grayish white, glistening, easily wiped-off warty growths on the valve surfaces.

4. **Thrombotic endocarditis** (Libman-Sacks) is a non-bacterial endocarditis with soft, coarse thrombi formed of platelets and fibrin. There is marked fibrinoid degeneration of the valvular tissue and a decided inflammatory reaction (Fig. 68). The lesions are found frequently in *acute disseminated lupus erythematosus* along with renal involvement (wire loop glomerular lesions).

5. **Thrombo-ulcerative and ulcerative endocarditis** (also called endocarditis lenta or sub-acute bacterial endocarditis, Fig. 70) are, in contrast to verrucous endocarditis, bacterial infections of the valves, usually Strep. viridans. There is usually marked leukocytic infiltration and destruction of the valves.

Macroscopically, there are valvular deformities and polypoid thrombi. *Complications of endocarditis:* 1. in non-bacterial endocarditis: arterial emboli, valvular defects; 2. in bacterial endocarditis: valvular deformities, metastatic pyemic abscesses, focal embolic nephritis (LÖHLEIN).

In **recurrent rheumatic endocarditis** (Fig. 69), low magnification shows thickening of the mitral leaflet due to a superimposed broad layer of red-staining eosinophilic material. Heart muscle (→ 1) is seen at the lower margin of the photograph, and the endocardium of the left ventricle at → 2. Medium magnification shows connective tissue thickening of the valve leaflet and numerous capillaries (→). The chordae tendinae show fibrous thickening (→ 3). The thrombus consists of eosinophilic material (blood platelets). From the fact that capillaries are present in the ground substance of the valve, it can be concluded that there was a previous episode of endocarditis.

Thrombo-ulcerative endocarditis (Fig. 70) *is a form of bacterial endocarditis with destruction of valve leaflets and superimposed, bacteria-laden thrombi.* Both low and medium magnification show aortic media (→ 1), and left ventricular myocardium (→ 2) covered by endocardium (→ 3) that has been thickened by fibrous connective tissue. Remnants of valvular tissue are still plainly seen (→ 4). A thrombus, composed of fibrin and platelets and containing bacterial colonies (→), sits on top of the valve. Calcification of the connective tissue fibers (x) at the base of the leaflet indicates that there had been previous inflammation with subsequent scarring.

Pericarditis

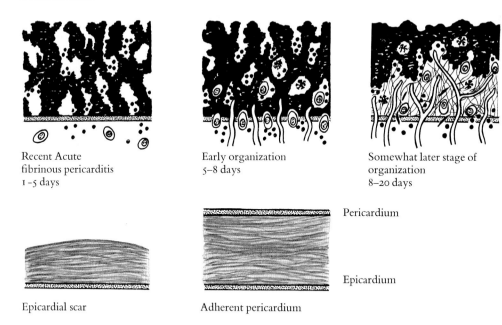

Recent Acute
fibrinous pericarditis
1–5 days

Early organization
5–8 days

Somewhat later stage of
organization
8–20 days

Pericardium

Epicardium

Epicardial scar

Adherent pericardium

Fig. 71. Diagram of the essential features and time sequences in pericarditis.

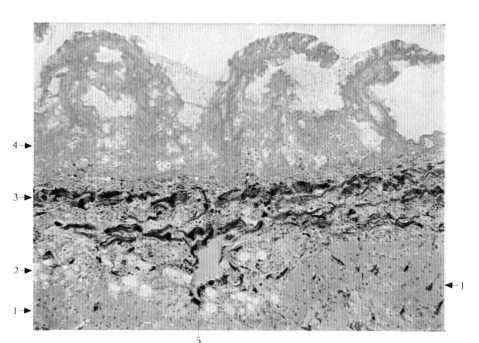

Fig. 72. Recent, acute, fibrinous pericarditis; van Gieson stain, 62 ×.

Pericarditis

Pericarditis is an inflammation of the serous coverings of the heart, including both the visceral or epicardial, and the parietal layers. All variants of the inflammatory reaction may occur (serous, fibrinous, purulent, hemorrhagic, chronic, granulomatous, etc.). *It can arise by metastasis*, for example, in sepsis or infectious diseases; *by direct extension*, for example, from the lung, pleura or esophagus; or as a *toxic response*, for example, in uremia; or as a result of *myocardial infarction.*

Any inflamed serosal surface (pleura, peritoneum, pericardium) will show the same histological changes and the same end results.

Figure 71 illustrates the **chief changes and the time sequence in fibrinous pericarditis.** The black areas are fibrin.

Recent acute fibrinous pericarditis (1–5 days): Fibrinogen and serum proteins have leaked from the pericardial capillaries and immediately polymerized to fibrin fibers. Irregularly shaped, tangled masses of fibrin are present on the surface of the pericardium (Fig. 72). The lining endothelial cells are in part destroyed and in part preserved, although swollen by irritation.

Early organization of acute fibrinous pericarditis (5–8 days): At this stage, granulation tissue (capillaries, histiocytes, fibroblasts) has begun to grow in from the epicardium and pericardium (Figs. 73 and 74), leading to destruction of the fibrin and its partial reabsorption by proteolytic enzymes of the histiocytes.

Later stage of organization of fibrinous pericarditis (8–20 days): Proliferation of granulation tissue has progressed, and increasing numbers of collagen fibers are forming from the fibroblasts in the deeper parts (Fig. 73).

In the end, a **pericardial scar** of collagenous tissue develops (eventually forming flat hyalinized fibrous plaques in the epicardium, known as soldier spots). If the inflammation has involved both the epicardial and parietal surfaces, the pericardial sac may be obliterated (*adhesive pericarditis, synechia pericardii*, see Figs. 71, 75).

Under certain conditions (possibly activation of fibrinolytic mechanisms), the fibrin is dissolved completely and the pericardium is restored to normal. If a large amount of fluid rich in serum proteins and fibrin is a feature of the inflammation, it is called *serofibrinous pericarditis.* Pericardial adhesions usually do not develop in this form.

Recent fibrinous pericarditis (Fig. 72). Examination of the section with either the unaided eye or a hand lens discloses three layers: a broad, compact layer of *heart muscle* stained yellow with van Gieson's stain (→ 1), a loose layer of *subepicardial fat tissue* (→ 2) and a shaggy outer *layer of fibrin* (→ 4). With medium magnification, the details can be better seen: the layer of muscle fibers, the layer of loosely arranged connective tissue (van Gieson red, → 3) and fat showing the usual round, optically empty spaces, and occasional infiltrated granulocytes and lymphocytes. The overlying fibrin is colored yellow with van Gieson's stain and appears as compact masses between which stretches a fine network of fibrin threads, which is seen especially well at the surface. A few leukocytes and erythrocytes are enmeshed in the fibrin network together with a pale yellow-stained, homogeneous, proteinacious material. Notice that only an occasional enlarged cell of the surface endothelium (mesothelium) can be seen (→). A small vein in the fat tissue shows plasma stasis (homogeneous yellow in the van Gieson stain, → 5).

Macroscopic: The surface is dull and shaggy (shaggy heart, cor villosum).

Note: Fibrinous inflammation commonly undergoes fibrous organization resulting in *fibrous adhesions.*

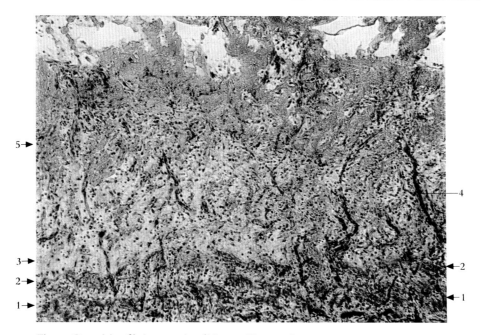

Fig. 73. Organizing fibrinous pericarditis; van Gieson stain, 99 ×.

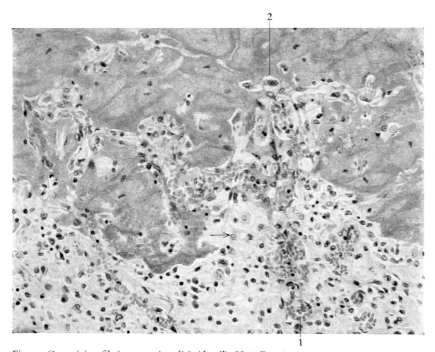

Fig. 74. Organizing fibrinous pericarditis (detail); H & E, 248×.

Organizing fibrinous pericarditis (Fig. 73). After about 5 days, granulation tissue begins to invade the fibrin. Examination of a microscopic preparation with a hand lens still shows preservation of the three layers (muscle, fat tissue, superficial layer of fibrin) described in Figure 72. Now, however, the subepicardial fat tissue is not clearly demarcated and is more densely infiltrated with cells and permeated with collagenous fibrous tissue. With medium magnification and a van Gieson preparation (Fig. 73), interlacing of the red-stained epicardial fibers can be seen (→ 1) as well as the infiltration of histiocytes, fibroblasts and lymphocytes (→ 2), which originate from the epicardium. This is followed by the appearance of granulation tissue composed of pale red newly formed connective tissue fibers (→ 3). The vascular sprouts in the connective tissue (→ 4) can be seen clearly to have their origin in the pericardium and from there to course perpendicularly to the surface. The granulation tissue shows fibroblast nuclei (cut longitudinally) and occasional lymphocytes. In the upper portion of the section, the remaining strands of fibrin (→ 5) resemble tongue-like projections into the granulation tissue. In many places, lacunae of various shapes have formed in the fibrin, where the histiocytes have brought about resorption.

Macroscopic: Surfaces covered with a grayish white, firmly adherent shaggy layer.

Figure 74, **organizing fibrinous pericarditis,** shows the boundary between the fibrin and the connective tissue at high magnification. In the lower portion of the figure, loosely arranged fibrin is being replaced by granulation tissue. Histiocytes (→, also see Fig. 27), lymphocytes and solitary fibroblasts can be seen (also see Fig. 28), as well as dilated capillaries filled with erythrocytes (→ 1). In the path of the advancing granulation tissue, wandering histiocytes are also found lying in spaces free of fibrin (resorption lacunae → 2).

Pericardial adhesions (Fig. 75) may be the end result of fibrinous pericarditis. In our illustration, heart muscle (→ 1) is seen at the bottom of the photograph, overlaid by a thin remnant of subepicardial fat tissue. Above it there is loosely arranged and richly vascularized new connective tissue which fills the space between the two layers of the pericardium. The compact connective tissue of the parietal layer (→ 2) and the mediastinal fat tissue (→ 3) occupy the upper half of the photograph. Mesothelial cells line clefts between the strands of connective tissue so that adenomatous structures may form, which must not be mistaken for metastases of an adenocarcinoma (also peritoneal and pleural adhesions).

Adhesions always carry the possibility of *obliteration* of the pericardial space. However, in most cases, fibrinous pericarditis is inconsequential and only scattered, delicate, easily freed fibrous adhesions are formed.

In *recurrent pericarditis*, additional new granulation tissue is laid down and cicatrized so that eventually a thick, tough, fibrous scar is formed which may sometimes become calcified (armored heart). Pleuritis or peritonitis may have a similar outcome (flat, hyalinized or calcified pleural scars; exuberant peritoneal fibrosis).

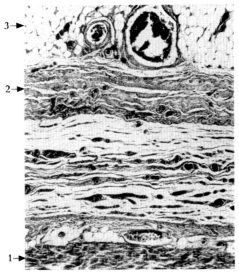

Fig. 75. Pericardial adhesion;
H & E, 30×.

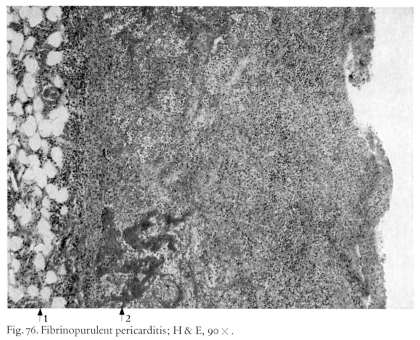

Fig. 76. Fibrinopurulent pericarditis; H & E, 90 ×.

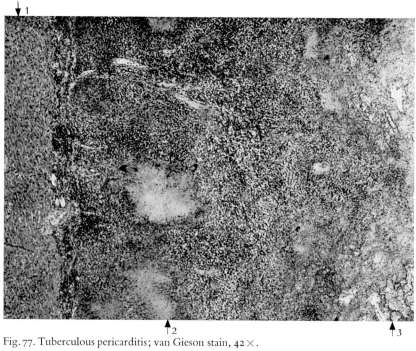

Fig. 77. Tuberculous pericarditis; van Gieson stain, 42 ×.

Fibrinopurulent Pericarditis (Fig. 76). As has been mentioned for other forms of pericarditis, naked-eye examination of a microscopic slide shows three distinct layers – heart muscle, subepicardial fat tissue and a layer of fibrinous exudate. Figure 76, which does not include heart muscle, shows subepicardial fat ($\rightarrow$ 1) covered with fibrin. Just as in non-purulent fibrinous pericarditis, examination with a hand lens shows that the fibrin layer on the surface has a distinctly bluish cast and the network-like structure of the fibrin is largely absent. This is because of dense infiltration of the fibrin with cells which, under high magnification, are seen to be polymorphonuclear leukocytes with typical lobulated nuclei. For the most part, the cytoplasm of these cells is poorly demarcated from surrounding fibrinous exudate. In this particular preparation (Fig. 76), only a few clumps of deeply eosinophilic fibrin lie directly on the epicardium ($\rightarrow$ 2). The superimposed, more homogeneous, red-staining masses in which the leukocytes are enmeshed consist of coagulated blood plasma, fibrin and erythrocytes. The loosely arranged fibro-adipose tissue of the epicardium on the left-hand side is likewise infiltrated with leukocytes.

Macroscopic examination shows a shaggy heart just as in fibrinous pericarditis, except it is usually not grayish white but rather grayish yellow. Creamy, cloudy or flocculent exudate fills the pericardial sac (specific gravity in excess of 1018).

Tuberculous Pericarditis (Fig. 77). As in fibrinous pericarditis, pericarditis caused by specific infections, such as tuberculosis, is remarkable for the degree of cellular infiltration ($\rightarrow$ 1). In addition, round or irregularly shaped granulomas are present that have red, eosinophilic, acellular centers ($\rightarrow$ 2) and are surrounded by a cellular zone. Medium magnification shows the typical features of such a tubercle (see p. 97 ff.):

1. Central *caseation necrosis* with either a homogeneous or finely granular appearance.
2. A zone of radially arranged *epithelioid cells* surrounding the caseous center. The cells are arranged side by side like epithelial cells; therefore, the term epithelioid.
3. *Langhans giant cells* with nuclei arranged in semi-lunar fashion and in such a way that the opening of the half moon is turned toward the necrosis.
4. A marginal zone of *connective tissue* containing lymphocytes which are scanty, however, in the adjacent tissue.

Between individual tubercles there is an exudate of fibrin and serum rich in leukocytes and lymphocytes. Fibrin can be seen to the right in the figure ($\rightarrow$ 3). At the myocardial edge ($\rightarrow$ 1), which is chiefly subepicardial fat tissue, numerous lymphocytes accompany the advancing granulation tissue, in which are seen empty double-contoured, capillary sprouts. Tuberculous pericarditis usually arises secondarily most commonly by way of lymphatics or blood vessels, and less commonly by direct extension from neighboring structures. Frequently, an adherent tuberculous bronchopulmonary lymph node is the most probable site of origin.

Macroscopically, the appearance is that of fibrinous pericarditis, but the layer of exudate is yellowish gray and caseous nodules are seen on the cut surfaces. Eventually, a dense adherent pericarditis develops, often with obliteration of the pericardial space, calcification and even constriction of the heart (constrictive pericarditis).

Arteriosclerosis

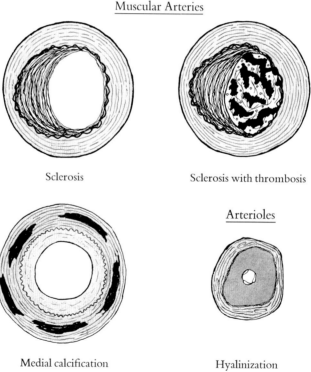

Fig. 78. Diagram of various forms of arteriosclerosis.

Blood Vessels

In order to evaluate the pathological changes that occur in blood vessels, it is first necessary to be clear as to the kind of blood vessel that is involved – arteries, veins or capillaries. With regard to arteries, which will chiefly interest us here, it is most important to keep in mind those structures in the vessel wall that control changes in the caliber of the lumen. **Arteries of elastic type** (e. g., aorta, subclavian and iliac arteries, etc.), the media of which contains elastic membranes and smooth muscle cells, are especially prone to intimal sclerosis and atherosclerosis (perhaps also medial necrosis, syphilitic medial inflammation). Arteriosclerosis in *large arteries* of **muscular type** (e. g., femoral, popliteal and brachial arteries), which have distinct internal and external elastic lamina, may show medial calcification in addition to intimal sclerosis or can present as an endarteritis obliterans (arteries of the legs). In *small arteries of muscular type*, such as the coronary arteries, the arteries at the base of the brain and those in the renal medulla, arteriosclerosis develops chiefly as focal semilunar zones of elastosis and sclerosis. These arteries, as well as the arterioles, are also attacked in periarteritis. In **arterioles**, arteriosclerosis takes the form of hyalin deposition (arteriolosclerosis). The malignant form of nephrosclerosis as well as periarteritis nodosa likewise involves arterioles.

Histological examination should take note of the thickness of the intima, alterations of the media (deposits, inflammatory infiltrates, structural changes) and any cellular infiltrate in the adventitia.

Survey of the various forms of arteriosclerosis (Fig. 78).

Arteriosclerosis is a chronic, progressive disease of arteries characterized by deposition of pathological metabolic products and accompanied by tissue proliferation and reconstruction of the vessel wall. Recent studies suggest that arteriosclerosis begins with **edema of the intima.** Because of this, the intima becomes swollen (glassy macroscopic appearance) with faintly staining protein material and fibrin situated between connective tissue fibers. This stage is fleeting and reversible. More easily recognized grossly are the **fatty flecks and streaks** – lipidosis – (Fig. 79) caused by deposition of fine droplets of fat (lipoprotein) between the connective tissue fibers of the intima and secondary phagocytosis of the fat droplets by macrophages (macroscopically, flat yellow flecks and streaks).

This stage is reversible, but it can also go on to the next stage – a **fibrous or sclerotic plaque** (Figs. 80, 82). At this stage, there is a great increase in the intimal connective tissue, which frequently is hyalinized (see Fig. 90), with simultaneous splitting of the elastic lamellae of the internal elastic membrane. The lipids then fuse into larger foci and, at the same time, *necrosis* develops, probably due to pressure from swelling (Fig. 80). As a result, anuclear zones develop with typical spear-shaped spaces corresponding to the shape of cholesterin crystals (**atheroma** with macroscopically visible yellowish white masses and glistening cholesterin crystals, Figs. 80, 81). Occasional phagocytic cells with vacuolated cytoplasm (foam cells) can be seen at the margins of the atheroma as a reaction to the deposition of fat.

An atheroma may ulcerate and a parietal thrombus form secondarily **(atheromatous ulcer with thrombosis).** Simultaneously with the development of sclerosis and atheromatosis of the intima, fibrous tissue and mucopolysaccharides are increased in the media (increased mucoid ground substance?, uncoupling of reactive groups of the mucopolysaccharides?) and fine deposits of calcium are laid down.

Complications: Thrombosis of ulcerated atheromatous plaques and possible arterial embolization; cholesterol crystal emboli, ectasia, aneurysms, intimal hemorrhages.

Medial calcification causes pipe-stem arteries in the extremities (detected by palpation).

Sclerosis of medium and small arteries (e. g., the coronary arteries) results mostly in semilunar narrowing of the arterial lumen and atrophy of the media. Hemorrhage into the atheromatous plaque and secondary thrombosis may develop (see Figs. 82, 83, 84).

Hyalinization of arterioles (arteriolosclerosis or arteriolarsclerosis) is characterized microscopically by homogenization of the vessel wall and consequent atrophy of the media (Fig. 32 and p. 152). The hyaline material lies between the intima and media.

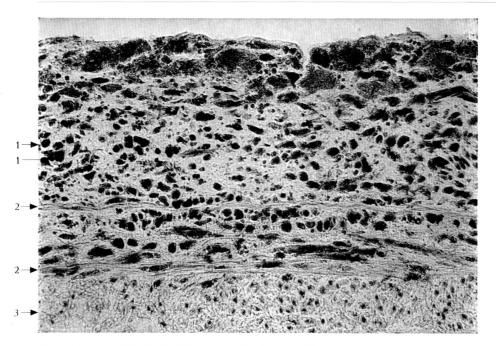

Fig. 79. Fatty streak (lipidosis) of the aorta; sudan–hematoxylin, 252×.

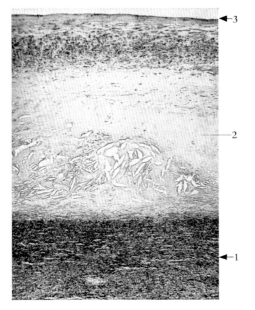

Fig. 80. Base of atheromatous plaque with
pressure necrosis due to swelling;
H & E, 40×.

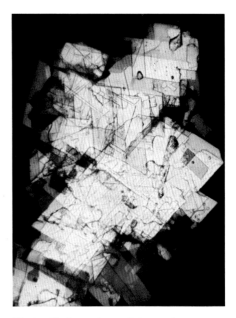

Fig. 81. Cholesterol crystals in an atheroma as
seen in the polarizing microscope;
unstained, 100×.

Arteriosclerosis of the Aorta

Fatty streak (lipidosis) of the aorta (Fig. 79). The earliest visible sign of aortic arteriosclerosis is *deposition of lipids and protein material in the intima*. The lipids persist, although frequently they are of no consequence. They can disintegrate or be carried away by the lymph stream (e. g., the so-called aortic milk-streaks of children). Thus, a fatty streak is not necessarily the same as arteriosclerosis. The disease process is initiated first by a mesenchymal reaction in the intima, and only after this is it progressive. Fatty streaks (lipidosis) are thus only an indicator of abnormal permeability of the vessel wall. The less readily visible protein material is probably the chief irritant of the mesenchymal tissues.

In sections stained for fat and examined with a scanning lens, the three layers of the aorta can be easily recognized: adventitia containing nutrient vessels, media which appears as a blue, homogeneous band and intima which shows cushion-like thickening and small, red focal deposits. With medium magnification (Fig. 79), the intima, in addition to the red-stained areas of fat, is seen to be stained pale blue and to contain collagen fibers and occasional longitudinally cut nuclei of fibrocytes. The intima is thickened in the region of the sudan-positive areas. In the uppermost layers of the intima, the lipids form large aggregates, while in the remaining portions of the intima the lipid is in the form of fine droplets contained in round or oval cells with marginally situated nuclei (histiocytes and phagocytes, → 1). These cells were first seen in 1852 by ROKITANSKY and later described more accurately by LANGHANS (1866). In Figure 79 the internal elastic membrane is already somewhat splintered (→ 2). The media is finely dusted with fatty material (→ 3 : muscle cells of the media). With polarized light, doubly refractive material (cholesterol) can be easily demonstrated (Fig. 81).

Macroscopic: Yellow, flat lesions, often streak-like.

Base of atheromatous aortic plaque with necrosis due to swelling (Fig. 80). The deposition of lipids and protein in the intima evokes fibroblastic proliferation and collagen fiber production and leads to fibrous thickening of the intima (→ 1 aortic media; → 3 endothelium). When great thickening develops, the intima may well be thicker than the media in some places. Under medium magnification, compactly arranged, eosinophilic, collagenous fibers and a few fibrocytes can be seen. Some areas are completely devoid of cell nuclei. The fibers appear homogeneous, strongly eosinophilic and can no longer be distinguished as separate cells as they fuse into an amorphous substance (necrosis following swelling → 2).

Cholesterol crystals are deposited in such areas and appear as spear-shaped spaces in paraffin sections (Fig. 80), whereas in smears examined with the polarizing microscope they appear as doubly refractive rhomboid plates (Fig. 81). The media contains increased amounts of mucopolysaccharides (blue staining, chromotropic ground substance) and frequently finely granular calcium deposits.

Macroscopic: Raised lesions which, on sectioning, show glistening cholesterol crystals (atheroma).

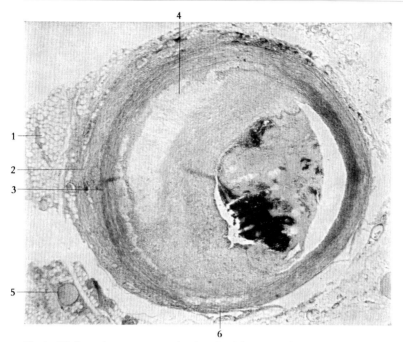

Fig. 82. High-grade coronary arteriosclerosis with a recent thrombus; H & E, 26×.

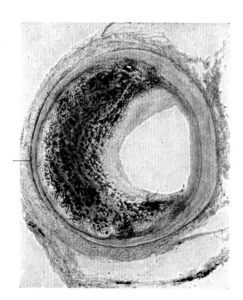

Fig. 83. Coronary arteriosclerosis with
atheroma formation;
sudan stain, 14×.

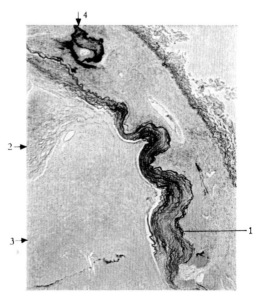

Fig. 84. Elastosis of a coronary artery filled
with an old thrombus;
elastica-van Gieson stain, 40×.

Coronary arteriosclerosis

Among the common diseases of the vascular system, coronary arteriosclerosis and its frequent sequel, a myocardial infarct, takes a foremost place. It arises like the other forms of arteriosclerosis from fat deposition and is followed by sclerosis. Sometimes, marked edema of the intima develops and the artery is suddenly obstructed (a cause of death in young persons). Complications include secondary thrombosis, bleeding in a sclerotic plaque or necrosis from excessive swelling, all of which may lead to sudden narrowing of the lumen of the vessel. Hyalinization of small intramural (myocardial) branches is also commonly seen.

High-grade coronary sclerosis with a recent thrombus (Fig. 82). The changes are well shown by examining a cross-section of a coronary artery. The coronary artery is embedded in subepicardial fat tissue ($\rightarrow$ 1). The loosely arranged adventitia ($\rightarrow$ 2) forms an outer mantle. The media appears as a red ring ($\rightarrow$ 3). The intima is thickened by a crescent-shaped layer of fibrous tissue with a lightly stained atheromatous base in which necrosis has occurred as a result of swelling ($\rightarrow$ 4). What remains of the lumen is filled with a preformed thrombus consisting chiefly of platelets, fibrin and erythrocytes (conglutination thrombus, see also Fig. 93). At $\rightarrow$ 5, a small nerve can be seen in the fat tissue. Interference with medial nutrition is suggested by a focus of cystic degeneration ($\rightarrow$ 6) in the media (medial necrosis). Note that the adventitia adjacent to the crescent-like area of intimal sclerosis shows an increase in collagenous connective tissue. Calcium may be deposited secondarily in both the intima and media.

Coronary arteriosclerosis with atheroma formation (Fig. 83). Fat stains show clearly the marked deposition of lipid in crescent-shaped areas of intimal thickening. The fatty material is partly within histiocytes and partly lying free in the tissues where it has fused (atheroma). The inner layer of the sclerotic plaque contains no lipid. Noteworthy is the marked atrophy of the media in the base of the plaque ($\rightarrow$), a finding that is almost always present (disturbed medial nutrition caused by the plaque).

Elastosis of a coronary artery filled with an old thrombus (Fig. 84). Sclerosis is always accompanied by more or less marked elastosis, that is, by splintering and proliferation of the elastic fibers. Figure 84 shows such splintering and increase of the elastic fibers ($\rightarrow$ 1) together with an old thrombus. The lumen of the artery is partly filled with collagenous connective tissue containing a few blood vessels (cicatrized granulation tissue, $\rightarrow$ 2). The yellow homogeneous mass ($\rightarrow$ 3) is the residue of the old thrombus. In the old scar tissue in the muscle of the media can be seen a few blood vessels ($\rightarrow$ 4) that have arisen in the adventitia and grown into the thrombus.

Macroscopic: Lipidosis: Yellow, flat deposits. *Sclerosis and atheroma:* lumen narrowed by grayish yellow or yellow plaques which are frequently focal. *New thrombus:* reduction or complete closing of the lumen by gray-red masses. *Old thrombus:* grayish brown to grayish white deposits on the vessel wall, often in a form resembling a rope ladder. Preferred localization of coronary arteriosclerosis: usually 1 cm. below the origin of the descending branch of the left coronary artery.

61

Vascular Inflammation

Periarteritis Nodosa

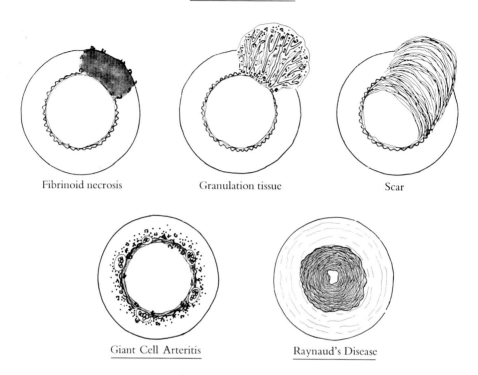

Fibrinoid necrosis   Granulation tissue   Scar

Giant Cell Arteritis   Raynaud's Disease

Thromboangiitis Obliterans

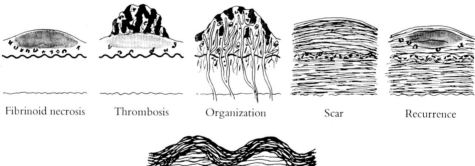

Fibrinoid necrosis   Thrombosis   Organization   Scar   Recurrence

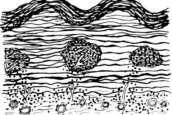

Syphilitic Mesarteritis

Fig. 85. Diagram of the different sorts of vascular inflammations.

Inflammations of Blood Vessels

Figure 85 on the opposite page shows the chief sorts of primary arteritis. The changes occurring in **periarteritis nodosa** (KUSSMAUL and MAIER, 1866) will serve as an example of their pathogenesis. The earliest change, or first stage, is *fibrinoid necrosis and leukocytic infiltration involving a segment of the intima and media of arterioles* (see Fig. 86). In the *second stage*, the fibrinoid material is reabsorbed and replaced by *granulation tissue* (see Fig. 87), with the result that discrete nodules form in the adventitia (periarteritis nodosa; in reality, a panarteritis). The *granulation tissue becomes cicatrized (third stage)*, with consequent narrowing of the lumen, which may be marked (see Fig. 88). As a consequence of the inflammation and scarring, circulatory obstruction and infarction may develop (e. g., anemic infarcts in the kidney and spleen).

Giant cell arteritis (granulomatous giant cell mesarteritis) manifests itself by *fibrinoid degeneration* and a *granulomatous reaction at the intimal-medial boundary* (see Fig. 89). The internal elastic membrane is destroyed by the inflammatory process and the fragments of the elastic fibers elicit a foreign-body response (foreign body giant cells).

Note: Fibrinoid degeneration is always followed by granulation tissue and scarring (examples: verrucous endocarditis, rheumatic fever, periarteritis nodosa, thromboangiitis obliterans, giant cell arteritis, etc.).

Thromboangiitis obliterans, also called **endarteritis obliterans** (Winiwarter-Buerger's disease), shows essentially the same inflammatory process that occurs in periarteritis nodosa. The disease process is initiated by fibrinoid necrosis and leakage of blood plasma into the intima. Organization is brought about by mobilization of histiocytes and granulation tissue. The disease affects chiefly the arteries of the lower extremities *(juvenile gangrene of the extremities)*. Occasionally, the cerebral, mesenteric or coronary arteries are involved.

The *earliest changes* in the disease consist of *fibrinoid degeneration (necrosis) of the intima*, with a sparse leukocytic reaction extending as far as the internal elastic membrane. *Thrombi* may or may not form on the injured intima. This is followed either by granulation tissue growing from the adventitia into the site of injury *(organization)* or by mobilization from the local connective tissue of fibrocytes and histiocytes which reabsorb the fibrinoid and thrombotic material. The *final residue* is an *intimal* or *intimal-medial scar* (see Fig. 90). Arteriosclerosis may develop secondarily. Recurrences localize in a previous scar.

Syphilitic mesaortitis begins with *inflammation around the vasa vasorum in the adventitia* and only *secondarily involves the media and destroys the elastica*. Shrinkage of the resulting scars leads to contracture of the intima over the scar sites (Fig. 91).

The vascular changes of **Raynaud's disease** (Raynaud's gangrene) do not properly belong in the group of inflammatory vascular diseases. The disease is seen chiefly in women and is a progressive disease of the arterioles of the fingers, knees and ear lobes and runs a chronic course. There is hypertrophy of the medial musculature (indicated by concentric lines in Fig. 85) and slight fibrosis of the intima. The malady is thought to be an angioneuropathy.

63

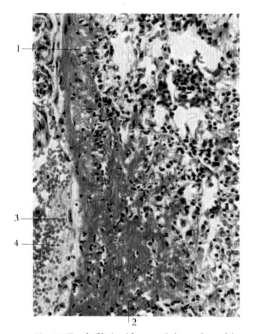

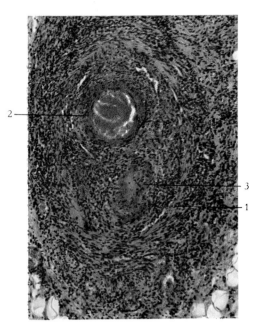

Fig. 86. Fresh fibrinoid necrosis in periarteritis nodosa;
H & E, 220×.

Fig. 87. Recurrent periarteritis nodosa;
H & E, 95×.

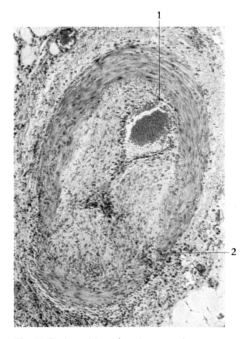

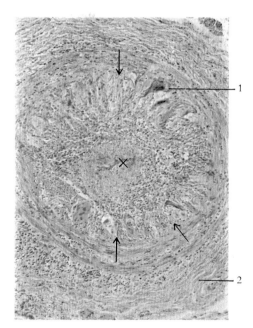

Fig. 88. Periarteritis nodosa (scar stage);
H & E, 74×.

Fig. 89. Giant cell arteritis;
H & E, 100×.

Periarteritis Nodosa (Panarteritis)

The *earliest stage* is shown in Figure 86 **(fresh fibrinoid necrosis in periarteritis nodosa).** *Fresh fibrinoid necrosis* (homogeneous, strongly eosinophilic) has developed in segments of the intima and media (→ 2). In the surrounding tissues there are leukocytes and a beginning granulomatous reaction. At → 1, slightly edematous but otherwise unaffected vascular media can still be seen. The intima is lifted off the area of fibrinoid necrosis (→ 3: endothelial cells) and a loose network of fibrin and erythrocytes lies on the intimal endothelium (→ 4).

Under very low magnification, it is seen that the vascular changes are nodular, being formed of red or bluish red, focal areas of exudate in the arterial wall. The appearance of a *fully developed lesion with superimposed subacute inflammation* is shown in Figure 87 **(recurrent periarteritis nodosa).** The lumen of the artery, with the exception of a small channel, is almost completely closed by granulation tissue which extends into a portion of the media and the adventitia. The granulation tissue consists of proliferated capillaries, fibroblasts, histiocytes and lymphocytes (infrequently plasma cells and eosinophils). The media is preserved in large part (→ 1). A new vascular space with a muscularis and containing erythrocytes has developed in the granulation tissue filling the original lumen (→ 2). Fresh fibrinoid necrosis (exacerbation?) is seen at → 3, the homogeneous eosinophilic material of which is invaded by histiocytes.

The **scar stage** (Fig. 88) resembles the appearances seen in Figure 87. Fibroblasts and young cellular scar tissue have reduced the lumen to a small channel (→ 1). The place where the artery has been breached by granulation tissue arising from the adventitia can be clearly seen (→ 2), as well as the collagenous scar tissue and occasional lymphocytes.

Macroscopic: Bead-like nodules 1–2 mm. in diameter especially well seen in the heart (beneath the epicardium) or mesenteric arteries.

The consequences of the vascular occlusions are multiple infarcts of the kidney and spleen, red infarcts of the liver and necrosis in the gastrointestinal tract with ulceration.

Practically any organ can be affected. Neuromuscular symptoms follow involvement of the arteries of the peripheral nerves and muscles. A biopsy of the skin or muscle may confirm the clinical diagnosis. The disease particularly attacks men 20–40 years old. The course is mostly subacute (1 year) and death results from uremia, myocardial necrosis, intestinal infarction or rupture of a blood vessel.

Giant cell arteritis (Fig. 89). This relatively benign form of periarteritis nodosa was once thought to affect chiefly the temporal artery of older women. However, more recent statistics indicate that man and women are equally affected. Next to the temporal artery in incidence comes involvement of the ophthalmic artery (blindness), brain, heart, liver, spleen, etc. Fibrinoid necrosis develops locally in the region of the intima, with destruction of the internal elastica. As Figure 89 shows, the involvement is preponderantly in the intima and media. In this particular vessel, the intima shows both inflammatory exudate and granulation tissue and only a small lumen remains (→ x). The boundary between intima and media is marked by the arrow. The internal elastica is broken into fragments that are surrounded by giant cells (→ 1). The media is diffusely infiltrated with lymphocytes and histiocytes. The exudate involves the adventitia only slightly (→ 2: adventitia).

Macroscopically and clinically, the temporal arteries are thick (pulseless) and the overlying skin is red; migraine-like headaches.

65

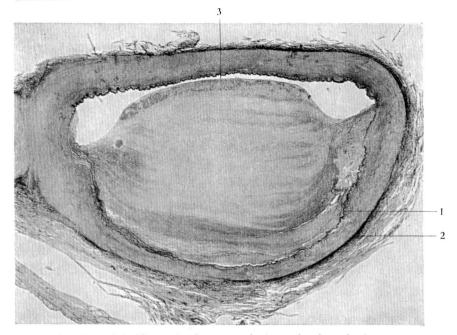

Fig. 90. Thromboangiitis obliterans in a leg artery; elastica–nuclear fast red stain, 19 × .

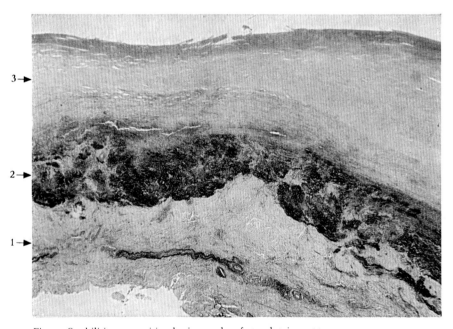

Fig. 91. Syphilitic mesaortitis; elastica–nuclear fast red stain, 32 × .

Thromboangiitis obliterans. Figure 90 is a very low magnification of a cross-section of an artery of the leg stained for elastica. The lumen is almost completely filled by poorly cellular fibrous tissue. The internal elastica ($\rightarrow$ 1) and the external elastica ($\rightarrow$ 2) show as black bands. The media appears as a red, homogeneous layer. The internal elastica is slightly split in several places. Proliferation of intimal connective tissue has almost completely filled the lumen of the artery. Fresh fibrinoid necrosis (exacerbation, $\rightarrow$ 3) can be seen in the upper portion in the form of red, band-like streaks.

Thromboangiitis obliterans may have various morphological appearances. The *earliest stage*, which is often fleeting, consists of *fibrinoid degeneration* and is seldom seen. The most frequently seen stage is of a *recurrent thrombus* showing organization and a *sclerotic base*. The final stage can often scarcely be differentiated from arteriosclerosis, especially if a secondary thrombus has formed on a sclerotic plaque (see Fig. 85).

The disease process attacks the arteries of the legs, is decidedly focal with cushion-like intimal thickening, fresh thrombosis and corresponding reduction in vessel lumen. Distal to the obstruction, the artery shows intimal proliferation, which may act as a sort of plug. The disease runs a course with many exacerbations and affects mostly a single lower extremity, particularly of young men (juvenile gangrene of the leg). Endarteritis of small arteries shows the same histological picture and attacks in particular the arteries of the brain (resulting in atrophy of the granular layer) and the renal, mesenteric and coronary arteries (myocardial infarct!).

Syphilitic Mesaortitis (Fig. 91). *This is an inflammation of the adventitia and media of the aorta developing in tertiary syphilis.* Figure 91, taken at low magnification, shows the typical "moth-eaten" pattern of the destruction of the medial elastica. The adventitia ($\rightarrow$ 1) shows an increase in collagenous fibrous tissue (scar formation). The greater part of the media ($\rightarrow$ 2) is irregularly replaced by nodular, sparsely cellular scar tissue. The intima ($\rightarrow$ 3) is greatly thickened by secondary arteriosclerosis. In the right hand side of the figure hyalinization of the intima has occurred. The disease process begins with a lympho-histiocytic and plasma cell inflammation around the vasa vasorum of the adventitia and creeps along the vessels into the media. The small medial arteries then show an endarteritis which results in medial ischemia (necrosis), formation of granulation tissue, destruction of elastica and replacement of the lost tissue by a scar. Since the scar tissue shrinks, the intima is pulled inward over the scar.

From this result the characteristic *macroscopic* ridges (wrinkles) or tree-bark appearance of the intima, especially prominent in the thoracic portion. In addition, the wall of the aorta is thin and the vessel dilated (ectasia). Frequently, the inflammation also encroaches upon the cusps of the aortic valve, causing widening of the commissures and formation of a channel between them. In addition, the cusps contract so that aortic insufficiency develops. Furthermore, the coronary ostia can become obstructed by intimal proliferation, so that death is not infrequently due to a myocardial infarct.

Medium and small sized arteries, in particular those at the base of the brain, can also be affected in tertiary syphilis, chiefly in the form of an endarteritis with intimal proliferation.

Thrombosis - Thrombophlebitis - Organization

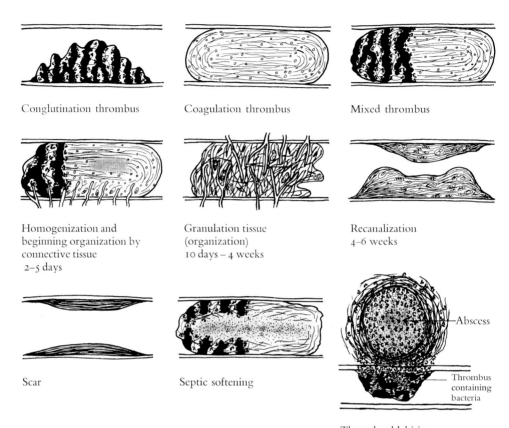

Conglutination thrombus

Coagulation thrombus

Mixed thrombus

Homogenization and
beginning organization by
connective tissue
2–5 days

Granulation tissue
(organization)
10 days – 4 weeks

Recanalization
4–6 weeks

Scar

Septic softening

—Abscess

Thrombus
containing
bacteria

Thrombophlebitis

Organization of a Thrombus

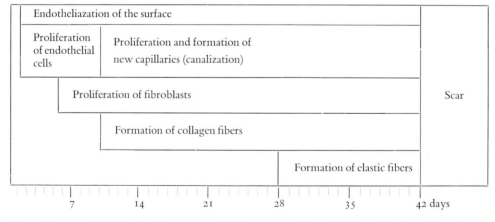

Endotheliazation of the surface					Scar
Proliferation of endothelial cells	Proliferation and formation of new capillaries (canalization)				
	Proliferation of fibroblasts				
		Formation of collagen fibers			
				Formation of elastic fibers	
	7	14	21	28	35	42 days

Fig. 92. Diagram of the histological structure of different sorts of thrombi, the results of secondary changes in a thrombus and the process of organization. Thrombophlebitis.

Thrombosis – Thrombophlebitis

Thrombosis is the intravascular coagulation of blood during life. Figure 92 illustrates in diagrammatic fashion the histological structure and fate of the different sorts of thrombi and the temporal events in the course of organization.

1. **A conglutination or agglutination thrombus,** shown adhering to the vessel wall (a mural or parietal thrombus) has a typical form. Conglutinated blood platelets are built up into a coral-like laminated scaffold. Fibrin surrounds and also lies between the columns of platelets, giving an appearance like that of a reinforced steel building. Leukocytes are enmeshed in the fibrin and accumulate like mantles around the blood platelets. Between the fibrin columns lie masses of erythrocytes (see Fig. 93).

Macroscopic: Rib-like projections of platelets are seen on the surface of the thrombus, giving it a rippled appearance crosswise to the direction of blood flow like the pattern on a wind-swept sand dune. Grayish red in color and friable.

2. A **coagulation thrombus** completely fills the vessel lumen and histologically consists of fibrin lamellae arranged parallel to the vessel wall. Between the lamellae stretches a delicate, irregularly constructed framework of fibrin in the meshes of which erythrocytes have become trapped. Platelets cannot be seen with the light microscope. There is a scanty sprinkling of leukocytes.

Macroscopic: A red, structureless column of coagulated blood.

3. A **mixed thrombus** consists of a headpiece, which has the structure of a *conglutination thrombus,* and a tailpiece, which has the structure of a *coagulation thrombus.* In the femoral vein, both conglutination and coagulation thrombi are frequently intermingled.

Macroscopic: Intermixed red and gray parts. *Postmortem clots,* in contrast to thrombi, have an elastic consistency (clots formed slowly are gray due to the buffy coat; clots formed quickly are red) and show no stratification or other signs of a structure.

4. In **septic thrombophlebitis,** there is a purulent inflammation of the vessel wall of bacterial origin. A thrombus containing bacteria forms at the site of the inflammation and histologically shows irregularly arranged masses of platelets and fibrin and bacterial colonies. If thrombotic material comes loose, then pyemic abscesses develop in the lung or elsewhere (see Fig. 113).

Macroscopic: Gray to grayish white, cheesy coating of the walls of veins.

5. **Hyalin thrombi** have a red homogeneous appearance in H & E sections and are composed of platelets and fibrin. They are found in capillaries and venules particularly in shock (see Figs. 160, 191).

Fate of Thrombi

1. *Emboli:* parts of a thrombus, or even the whole thrombus, may become detached and circulate with the blood. The danger of embolism is reduced when the thrombus has become organized (10 days). 2. *Alterations in the structure of the thrombus (homogenization):* In the course of disintegration, the contained erythrocytes, granulocytes and platelets fuse with the fibrin and cell fragments and form a homogeneous mass. This process of homogenization begins in the center of the thrombus as early as the second day and proceeds continuously. Homogenized portions of a thrombus are resistant to the lytic action of streptokinase (see thrombolysis below). 3. *Dissolution of the thrombus:* a) *by granulocytes* (putrid softening). When the proteolytic enzymes of the granulocytes are released they dissolve the fibrin, erythrocytes and platelets, especially in the center of the thrombus. A pus-like fluid results that is flushed away by the blood stream. b) *by the fibrinolytic system* (thrombolysis): By the conversion of plasminogen to plasmin, the fibrin in the thrombus can be dissolved by proteolysis (plasmin has a high specificity for fibrin, but does not lyse platelet masses). Plasminogen is present in flowing blood and is adsorbed by the fibrin fibers in the thrombus. The fibrinolytic system can be activated by bacterial products (streptokinase). Homogenized portions of a thrombus, however, are not dissolved by streptokinase (inactivation of plasminogen). c) *by granulation tissue* (organization). Endothelialization of a thrombus begins as early as one day after it starts to form (adjacent vascular endothelium grows onto the surface of the thrombus). Sprouts of vascular endothelial cells grow into the base of the thrombus (vascular endothelial cells have fibrinolytic activity). Capillaries from the endothelial

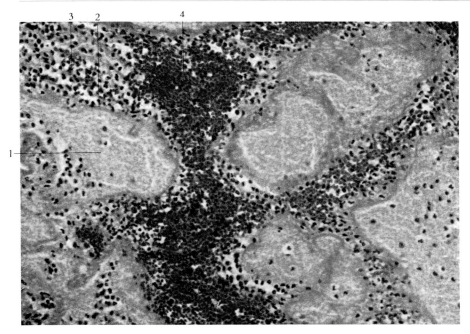

Fig. 93. Conglutination (agglutination) thrombus; H & E, 246 ×.

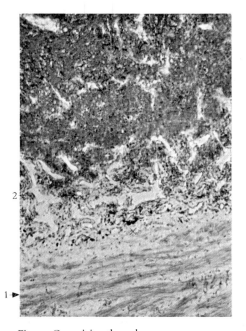

Fig. 94. Organizing thrombus;
H & E, 101 ×.

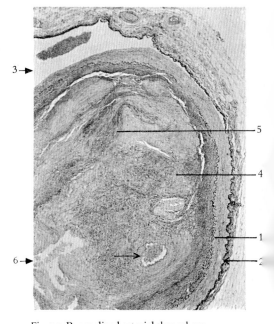

Fig. 95. Recanalized arterial thrombus;
elastica-van Gieson stain, 40 ×.

cell sprouts (about day 10), and ramify in the thrombus. About day 5 fibroblasts invade the base of the thrombus. About day 10 they form collagen fibers and later a lesser number of elastic fibers. Thus the cellular response of the vessel wall is formation of granulation tissue. Such granulation tissue, by virtue of its contained proteolytic enzymes, has the ability to dissolve a thrombus including the homogenized portions and replace it with connective tissue. In this way a scar may be formed after 4–6 weeks. The new capillaries bring about recanalization of the formerly thrombosed blood vessel.

Special Sorts of Organization: The newly formed connective tissue may become calcified or ossified (phleboliths). The new blood channels in the thrombus can be especially large and numerous (cavernous.) Involvement of the valves of the veins in the process of organization of thrombi in the leg veins may be very important in the development of post-thrombotic syndromes (e. g. varicosities, stasis ulcers). 4. *Propagation or "growth" of thrombi:* Simultaneously with the processes of dissolution, a thrombus can also increase in size through the addition of new thrombus. Such propagation of a thrombus occurs particularly in the veins of the lower extremities (calf veins – femoral, iliac) and always carries a high risk of embolization.

Conglutination (agglutination) thrombus (Fig. 93). When a section of such a thrombus is examined under very low magnification, the vessel wall is seen to be covered with a thrombus having a rough, undulating surface. Projecting columns of platelets fill the spaces between erythrocytes. Under medium magnification (Fig. 93), the coral-like structure of the platelet masses ($\rightarrow$ 1) is easily recognized. Under high magnification, the platelets appear as finely granular material. Fibrin appears as homogeneous bands ($\rightarrow$ 2) which envelop the platelets. Outside the bands of fibrin is a zone of leukocytes ($\rightarrow$ 3). In the spaces between the platelet columns there are thickly massed erythrocytes ($\rightarrow$ 4) and a loose fibrin network. In old thrombi it may be difficult to distinguish between platelets and fibrin. Azan stains are helpful, since platelets stain blue, whereas fibrin stains red.

Organizing thrombus (Fig. 94). The early stages of resorption and organization begin from the vessel wall and are already under way at two to four days after the onset of thrombosis. Very low magnification shows red material completely filling the lumen. The wall of the vein ($\rightarrow$ 1) appears as a light red band. Low-power magnification discloses a brighter red, sparsely cellular zone in the vessel wall near the thrombus. Medium magnification (Fig. 94) shows granulation tissue developing in this zone of the vessel wall where markedly dilated capillaries ($\rightarrow$ 2) and erythrocytes are clearly visible. In between lie fibroblasts and histiocytes, and formation of new connective tissue fibers has already started. Vessels are still sparse in the interior of the thrombus. Isolated histiocytes (precursors of granulation tissue) are present, lying in part around empty spaces ($\rightarrow$) (for another example, see pp. 40, 52). The brownish black granules ($\times$) in the organizing tissue are intracellularly situated products of hemoglobin-hemosiderin.

Macroscopic: Firmly attached, grayish red to brown layer. Fresh coagulation thrombi are only loosely attached to the vessel wall.

Recanalization of an arterial thrombus (Fig. 95). The microscopic appearance depends on the age and mass of the thrombus and the degree of recanalization. In Figure 95, the internal elastic lamina ($\rightarrow$ 1) and external elastic lamina ($\rightarrow$ 2) are present. The former is partly split and fragmented. At $\rightarrow$ 3, the external elastic lamina is lifted off the media and blood fills the breach (artifact of preparation). The true lumen of the blood vessel is obstructed by connective tissue of different ages (richly cellular young granulation tissue $\rightarrow$ 4: older fibrous connective tissue $\rightarrow$ 5). In the midst of the connective tissue there are spaces lined by endothelium and containing erythrocytes ($\rightarrow$ 6 and arrow). These dilated blood vessels pass through the organized thrombus and have terminations in the main lumen of the artery, both before and behind the thrombus.

Macroscopic: Depending upon the stage of organization and recanalization, any of the following may be seen: a mural scar, web-like adhesions (particularly in thrombi of leg veins) and sinusoidal transformation of blood vessels (e. g., thrombosis of the portal vein). Usually, the surrounding tissues are stained brownish (hemosiderin). A less frequent consequence of the organization of a thrombus is the formation of phleboliths or of a so-called myxoma (organization of thrombi in the heart).

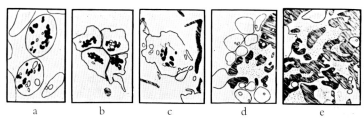

Fig. 96. Schematic representation of the pathogenesis of thrombosis (after RODMAN et al., 1963).

Thrombus formation starts with agglutination of thrombocytes, which is associated with loss of granulation (so-called *viscous metamorphosis*). Later, fibrin accumulates. The results of studies with the electron microscope show that this viscous metamorphosis takes place in four stages (Fig. 96). Normal thrombocytes (Fig. 96a) consist of a *clear* portion (ground substance) and a *granular* portion containing the cellular organelles. In the *first stage* of agglutination (preagglutination), the thrombocytes *swell* (membrane injury?), form *pseudopods* and stick together (Fig. 96 b). The existing ATP begins to disintegrate (because of ATPase activity). The integrity of the outer membranes of the thrombocytes is probably preserved through the mediation of ADP and calcium. In the *second stage* of agglutination, the outer membrane of individual thrombocytes is still largely intact (Figs. 96 b, 97). The granular ground substance disappears from the center of the platelets (Fig. 97). During the *third stage (thrombocytic rhexis)*, the outer membranes of the thrombocytes disintegrate (Fig. 96 c, d). In the center, the various constituents of the granular ground substance deteriorate. At the outer margin, protrusions are formed. Now, for the first time, fibrin is visible at the margins of the aggregates (Fig. 96 d). In the last stage, that of *thrombocytolysis* (Fig. 96 e), the thrombocytes disintegrate completely into granular material and membrane fragments. A large amount of fibrin is intermingled with this remaining wreckage. During this stage of viscous metamorphosis, the thrombocytes give up the following substances: 1. those effecting plasma coagulation (factor 3 = thromboplastin (thrombokinase) and factor 4 = calcium); 2. those effecting fibrinolysis – platelet proactivator antiplasmin; 3. those with an effect on the blood vessel wall – adrenalin, noradrenalin, serotonin.

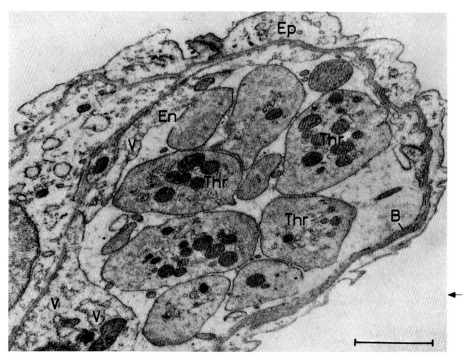

Fig. 97. Lung capillary with agglutinated thrombocytes (Thr) in the lumen (histamin shock, rabbit). The platelets are heaped on one another, the granular ground substance has concentrated in the center. The endothelium (En) shows numerous vesicles (V), as does the alveolar epithelium (Ep) (accumulation of fluid in vacuoles). B = basement membrane, → alveolar clearing. 20,000 × (NIKULIN et al., 1965).

Electron Microscopy of Thrombi

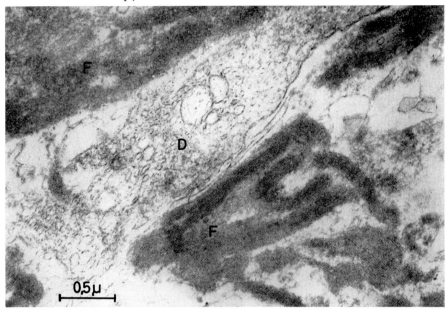

Fig. 98. Experimental coagulation thrombus (rabbit) showing bundles of fibrin threads (F) (cross-bands are not visible) and platelet detritus (D). 30,000× (Dr. KLEINSCHMIDT).

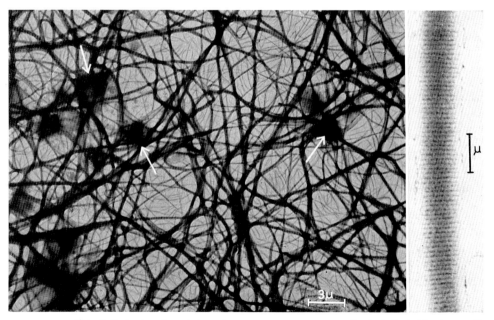

Fig. 99. a) scaffold of fibrin threads and thrombocytes (→) in spontaneously shed, fresh blood (metallic shadowing). Fibrin fibers have formed in both thick bundles and a fine network. b) shows a single fibrin fiber with distinct cross-bands (periodicity of 230 Å). Magnifications, a) 3,000×, b) 100,000× (see KÖPPEL, 1962).

73

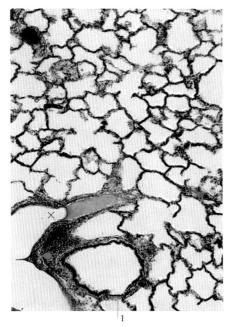

Fig. 100. Normal lung;
H & E, 53×.

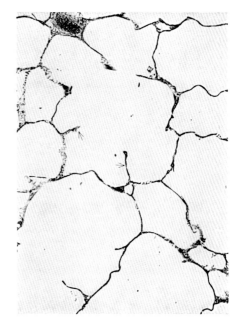

Fig. 101. Emphysema;
H & E, 53×.

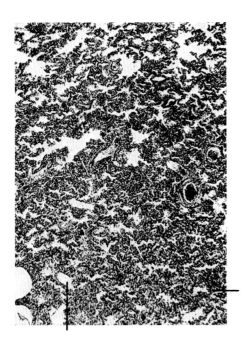

Fig. 102. Atelectasis;
H & E, 53×.

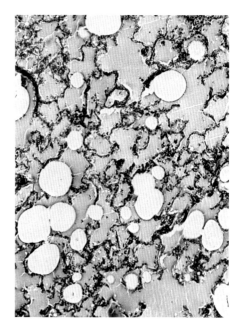

Fig. 103. Pulmonary edema;
H & E, 53×.

Lung

Histological evaluation of lung sections is often difficult for the beginner, particularly so when the disease has altered the normal architectural pattern of the lung. Frequently, in inflammatory processes, the alveolar spaces can no longer be recognized as empty sacs. Therefore, in order to identify the organ it is necessary to search for the bronchi (→ 1 in Fig. 100, normal lung) with their characteristic tall cylindrical epithelium, annular muscular wall and bronchial cartilage, and to look as well for the branches of the pulmonary arteries which lie adjacent to bronchi (x in Fig. 100: an artery partly filled with blood plasma).

The answers to the following questions will provide *clues* to the pathological diagnosis: Is the lung affected focally or diffusely? Does the lesion involve the alveolar or bronchial spaces, or their walls? Are the alveolar or bronchial spaces distended or not? Is the lung tissue preserved or destroyed? When such questions are properly answered, then a correct interpretation will be reached.

Vesicular emphysema (Fig. 101). *The pulmonary alveoli are enlarged because of atrophy and destruction of the alveolar septa.* In comparison to normal lung tissue (see Fig. 100), there are large, optically empty spaces bounded by thin, ruptured alveolar septa. The stump-like remnants of the septa (→), which project into the alveolar spaces, are noteworthy. In contrast to acute insufflation of the lung, emphysema shows actual destruction of the septa. Examination under high magnification of tissue stained for elastica demonstrates degenerative changes in the elastic fibers such as thinning, fusion, increased staining, etc.

Macroscopic: Small, medium or large vesicles. Bullous emphysema is particularly noticeable just beneath the pleura.
Complications: Rupture of vesicles and spontaneous pneumothorax; hypertrophy of the right ventricle of the heart.

Pulmonary atelectasis (Fig. 102). *This consists of alveolar collapse with diminished pulmonary air capacity and is usually coextensive with the territory supplied by a bronchus (e. g., reabsorption atelectasis).* Microscopic examination shows alveoli with such closely placed walls that the cellular content of the lung tissue appears to be increased. The arrow in Figure 102 indicates the slit-like alveolar spaces. The capillaries are mostly dilated.

Histologically, the various **forms** of atelectasis [compression atelectasis (e. g., in pneumothorax, or pleural effusion), obstructive or reabsorption atelectasis (e. g., with bronchial tumors)] all have the same appearance. In fetal atelectasis, the development and differentiation of the lung is defective.

Macroscopic: The entire lung may be dark bluish red or there may be sharply delimited, depressed zones of firm, rubbery consistency. The tissue does not float in water.

Pulmonary edema (Fig. 103). *Fluid exudate has escaped from the blood stream into the alveoli* (see Figs. 109, 110). Microscopically, the alveoli are seen to be filled with homogeneous, eosinophilic, cell-free fluid. A few solitary exfoliated alveolar epithelial cells are present. The capillaries are congested. In some places, the alveolar fluid has been lost during preparation of the section, so that empty spaces have resulted (artifacts).

Macroscopic: Heavy lungs, the cut surfaces of which exude frothy fluid.
The *pathogenesis* is concerned with an increase in pressure in the pulmonary circulation accompanied by altered permeability of the terminal vascular channels (due to toxins or dxygen lack).

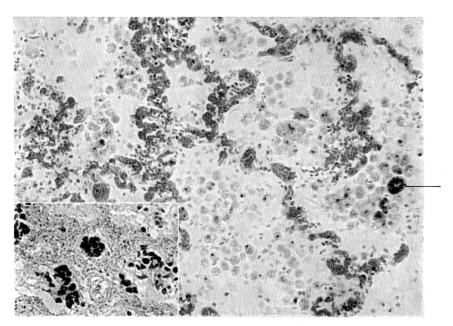

Fig. 104. Congestion of the lung (passive hyperemia, stasis); H & E, 240 × – the inset in the lower left corner shows the Berlin-blue-reaction, 132 × .

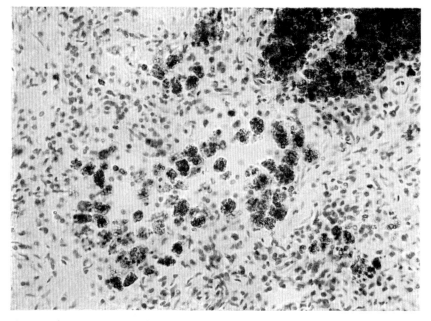

Fig. 105. Chronic congestion of the lung (chronic passive hyperemia or stasis); Nuclear fast red stain, 330 × .

Congestion of the Lungs

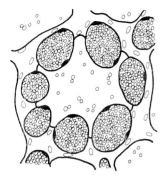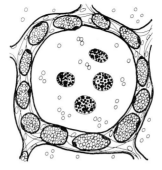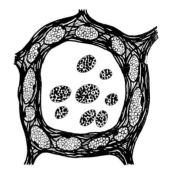

| Hyperemia | Beginning induration | Chronic congestion |
| Acute | Subacute | (Stasis) of lung |

Fig. 106. Different stages of congestion of the lung.

Passive congestion of the lungs *results from obstruction to the flow of blood from the left side of the heart (e. g., in mitral stenosis). The condition is therefore one of passive hyperemia with morphological alterations corresponding to the severity of the congestion or stasis.* In the **acute stage** (Fig. 106), there is simple hyperemia, the dilated capillaries projecting into the alveolar spaces in knot-like fashion. The capillaries are filled with thickly packed erythrocytes.

Macroscopic: Large, heavy, often bright red lungs, so-called red induration.

Passive congestion of longer duration (subacute to subchronic) (Figs. 104, 106) leads to increased extravasation of erythrocytes into the alveoli which are phagocytosed by alveolar epithelium and the hemoglobin converted into *hemosiderin* (heart failure cells laden with brown intracytoplasmic pigment, see Fig. 108). An increase in connective tissue and the basement membrane thickens the alveolar walls.

Chronic passive congestion (brown induration) (Figs. 105, 106) is manifest by greatly thickened alveolar septa (collagenous fibrosis), thickening of the basement membrane, see Figure 107, and heavy loading of the alveolar epithelium with hemosiderin (heart failure cells may appear in the sputum). Iron is liberated and may be deposited along with calcium in both the connective and elastic tissue (iron-calcium incrustations).

Macroscopic: Heavy, cinnamon-brown or brick-red lungs.

Congestion of the lung. Figure 104 shows a subacute stage with marked hyperemia of the capillaries so that they project into the alveolar spaces. The alveolar walls are not fibrotic or thickened. The alveolar spaces contain exfoliated alveolar epithelial cells, the cytoplasm of which contains finely granular, brown, refractile hemosiderin pigment. The Berlin-blue reaction (inset in the lower left-hand corner) shows that the pigment is an iron-containing product of hemoglobin breakdown.

Chronic passive congestion of lung (Fig. 105). Inspection under very low magnification shows a thicker lung framework than normal. Alveolar spaces appear narrow because of great thickening of the walls by collagenous tissue. The cell content, however, is not substantially increased (compare with interstitial pneumonia, Fig. 465). Numerous heart failure cells, with clearly visible brown pigment, are found in the alveolar spaces. In many cases there is also an increase in smooth muscle (see Figs. 107, 108).

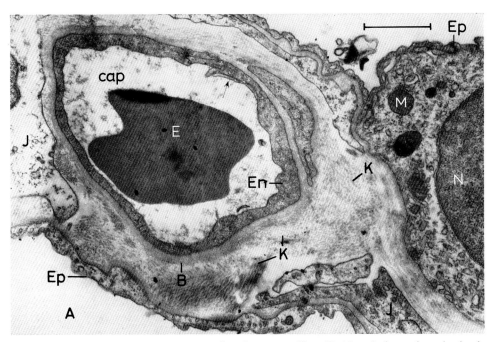

Fig. 107. Human chronic pulmonary congestion. The pulmonary capillary (Cap) is pushed away from the alveolar surface by collagen fibers (K) and the cytoplasmic processes of the interstitial cells (J). (The normal distance between the blood and air spaces is 0.3–0.5 μ; in this case, it is 1.5 μ.) In addition, the basement membrane (B) is greatly thickened (normal 0.01–0.1 μ; here, it is 0.2 μ). The cytoplasm of the endothelial cells (En) is also thickened. The endothelial cells overlap like tiles on a roof (→). An erythrocyte (E) is seen in the capillary lumen. On the right-hand side of the picture there is an alveolar lining cell (Ep) with its nucleus (N) and mitochondria (M). The outstretched cytoplasmic processes of the lining cells (Ep) contain small vesicles. A = the alveolar lumen. 18,000 × (Dr. GIESEKING).[1]

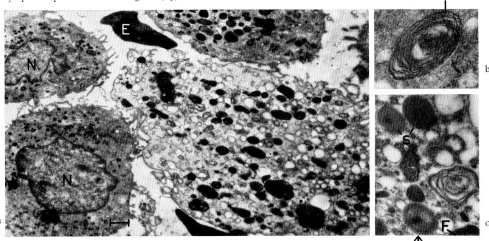

Fig. 108. a) Detached alveolar epithelium from a chronically congested lung showing numerous small cytoplasmic inclusions consisting for the most part of siderosomes (compare Fig. 13). b) and c) higher magnification of the cytoplasmic inclusions in the alveolar epithelial cells: myelin figure (→: small osmiophilic laminated bodies, finger print. Remnants of disintegrated erythrocytes?), lysome→, siderosome (S), fat droplet (F). Magnifications: Fig. 108 a, 5,000 × ; b and c, 25,000 × (Dr. GIESEKING).

1) Literature: SCHULZ, 1959; MEESEN, 1960; GIESEKING, 1958, 1959, 1960.

Electron Microscopy of Lung Diseases

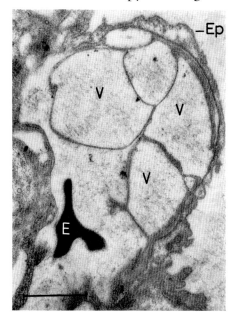

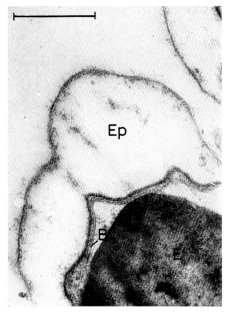

Figs. 109 (left) and 110 (right). *Acute pulmonary edema* (rat lung following intratracheal injection of adrenalin). Figure 109 shows marked swelling of the endothelium and formation of large cytoplasmic vacuoles that contain blood plasma (V = endothelial vacuole). With more marked swelling, the cytoplasmic border of the base of these endothelial vacuoles may burst, and the edema fluid flow into the interstitial tissue of the alveolar septum and thence into the cytoplasm of the processes of the overlying alveolar lining cells (Ep). In Figure 110, the process of the lining cell is already considerably blown up by the marked intracellular edema (Ep). B = basement membrane. Magnifications: Figure 109, 18,000×, Figure 110, 22,000× (Dr. GIESEKING).

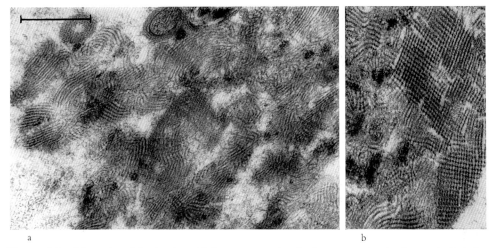

a   b

Fig. 111. a) Special reaction of the alveolar epithelium to quartz dust (rat lung, 3 months after intratracheal administration of quartz dust). There is a crystal-like lamellar system in the cytoplasm of the alveolar epithelium. b) higher magnification of a portion of the same area.
Magnifications: a) 18,000×, b) 35,000× (Dr. GIESEKING).

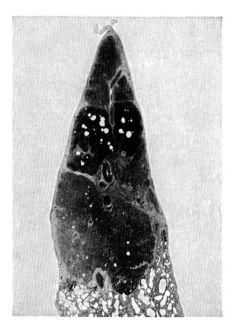

Fig. 112. Hemorrhagic infarct of lung;
H & E, 5×.

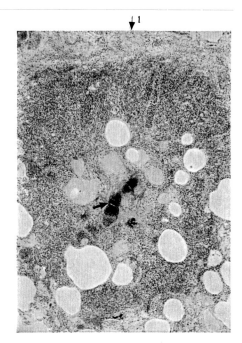

Fig. 113. Pyemic lung abscess;
H & E, 42×.

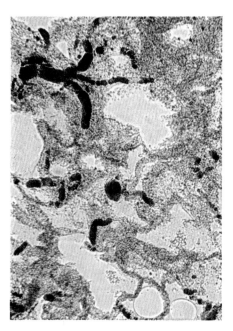

Fig. 114. Fat emboli in the lung;
Sudan stain, 58×.

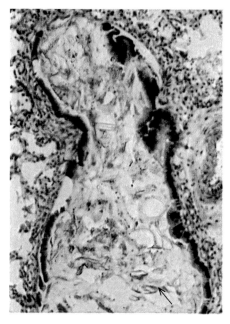

Fig. 115. Bronchial aspiration of amniotic fluid;
H & E, 162×.

Hemorrhagic Infarct of lung (Fig. 112). *This denotes focal necrosis and hemorrhage of lung tissue following embolic occlusion of a branch of the pulmonary artery in the presence of passive hyperemia of the bronchial circulation.* Naked eye inspection of a section usually shows a wedge-shaped, red, homogeneous lesion. The tissue in Figure 112 is from the lingula of the lung so that the wedge shape of the infarct is fortuitous. The embolic occlusion (→) of the nutrient branch of the pulmonary artery can be easily seen. Medium and high magnification disclose a monotonous picture: the alveolar spaces are filled with densely packed erythrocytes. In older infarcts, these show only as shadowy forms or are disintegrated into crumbled, eosinophilic, homogeneous, dingy, reddish brown masses. The alveolar septa can scarcely be distinguished from the contents of the alveoli. Septal nuclei have disappeared (evidence of *necrosis*).

Infarcts must be *differentiated from aspirated blood*, in which necrosis is lacking.
Macroscopic: Subpleural, wedge-shaped, firm, dark red masses which project above the surface of the lung and show fibrinous pleurisy.
Outcome: Leukocytic demarcation, organization and scar formation. Eventually, sequestration, abscess or gangrene may develop.

Pyemic lung abscess (Fig. 113). *This occurs if a branch of a pulmonary artery is obstructed not by a bland embolus but by a bacteria-containing embolus arising from a purulent thrombophlebitis (pyemia). A subpleural abscess then develops in the tissue supplied by the obstructed artery.* Low-power magnification again shows a wedge-shaped, compact mass (→ 1 : pleura) that has a blue-stained appearance because of its high cellular content. Medium magnification shows that the alveoli are crowded with leukocytes. The nutrient branch of the pulmonary artery is filled with an embolus containing large, bluish black bacterial colonies (→) and many leukocytes. At the center of the lesion, the alveolar septa are necrotic and there is beginning dissolution of lung tissue (*abscess* formation) (compare with purulent thrombophlebitis, pp. 68, 87).

Macroscopic: In the early stages there is no tissue softening: instead, there are grayish yellow, raised, firm subpleural masses with overlying fibrinous pleuritis and pleural necrosis (pleura is white). After *softening:* abscesses from which grayish yellow material discharges. Secondary empyema.

Fat embolism (Fig. 114). *Release of fluid fat from bone marrow (also from subcutaneous fat tissue or a fatty liver) after trauma (e.g., burn injury) may cause obstruction of the pulmonary capillaries and eventually escape into the arterial circulation.* Low magnification reveals small red flecks in the lung parenchyma. Medium magnification shows sudan-positive material in the capillaries, which have a stag-horn or small round disk shape (cross section). There is usually hyperemia and pulmonary edema also.

Fat embolism must be *differentiated from hyperlipemia* (diabetes, a fat-rich meal), which is much more common.

Aspiration of amniotic fluid (Fig. 115). *This occurs during premature, intrauterine respiration.* Microscopically, the signs of aspiration consist of golden brown or greenish amniotic fluid and meconium in small bronchi and in occasional alveoli. Figure 115 shows a small bronchus, the lumen of which contains abundant squames (→). These consist of cross-sectioned desquamated squamous epithelium of the vernix caseosa. The masses stained golden brown (bilirubin) consist of meconium. The small round bodies are known as meconium bodies (probably desquamated colonic cells of the fetus). Secondary aspiration pneumonia may develop (infected amniotic fluid) in which maternal leukocytes participate. Aspiration of amniotic fluid occurs chiefly in premature births.

Bronchitis

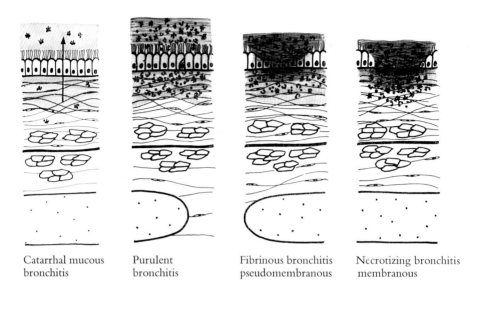

Catarrhal mucous
bronchitis

Purulent
bronchitis

Fibrinous bronchitis
pseudomembranous

Necrotizing bronchitis
membranous

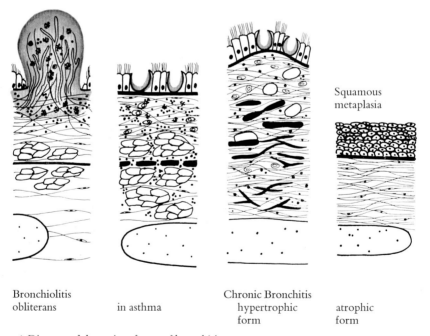

Squamous
metaplasia

Bronchiolitis
obliterans

in asthma

Chronic Bronchitis
hypertrophic
form

atrophic
form

Fig. 116. Diagram of the various forms of bronchitis.

Bronchitis - Tracheitis

Figure 116 shows the different forms of bronchitis in diagrammatic form. Acute **sero–mucous catarrh** shows edema and hyperemia of the tunica propria as well as a layer of mucus containing a few leukocytes. The exudate contains mucus mixed with protein material, occasional leukocytes and shed epithelium. **Purulent catarrh** is recognized by its richly cellular exudate. Erythrocytes appear in **hemorrhagic inflammation**. In **fibrinous inflammation,** grayish white, cohesive, detachable membranes *(pseudo–membrane)* develop which often extend widely (bronchial casts may be formed, e.g., in *diphtheria*), whereas **membranous necrotizing inflammation** (true membrane) is distinguished by a patchy, tightly adherent, putty-like layer. In the first case, the fibrin is superficial, lying on top of the epithelium, and the connective tissue is unchanged. In the second case, the fibrin infiltrates both the epithelium and the underlying necrotic connective tissue (deeply penetrating fibrinous necrosis). Necrotizing fibrinous inflammation is always followed by proliferation of granulation tissue. When bronchioles are affected in this way, the result is **bronchiolitis obliterans. In chronic bronchitis,** all coats are infiltrated by cells and the goblet cells are increased in number. Metaplasia of the epithelium often becomes prominent (see also p. 85).

Fibrinous tracheitis in diphtheria (Fig. 117). A cross-section of the trachea viewed under low magnification shows the cartilagenous rings which stain blue. Medium magnification (Fig. 117) shows the hyperemia and edema of the tunica propria ($\rightarrow$ 1). The ciliated epithelium is lacking. The basement membrane ($\rightarrow$ 2) is overlaid with densely packed bundles of fibrin fibers ($\rightarrow$ 3) (see also Fig. 126).

Necrotizing tracheitis in influenza (Fig. 118). In contrast to diphtheria, the fibrin layer is scaly and less marked. The basement membrane is no longer recognizable ($\rightarrow$ 1). Homogeneous material (fibrin and necrotic tissue) extends into the outer layers of the tunica propria ($\times$ in the picture). Bacterial colonies are seen in the necrotic material ($\rightarrow$ 2). The cellular reaction (leukocytes, lymphocytes) is more marked than in diphtheria. Accumulated secretion in the excretory duct of a mucus gland is shown at $\rightarrow$ 3 ($\rightarrow$ 4 is cartilage).

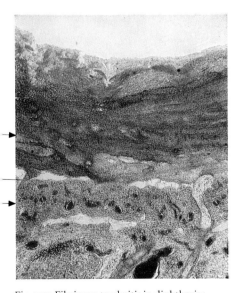

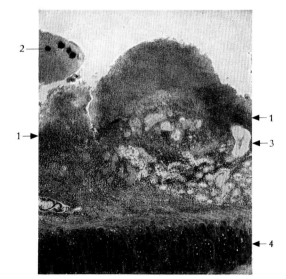

Fig. 117. Fibrinous tracheitis in diphtheria;
H & E, 41×.

Fig. 118. Necrotizing tracheitis in influenza;
H & E, 42×.

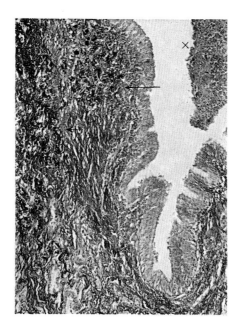

Fig. 119. Chronic bronchitis;
elastica–van Gieson stain, 100×.

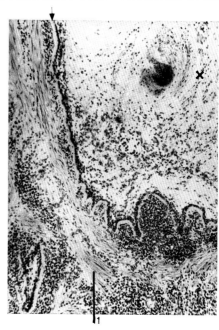

Fig. 120. Chronic mucous bronchitis in asthma;
H & E, 120×.

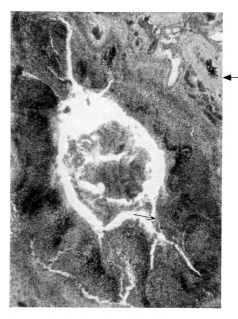

Fig. 121. Severe chronic proliferative
bronchitis;
H & E, 32×.

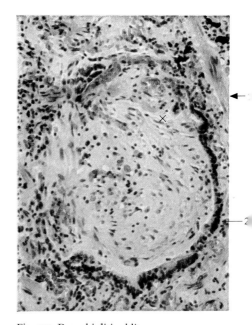

Fig. 122. Bronchiolitis obliterans;
H & E, 195×.

84

Chronic bronchitis (Fig. 119). Histologically, there is moderate infiltration of the bronchial wall by lymphocytes, plasma cells and polymorphonuclear leukocytes. In the figure, the ciliated epithelium is intact and slightly hypertrophic. The lumen of the bronchus contains numerous polymorphonuclear leukocytes and mucus ($\times$). The excessive production of mucus is due to an increased number of goblet cells in the mucosa as well as enhanced secretion by the seromucous glands. Elastic stains show an increase in elastic fibers (black in the photograph), which, moreover, show splitting ($\rightarrow$) and degenerative granular fragmentation. In addition, there is a decrease in the number of collagen fibers. The muscle may show hypertrophy (see Figs. 116, 120). If the elastic membranes and muscle are destroyed, the bronchial lumen will dilate *(bronchiectasis)*.

Macroscopic: The mucous membrane is red, thickened and velvety with longitudinal and cross ripples, especially in *hypertrophic bronchitis* (increase in connective tissue, elastica and muscle fibers, see Fig. 116). In *atrophic bronchitis*, which is essentially the end-stage of chronic hypertrophic bronchitis, the mucosa is grayish white and smooth (atrophy of the supporting elements of the bronchial wall, see Fig. 116). *Complications:* cor pulmonale, pulmonary emphysema, bronchiectasis and brain abscess, amyloidosis, recurrent pneumonias.

Chronic mucous bronchitis in asthma (Fig. 120). *This is an allergic bronchitis, which is accompanied during the attacks by increased secretion of tenacious, highly viscous mucus.* Figure 120 shows the bronchial lumen filled by mucus which has formed a whirling spiral with a dark blue center *(Cushman's spiral, $\times$).* Both the mucus and the bronchial wall are infiltrated with eosinophils. In addition, there is a lymphocytic infiltrate in the wall. The basement membrane ($\rightarrow$) is thickened and the bronchial muscle hypertrophied ($\rightarrow$ 1). Frequently, lance-shaped eosinophilic crystals are found in the mucus and these arise from the destruction of leukocytes *(Charcot-Leyden crystals).*

Macroscopic: Stringy, glistening mucus that can be pulled from the opened bronchi.

Severe chronic proliferative bronchitis (Fig. 121). Under low magnification, the thickened bronchial wall appears blue (increased cell content) and the breadth of the peribronchial connective tissue is greater than normal. A bronchial cartilage is shown at $\rightarrow$. The tunica propria of the bronchus is greatly widened and partially projects into the lumen. The thickening of the bronchial wall is due to granulation tissue which has completely destroyed the muscle and mucous glands. The granulation tissue is particularly well developed in the inner layers of the wall and is heavily infiltrated with granulocytes, lymphocytes and plasma cells. The bronchial epithelium is largely lacking, being replaced by flat ulcers covered with fibrin ($\rightarrow$). Mucus and leukocyte-rich exudate fill the lumen.

Macroscopic: Thickened bronchial walls; narrowed lumens; secondary bronchial stenosis.

Bronchiolitis obliterans (Fig. 122). *In pseudomembranous, necrotizing bronchiolitis, the necrotic tissue and fibrin are replaced secondarily by granulation tissue. In this way, a web of tissue is formed which can completely fill the bronchi and bronchioles. Such a plug of granulation tissue can also form in proliferative bronchiolitis.* Under low magnification, single bronchioles are seen to be filled with cellular granulation tissue. Medium magnification shows that the ciliated epithelium ($\times$) is partly denuded. The lumen is filled with a plug of granulation tissue (fibroblasts, fibrous tissue, capillaries and lymphocytes). The wall of the bronchus shows a chronic inflammatory infiltrate. At $\rightarrow$ 1 can be seen the smooth muscle of the bronchial wall ($\rightarrow$ 2: ciliated epithelium).

Macroscopic: The cut surfaces of the lung show a very fine, white stippling.

Inflammation of the Lung (Pneumonia, Pneumonitis)

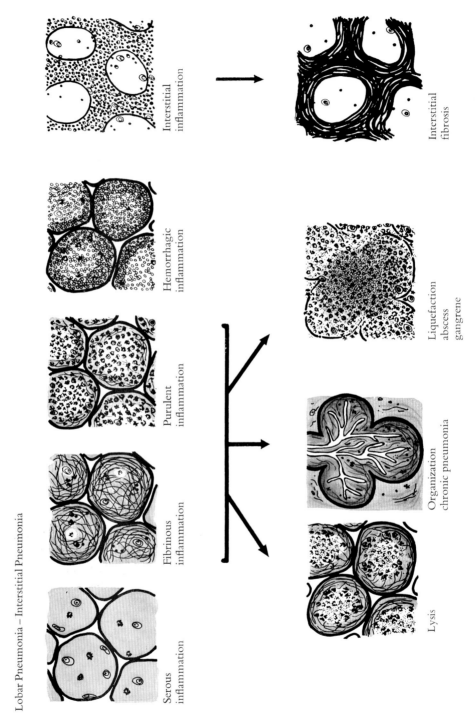

Interstitial inflammation

Interstitial fibrosis

Hemorrhagic inflammation

Liquefaction
abscess
gangrene

Purulent inflammation

Organization
chronic pneumonia

Fibrinous inflammation

Lysis

Serous inflammation

Lobar Pneumonia – Interstitial Pneumonia

Fig. 123. Summary of the various sorts of inflammation of the lung, the results of healing and the complications that may develop.

Inflammation of the Lung (Pneumonia, Pneumonitis)

Two large groups of inflammations of the lung can be distinguished (Fig. 123):

1. **Pneumonias characterized by an intra-alveolar exudate.**

2. **Pneumonias characterized by interstitial inflammation** (alveolar or connective tissue septa).

1. **Pneumonias characterized by an intra-alveolar exudate** are commonly *focal;* called *bronchopneumonia* or lobular pneumonia, since the inflammation arises within the bronchi (see Figs. 124, 125). *Peribronchial lobular pneumonia* is characterized by a zone of peribronchial exudate (see Figs. 124, 126).

When a *whole lobe of a lung* is affected, it is called *lobar pneumonia*. Lobar pneumonia (see p. 90) involves all the alveoli of a lobe of the lung. The exudate is of uniform appearance, at first serous, then fibrinous and finally purulent. In *bronchopneumonia*, by comparison, the inflammatory foci are in different stages of development (serous, purulent or fibrino-purulent). Moreover, fibrinous or purulent exudate is often found in the central portion, whereas at the periphery the exudate is serous.

The character of the alveolar exudate varies (Fig. 123). A *serous exudate* may be present (inflammatory edema = blood serum and a small amount of fibrin with a few leukocytes; for example, the stage of congestion in lobar pneumonia which must be distinguished from pulmonary edema). Or, again, there may be a *fibrinous exudate* with large amounts of fibrin in the alveoli, usually intermixed with a few leukocytes and alveolar epithelial cells (e. g., uremic pneumonia), or *purulent exudate* (with little fibrin) or *hemorrhagic exudate* (e. g., in influenza).

2. **Interstitial pneumonia** (Figs. 123, 134, 465) shows accumulations of lymphocytes, plasma cells or histiocytes in the alveolar walls.

Results of pulmonary inflammations. a) **Usual result:** lysis of the exudate by leukocytic proteolytic enzymes. Complete restitution of the lung to normal. b) **Organization by granulation tissue** (chronic pneumonia, carnification). c) **Liquefaction** (abscess or gangrene, finally sequestration). d) **Interstitial fibrosis** following incomplete healing of an interstitial pneumonia (Fig. 134).

Various Forms of Focal (Patchy) Pneumonia

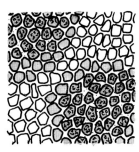

Bronchopneumonia
(lobular pneumonia)

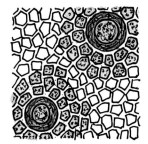

Peribronchial
focal pneumonia

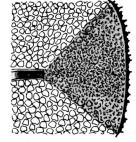

Pyemic
lung abscess

Fig. 124. Focal pneumonias.

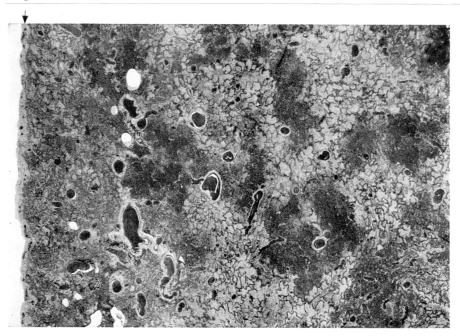

Fig. 125. Bronchopneumonia; H & E, 12.5 ×.

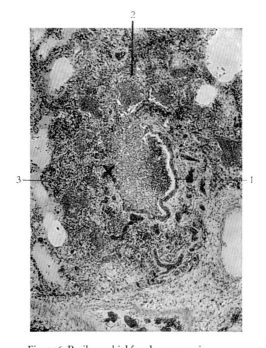

Fig. 126. Peribronchial focal pneumonia;
H & E, 64×.

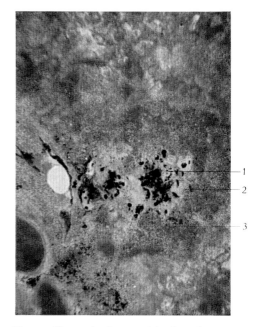

Fig. 127. Hemorrhagic necrotizing bronchopneumonia;
H & E, 36×.

Focal (Patchy, Lobular) Pneumonia

Focal pneumonias may have a variety of causes and their pathogenesis may be different (endo-bronchial, peribronchial, hematogenous). Common to all forms is the spread from multiple small foci to the rest of the lung tissue.

Bronchopneumonia (Figs. 124, 125). *There is patchy inflammation of lung tissue with involvement of single groups of alveoli and not sharply limited to the anatomical units (lobules).* With low magnification, irregular, poorly defined, blue staining foci are seen in the lung (→ pleura). The alveoli between these foci contain palely stained red exudate. If the center of one of the nodules is examined with higher magnification, the alveoli will be seen to be thickly packed with polymorphonuclear cells. Alveolar walls are preserved and the capillaries are hyperemic. The further one looks toward the periphery the fewer the number of leukocytes and fibrin threads that can now be seen. Adjacent alveoli are filled with inflammatory edema, shed alveolar epithelium and a few polymorphonuclear leukocytes *(focal inflammatory edema)*. The bronchi contain purulent exudate and shed ciliated epithelial cells.

Macroscopic: The cut surface shows grayish red to gray, slightly raised nodules with a firm consistency, which can often be better felt than seen. The lung tissue is easily torn. If the nodules have fused with one another, a confluent pneumonia arises. Staphylococci, pneumococci, streptococci and gram-negative organisms are common causes.

Peribronchial focal pneumonia (Figs. 124, 126). *In this type, the inflammation extends from the bronchial wall into adjacent lung tissue so that mantle-like peribronchial lesions develop.* Low-power magnification shows blue-stained lesions, in the center of which lies a small bronchus. With medium magnification, the bronchus can be recognized by its ciliated epithelium (→ 1), which is missing in one place (×) in the illustration. Reddish fibrinous membranes can be seen in the bronchi (pseudomembranous inflammation). During the healing process, such an area may develop into bronchiolitis obliterans (see Fig. 122). The lumen of the bronchus is filled with leukocytes and the wall is densely infiltrated with them. The blood vessels are hyperemic. The adjacent alveoli contain fibrin (→ 2) and leukocytes (→ 3). More distant alveoli are filled with inflammatory edema fluid.

Macroscopic: Small gray nodules with centrally situated bronchi. It occurs in measles, scarlet fever, diphtheria and influenza, chiefly because of superimposed streptococcal or staphylococcal infection.

Hemorrhagic necrotizing bronchopneumonia (Fig. 127). *Lobular or focal peribronchial pneumonia with hemorrhagic exudate occurs chiefly in infectious diseases (e. g., in influenza) caused by a mixture of etiologic agents (a virus plus influenza bacilli or various cocci).* The microscopic picture is variegated. Low magnification shows large, irregularly shaped, red and blue focal lesions. Bacterial colonies (→ 1) are seen in the center of the lesion. The surrounding lung tissue is necrotic (→ 2). Outside of this lies a zone of leukocytes (→ 3) mixed with exuded erythrocytes. Farther toward the periphery, the exudate is entirely hemorrhagic.

In very acute and toxic cases of influenza there is only hemorrhagic edema with hemorrhagic infarction and hyalin vascular thrombi.

Macroscopic: An extremely variegated bronchopneumonia with nodular foci of red, gray and grayish yellow color. Necrosis may develop, particularly in mixed streptococcal infections.

89

Lobar Pneumonia

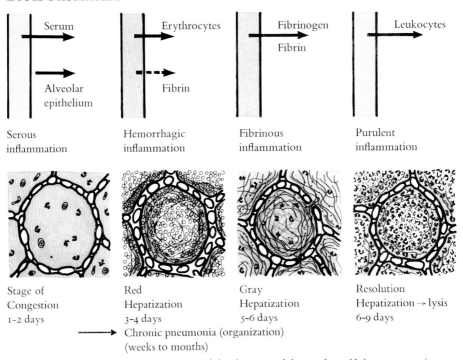

Serous inflammation	Hemorrhagic inflammation	Fibrinous inflammation	Purulent inflammation
Serum → Alveolar epithelium	Erythrocytes → Fibrin	Fibrinogen → Fibrin	Leukocytes →

Stage of Congestion
1–2 days

Red Hepatization
3–4 days

Gray Hepatization
5–6 days

Resolution
Hepatization → lysis
6–9 days

→ Chronic pneumonia (organization)
(weeks to months)

Fig. 128. Schematic diagram of the course and the character of the exudate of lobar pneumonia.

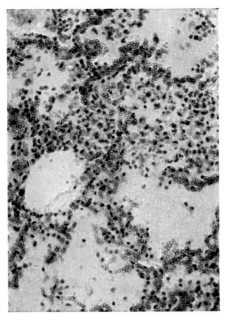

Fig. 129. Lobar pneumonia: stage of congestion;
H & E, 190×.

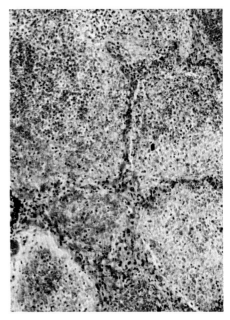

Fig. 130. Lobar pneumonia: stage of red hepatization;
H & E, 148×.

Lobar Pneumonia

This acute inflammation of a whole lobe of a lung is initiated by pneumococci and both clinically and pathologically follows a progressive course with definite stages. In contrast to focal pneumonia, an entire lobe of a lung (occasionally only a part of a lobe) suddenly becomes inflamed. This occurs in such a way that the different stages of the inflammation do not occur together, but rather follow one another in orderly succession. It is generally supposed that an allergic host reaction plays a part in the development of lobar pneumonia whereby a previous, banal pneumococcal infection acts as a sensitizing agent (Lauche).

Figure 128 shows the different stages of the disease in diagrammatic form. In the **stage of congestion or engorgement** (Fig. 129) the alveoli are filled with a *serous exudate*. The capillaries are hyperemic. The exudate contains shed alveolar epithelium and occasional leukocytes. Next follows the stage of **red hepatization** (Fig. 130), in which the hyperemia increases further and erythrocytes and fibrin appear in the alveoli. **Gray hepatization** (Fig. 131) is marked by the appearance of fibrinous exudate. Leukocytes are especially increased in number and dominate the picture. Later, they undergo fatty degeneration and are destroyed (**resolution,** Fig. 132). At the same time, proteolytic enzymes are liberated which digest the fibrin (**lysis,** 9–28 days). If the fibrin is not digested, organization by granulation tissue occurs (**chronic pneumonia,** Fig. 133). All forms of pneumonia may be accompanied by pleuritis (**pleurisy**).

This strict division into stages naturally is not valid in every case, since estimates of the time intervals of the various stages are uncertain and different authors have differing opinions about them. Congestion and red hepatization often fuse into a single stage; there are also various opinions about the sequence of red, gray and yellow hepatization. Understandably, there are also transitional forms such as red–gray hepatization and gray–yellow hepatization.

Lobar pneumonia : stage of engorgement (Fig. 129). This very early stage is seldom seen at autopsy, since death usually occurs during red or gray hepatization. Microscopic examination shows alveoli filled with an inflammatory exudate, similar to the focal edema we have already seen in bronchopneumonia (Figs. 125, 126). There is a finely granular or homogeneous protein precipitate in the alveoli as well as abundant shed alveolar epithelium, but only a few leukocytes and erythrocytes. The capillary hyperemia is striking, and many of the capillaries project into the alveolar lumen in nodular fashoin.

Macroscopic: Red, bloody, moist cut surfaces from which reddish, frothy fluid can be scraped off (prune-juice sputum, rusty sputum).

Lobar pneumonia : Stage of red hepatization (Fig. 130). In this stage, the most prominent feature under low magnification is the red color caused by extravasated erythrocytes. The firm consistency (like liver = hepatization) is caused by the fibrin. Both medium and high-power magnification show great numbers of erythrocytes, between which lie clusters of numerous leukocytes and alveolar epithelium. In the H & E stain, the thick network of fibrin fibers can be seen only when the condensor diaphragm is closed as much as possible. In the illustration, the hyperemia of the alveolar septa has already disappeared (compressed by the intra-alveolar fibrin). Fibrin thrombi may develop in the capillaries.

Macroscopic: The cut surfaces are red, firm, friable. As the exudation of fibrin increases, the lungs lose their red color and become gray.

91

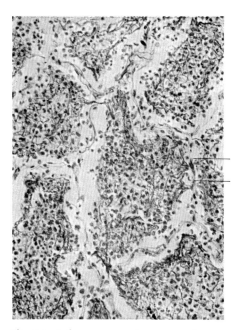

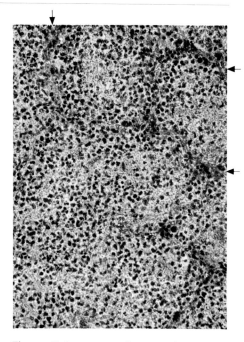

Fig. 131. Lobar pneumonia: stage of gray hepatization;
Stained by WEIGERT's method (fibrin), 263×.

Fig. 132. Lobar pneumonia: stage of resolution: van Gieson stain, 255×.

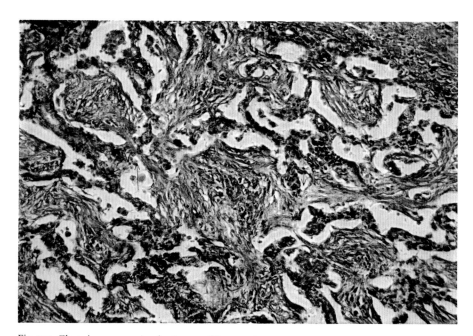

Fig. 133. Chronic pneumonia, elastica-van Gieson stains, 152×.

Lobar pneumonia: Stage of gray hepatization (Fig. 131). This stage begins after about 5–6 days and is recognized by the intense exudation of fibrinogen which polymerizes to fibrin in the alveoli. Microscopically, under low power and with H & E stains, the alveoli are seen to be filled by a network of red-stained fibers. With Weigert's method for demonstrating fibrin, they stain blue. Medium and high magnification show delicate, interlacing threads and bundles of threads which almost completely fill the alveoli. In several places, the plugs of fibrin are detached from the alveolar walls as a result of fixation. It should be noted that the fibrin threads extend through the pores of Kohn (KOHN, 1893) in the alveolar wall and fuse with those in neighboring alveoli. (Both the lines in Fig. 131 lie beside such a fibrin bridge so as not to obscure it.) Counter-staining with nuclear-fast red permits recognition of the numerous granulocytes. The capillaries are nearly empty, the erythrocytes present in the stage of red hepatization have been dissolved.

Macroscopic: The consistency of the lung is increased. The cut surfaces are friable, dry and finely granular (due to fibrin plugs projecting from the alveoli). The gray color comes from the scattering of light by the fibrin (Tyndall effect).

Lobar pneumonia: Stage of resolution (Fig. 132). Inspection under low magnification shows a homogeneous appearance. In H & E sections, all the alveoli are filled with blue-stained material. Figure 132 shows a section stained by van Gieson's method. The alveolar septa are clearly seen (→) which indicates that destruction of lung tissue (abscess) has not occurred. The septa surrounded by cellular exudate can be seen also in H & E stains. The figure likewise shows the great numbers of granulocytes and the yellow-stained fibrin bundles.

Macroscopic: Soft, yellow cut surfaces. The more extensive the lysis from digestion of the fibrinous exudate by proteolytic leukocytic enzymes, the more intense the yellow color of the lung tissue and the greater the amount of creamy, yellowish red fluid that can be scraped from the cut surfaces (turbid, mucopurulent expectoration). The lung tissue is easily torn.

A *fibrinous pleurisy* is found in all stages of lobar pneumonia and the regional lymph nodes are swollen *(non-specific lymphadenitis).* There is usually an accompanying infectious *splenomegaly* and frequently toxic *cloudy swelling* of the kidneys and liver (may result in hepatocellular jaundice). *Pericarditis, enteritis* and *pneumococcal meningitis* are less common complications. In addition, thrombotic occlusion of vessels can lead to complications such as *aseptic ischemic necrosis* with *sequestration* of a pulmonary segment, *lung abscess* (following secondary infection with streptococci or staphylococci) or *gangrene.*

Clinically, lobar pneumonia begins suddenly with shaking chills. With lysis (dissolution of the exudate), profuse sweating occurs and the fever falls (crisis). Simultaneously, there is increased excretion of uric acid (from destruction of leukocytes).

Chronic pneumonia (Fig. 133). If a crisis fails to develop, the fibrinous exudate becomes organized by granulation tissue. This arises from the respiratory bronchioles and invades the alveoli. Histologically, the changes can best be seen with van Gieson's stain, which clearly shows the red or reddish yellow plugs that fill the alveoli. Higher magnification shows the young (yellow-stained) and older (red-stained) collagenous fibers and, lying between them, angioblasts, newly formed capillaries, fibroblasts and histiocytes. The granulation tissue replaces the fibrin bridges *(pores of Kohn),* thus connecting the plugs of granulation tissue in neighboring alveoli (→). The alveolar septa are infiltrated with lymphocytes and histiocytes. The gaps next to the alveolar wall are due to cicatricial contraction of the granulation tissue. The clefts so produced can be secondarily covered with alveolar cuboidal epithelium forming pseudoglandular spaces. An increase in smooth muscle can also be seen *(muscular cirrhosis).*

Macroscopic: The lungs have a fleshy consistency (carnification). At first, the lungs are red and later grayish-white and shrunken.

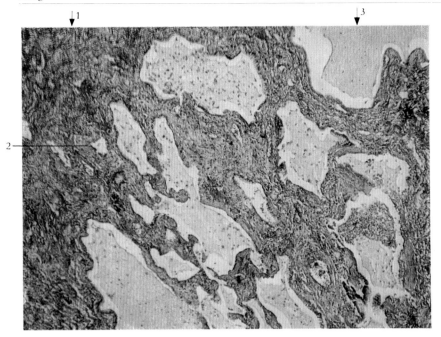

Fig. 134. Interstitial pulmonary fibrosis; van Gieson stain, 100×.

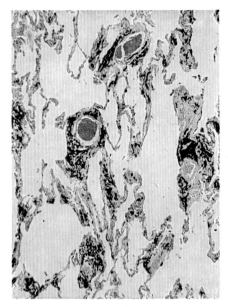

Fig. 135. Anthracosis of the lung;
H & E, 48×.

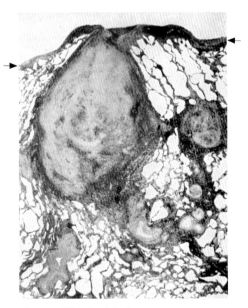

Fig. 136. Silicosis of the lung;
H & E, 15×.

Interstitial pulmonary fibrosis (Hamman-Rich) (Fig. 134). *This is a non-specific inflammation of the lung of unknown etiology, which runs its course in the interalveolar septa and leads to diffuse fibrosis of the lung.* The disease begins with serous inflammation of alveolar septa. Later, the septa become preponderantly infiltrated with lymphocytes and plasma cells. This is followed by proliferation of connective tissue (chiefly fibroblasts, lymphocytes and plasma cells).

Figure 134 shows this later stage. There is proliferation of richly cellular granulation tissue (→ 1) which has arisen from the alveolar septa. The alveoli are thereby considerably narrowed. Only remnants of the alveolar spaces remain and these are lined with cubical epithelium (→ 2). Granulation tissue gradually replaces the normal lung tissue so that, eventually, only collagenous fibrous tissue is visible. In isolated places, compensatory overdistention (→ 3) of the less-affected alveoli has occurred (emphysema). These distended alveoli are filled with protein-containing material (edema).

Macroscopic: Grayish white, firm, elastic consistency.

Anthracosis of the lung (Fig. 135). *In this condition, coal pigment is deposited in the interstitial tissues.* Coal dust reaching the alveoli is phagocytosed by alveolar epithelium. Since the coal dust is insoluble, it enters the lymphatics and accumulates there. The host reaction consists of slight fibrosis of the perilymphatic connective tissue. Figure 135 shows the black pigment (the differential diagnosis of various pigments is given on p. 9) and the slight perivascular fibrosis and lack of cellular infiltration. Occasionally, the deposits fuse into nodules.

Macroscopic: There are fine black cords and small nodules, particularly well seen beneath the pleura.

Silicosis of the lung (Fig. 136). Particles of quartz dust (1-5 μ in size) entering the lung are phagocytosed and deposited in the lymphatics. The electron photomicrograph in Figure 111 shows the early reaction of the alveolar epithelium to quartz dust. It is thought that the liberated silicates induce histiocyte formation and proliferation of reticular fibers, which later hyalinize, resulting in acellular fibrous nodules. In Figure 136 can be seen several large, concentrically arranged, fibrous nodules which are raised above the surface of the lung (→: pleura). Histiocytes containing coal pigment can also be seen at the periphery of the silicotic nodule. Because of their high refractive index, the quartz particles can be detected readily in histological preparations mounted in water and examined with polarized light. Emphysema is present in the areas adjacent to the silicotic nodules. Similar changes are observed in the hilar lymph nodes of the lung.

Macroscopic: Firm, gray, dry, round nodules.

Pulmonary emphysema, chronic bronchitis and cor pulmonale are the common *complications. Tuberculosis* commonly accompanies silicosis (30-60% of cases). Silicosis and silico-tuberculosis are recognized as compensatory diseases under Workmen's Compensation Laws. Most studies indicate no association with bronchial carcinoma.

Asbestosis of the lung (Fig. 137). Asbestos acts as a nidus for the formation of silicate spicules composed of magnesium, silica and iron. The asbestos dust elicits diffuse pulmonary fibrosis, in which are seen dumbbell- or club-shaped asbestosis needles encrusted with protein and iron (brown color). In Figure 137, typical asbestos bodies are seen in poorly cellular scar tissue.

Macroscopic: Diffuse fibrosis of the lung. Rather commonly, there is also secondarily a bronchogenic carcinoma.

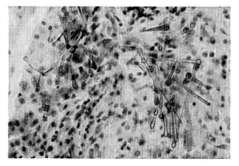

Fig. 137. Asbestosis; H & E, 255×.

Tuberculosis

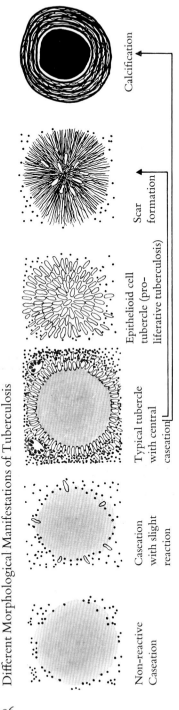

Different Morphological Manifestations of Tuberculosis

Calcification

Scar formation

Epithelioid cell tubercle (proliferative tuberculosis)

Typical tubercle with central caseation

Caseation with slight reaction

Non-reactive Caseation

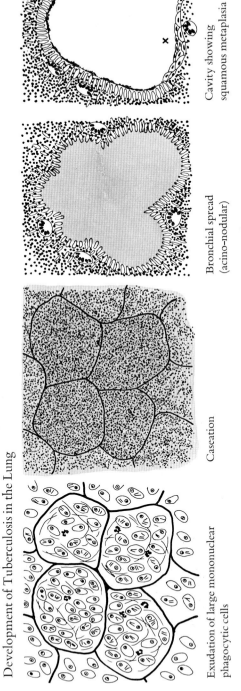

Development of Tuberculosis in the Lung

Cavity showing squamous metaplasia

Bronchial spread (acino-nodular)

Caseation

Exudation of large mononuclear phagocytic cells

Fig. 138. Various histological manifestations of the tubercle. Development of pulmonary tuberculosis.

Tuberculosis

Figure 138 illustrates the **various histological appearances of a tubercle.** The *"typical"* *tubercle* consists of a *necrotic center (caseation)*, a zone of *epithelioid cells* (modified histiocytes) *Langhans cells* and *granulation tissue*, and a more or less well-marked outer margin of *lymphocytes*. In lymph nodes and in certain diseases *(Boeck's sarcoid)*, the principal manifestation of tuberculosis may be proliferative, i. e., the formation of a *tubercle composed of epithelioid cells* and showing no central caseation. Occasionally Langhans giant cells are present as well as slight secondary caseation (see pp. 26, 27, 54, 174).

All the manifestations of the tubercle shown to the *right* in the diagram (Fig. 138) indicate a *defense reaction* by the host (productive tuberculosis). Epithelioid cell–tubercles as well as caseous tubercles heal by removal of the necrotic material and increased production of collagen fibers and scar formation (e. g., hyalin scars in lymph nodes, indurated slate-colored nodules in the lung). The caseous material may calcify secondarily *(calcified nodules)*.

The manifestations to the *left* in Figure 138 arise when there is reduced host resistance (exudative tuberculosis). In these cases, the caseation is progressive. Epithelioid cells are always scanty and the chief host reaction is necrosis. Finally, acute bacteremia and sepsis develop with non-reactive necrosis (fulminant tuberculous sepsis).

In the **development of tuberculosis in the lung** (Fig. 138), there is an exudative preliminary stage consisting of an acute serous inflammatory exudate containing many large mononuclear phagocytic cells (Fig. 139). Alveolar epithelial cells with ingested tubercle bacilli fill the alveoli. Necrosis then ensues very rapidly *(caseation)*. *Cavities* develop as a consequence of the tissue destruction (i. e., softening of the caseous necrosis) and may lead to bronchial spread with development of *acino-nodular tuberculosis* characterized by cockade-shaped areas of necrosis and typical tuberculous granulation tissue.

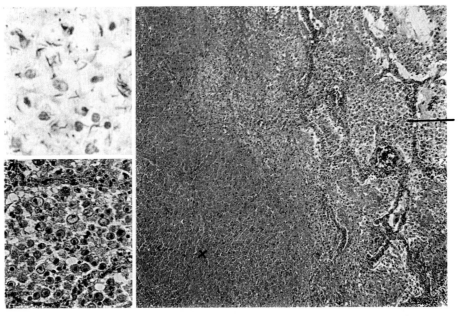

Fig. 139. Pulmonary tuberculosis, showing fresh caseation necrosis and exudation of large mononuclear phagocytic cells. H & E, 82 ×. Upper left: tubercle bacilli in alveolar epithelial cells. Ziehl-Neelsen stain, 1,000 ×. Lower left: exudate with numerous mononuclear macrophages. H & E, 195 × (see description on p. 99).

97

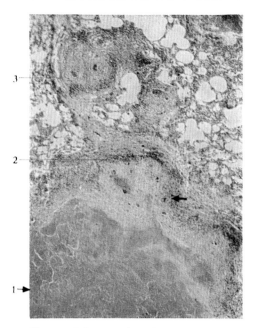

Fig. 140. Primary tuberculous nodule (Gohn tubercle) with lymphatic spread; H & E, 32×.

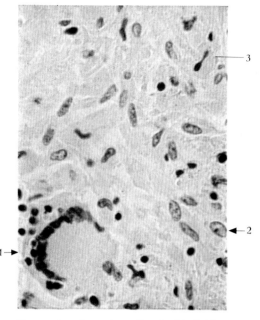

Fig. 141. Langhans giant cell and epithelioid cells; H & E, 576×.

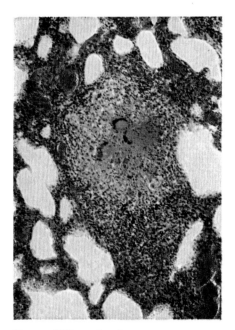

Fig. 142. Miliary tubercle; H & E, 99×.

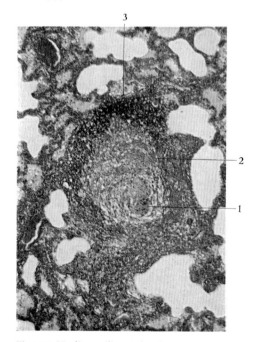

Fig. 143. Healing miliary tubercle; elastica–van Gieson stain, 56× (see description on p. 101).

Pulmonary tuberculosis, showing fresh caseation necrosis and exudation of large mononuclear phagocytic cells (see Fig. 139, p. 97). Examination with very low magnification shows a large, irregularly bordered, blue to bluish red area and an adjacent red zone. Medium and high magnification reveal that the blue area consists of crumbled, finely granular, bluish red material (×: necrotic tissue and nuclear fragments). The alveolar walls cannot be seen, but the elastic fibers can still be distinguished with elastica stains. There is a gradual transition without cellular demarcation from the necrosis to the zone containing the exudate of macrophages. In this area, the alveoli are completely filled with alveolar epithelial cells (→). Nearby there is seen a granular, proteinaceous exudate with fibrin and leukocytes. The inset in the upper left corner of Figure 139 shows *tubercle bacilli* (red rods) which have been phagocytosed by alveolar epithelial cells. In the lower left corner of the picture, the *macrophages of the exudate* are seen under high magnification. The alveolar epithelial cells are spherical and have abundant cytoplasm and round, eccentrically placed nuclei. The cytoplasm in many cells is finely granular and vacuolated.

Macroscopic: Grayish yellow, gelatinous lesions.

Primary tuberculous nodule with lymphatic spread (Fig. 140). *At the time of the first infection with tubercle bacilli, a primary nodule develops at the site of entry. In the lung, the primary nodule is beneath the pleura. In extrapulmonary primary tuberculosis, for example in the intestine, the primary nodule is in the intestinal mucosa (see Fig. 172). Extension from the primary nodule occurs by way of a tuberculous lymphangiitis to the nearest draining lymph node (hilus of the lung). The lung tubercle and tuberculous lymph node together constitute the primary tuberculous complex.*

Air-borne bacilli lodge in the lung and are taken up by alveolar epithelial cells (see Fig. 139). Liberation of toxins may then evoke a serous inflammatory reaction *(macrocytic exudation, desquamative macrocytic pneumonia)*. The resulting caseous necrosis becomes walled off by tuberculous granulation tissue. Histologically, at low magnification, round, red, anuclear lesions (blue if calcified) can be seen in the lung with small satellite lesions nearby. Medium magnification (Fig. 140) shows the tuberculous necrosis (→ 1), bounded by partially cicatrized granulation tissue (→ 2) containing many Langhans giant cells (→). Air-containing alveoli and a small satellite tubercle can be recognized in the neighboring portions of the lung (→ 3: a nodule arising from lymphatic spread and showing central necrosis and a broad capsule of granulation tissue and lymphocytes). Examination of the margin of the necrotic zone under high magnification (Fig. 141) discloses *epithelioid cells* and typical *Langhans giant cells* (→ 1 in Fig. 141, see also pp. 26, 27, 28). The nuclei of the giant cells are arranged in the shape of a crescent with the opening of the crescent facing the necrosis. The cytoplasm is finely granular. The giant cells arise chiefly by coalescence of epithelioid cells. *The epithelioid cells present two morphological forms:* plump epithelioid cells (→ 2) with poorly defined cytoplasm, oval nuclei and small nucleoli; or as shrunken cells with nuclei resembling a cat's tongue (slipper shaped → 3).

Macroscopic: Yellowish, map-like, subpleural nodules about 1 cm. in diameter, frequently with neighboring miliary tubercles.

Miliary tubercle (Fig. 142). *These are millet seed sized tubercles of lymphogenous or hematogenous (miliary tuberculosis) origin.* In miliary tuberculosis, low magnification shows numerous small, richly cellular nodules scattered throughout the lung tissue. Higher magnification shows a small central zone of necrosis surrounded by epithelioid cells and lymphocytes. In the illustration, many Langhans giant cells can be seen at the edge of the necrotic zone.

Macroscopic: Firm, gray, glassy nodules of pinhead size are present in both lungs.

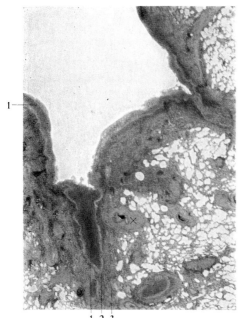

Fig. 144. Tuberculous cavity;
H & E; 8×.

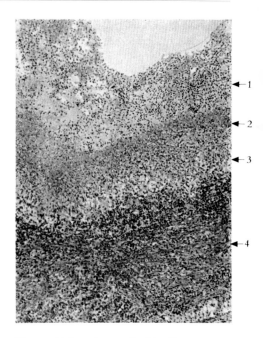

Fig. 145. Tuberculous cavity (detail);
van Gieson stain, 82×.

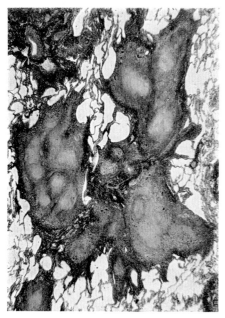

Fig. 146. Bronchial spread (acino-nodular)
in pulmonary tuberculosis;
van Gieson stain, 21×.

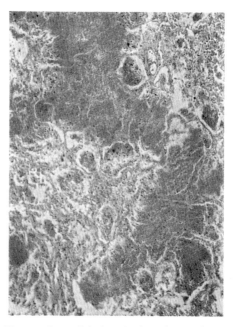

Fig. 147. Acute (fulminant) tuberculosis with
extensive caseous necrosis;
H & E, 66×.

Healing miliary tubercle (Fig. 143). Under the influence of tuberculostatic drugs (e. g., streptomycin), miliary tuberculosis can heal fairly quickly. In such a situation, small nodules of epithelioid cells are seen, in the center of which remnants of caseation still persist (yellow in van Gieson's stain → 1) walled off by a broad zone of red fibrous tissue (→ 2). The epithelioid cells have been transformed into histiocytes and fibrocytes and have formed mature reticular and collagenous fibers. In the illustration, there is an increase of elastic fibers at the margin of the tubercle (→ 3). Adjacent lung tissue shows slight emphysema.

Macroscopic: Completely healed tubercles are small white stellate scars.

Tuberculous cavity (Figs. 144, 145). *As a result of enzymatic digestion of the caseous material (leukocytic enzymes) and removal of the liquefied material by way of a draining bronchus, a cavity may develop in the wall of which three layers can be recognized histologically* (Fig. 144). The innermost layer (→ 1) consists of a narrow band of homogeneous, eosinophilic, *necrotic tissue* (yellow in van Gieson's stain), next comes a dark blue layer in which *cellular granulation tissue* and epithelioid cells (→ 2) can be seen under high magnification. Finally, the third and outside layer consists of *cicatrized granulation tissue* (→ 3) infiltrated with nodular collections of lymphocytes. Notice that the blood vessels in the region of the cavity (×) are nearly completely obstructed by intimal proliferation. At a distance from the cavity there are small and large caseous nodules.

Still **higher magnification** (Fig. 145) shows the **cavity wall in more detail.** Fibrin is present in the innermost zone (→ 1). Then comes a necrotic zone (→ 2), infiltrated and bordered by epithelioid cells (→ 3). A layer of granulation tissue exhibits numerous vessels and lymphocytes. In the outer portions there is cicatrized granulation tissue (→ 4), with red-staining connective tissue fibers (van Gieson's stain).

Macroscopic: 1. *Fresh cavities:* irregular, grayish white, shaggy wall. 2. *Old cavities:* shiny, grayish yellow or grayish white wall, often showing squamous metaplasia. Scarred, strand-like vessels and bronchi may traverse the cavity.

Bronchial spread in pulmonary tuberculosis (acino-nodular tuberculosis) (Fig. 146). *The lesions give a characteristic appearance as they cluster around the bronchial passages.* The tubercle bacilli either lodge in the territory served by a terminal bronchus (pulmonary acinus) or cause peribronchial inflammation, a focal peribronchial pneumonia. As a result, many closely grouped caseous nodules are found, some of which have fused, while others are completely enveloped by fibrous tissue. Higher magnification shows all the typical features of a tubercle (necrosis, a collar of epithelioid cells, Langhans giant cells, and granulation tissue). Figure 146, which is stained with van Gieson's method, shows the yellow, central area of necrosis, surrounded by red collagenous connective tissue and peripheral lymphocytes. Numerous giant cells are seen. Notice the emphysema next to the nodules.

Macroscopic: Yellow nodular lesions arranged in grape-like clusters, decreasing in size and extent from the apex to the base of the lung.

Acute (fulminant) tuberculosis with extensive caseous necrosis (Fig. 147). *Acute tuberculosis results from marked reduction of host resistance (or increased virulence of the infectious agent). It is sometimes seen as a terminal stage in the treatment of tumors with cytotoxic drugs or in advanced cachexia.* Histologically, there are eosinophilic, map-like areas of necrosis without significant cellular reaction. The illustration shows necrotic pulmonary lesions with serofibrinous exudate and occasional lymphocytes. The alveolar septa are destroyed or indistinct.

Macroscopic: Miliary and larger than miliary-sized, gray, poorly defined, map-like lesions.

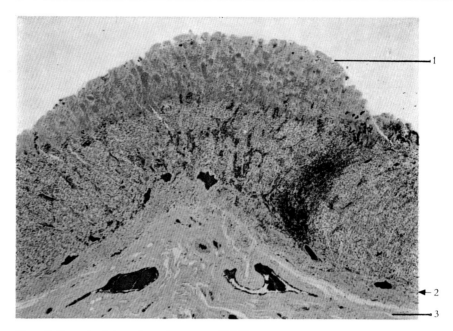

Fig. 148. Corrosive injury of gastric mucosa; H & E, 50×.

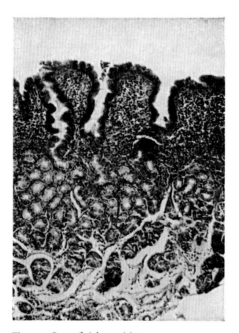

Fig. 149. Superficial gastritis;
H & E, 90×.

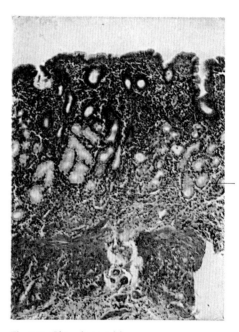

Fig. 150. Chronic gastritis;
H & E, 90×.

Alimentary Tract

A knowledge of the normal architecture of the alimentary tract is helpful in interpreting histopathological appearances (mucosa: squamous epithelium-cylindrical epithelium-glands; character of the villi; tunica propria, muscularis mucosa, submucosa, muscularis propria and subserosa). It is important to note the cellular constituents of the individual coats and any defects in the mucosa or atypical proliferation of the glands.

Corrosive injury of the gastric mucosa (Fig. 148). Corrosive acids cause coagulation necrosis of the gastric mucosa, while lye causes liquefaction necrosis. Figure 148 shows an area of fresh corrosion of the gastric mucosa due to HCl. The necrosis (coagulation necrosis → 1) can be seen on the surface. The cytoplasm of the necrotic cells in the glands is stained more strongly with eosin than the cells that lie deeper. The cells in the necrotic area lack nuclei. The necrotic zone is bordered by a narrow rim of granulocytes, scant numbers of which are also present in the submucosal stroma. With the passage of time, the necrotic mucosa sloughs off and an ulcer results. → 2 muscularis mucosae, → 3 submucosa.

Macroscopic: In the early stage of scab formation, there are different colors, depending upon the kind of corrosive: sublimate ($HgCl_2$)-grayish white, HNO_3-yellowish, H_2SO_4 and HCl-dark brown. The following sequelae may develop: perforation, cicatricial stricture (e. g., in the esophagus).

Gastritis

Superficial gastritis (Fig. 149), the most inconsequential form of gastritis, presents a histological picture of cellular infiltration in the superficial third of the gastric mucosa. The tips of the villi are large and broad and it is here that the cellular infiltration of lymphocytes, histiocytes and plasma cells is seen. In acute gastritis, polymorphonuclear leukocytes predominate.

In **chronic atrophic gastritis** (Fig. 150), the mucosal architecture is altered considerably. The chief and parietal cells of the fundus of the glands disappear and are partially replaced by mucous glands (→). Figure 150 shows the greatly reduced mucosa and the dense infiltration of lymphocytes and plasma cells extending to the muscularis. The muscularis itself is unchanged. Goblet cell metaplasia occurs frequently.

Macroscopic: Thin, gray, shiny, compact mucosa.

Chronic hypertrophic gastritis (Fig. 151) shows, even at low magnification, the mucosal thickening and marked mucosal folding caused by fibrosis of the submucosa.

Macroscopic: Mamillated elevations-état mamelonné. The clinical diagnosis of gastritis may be confirmed by gastric biopsy.

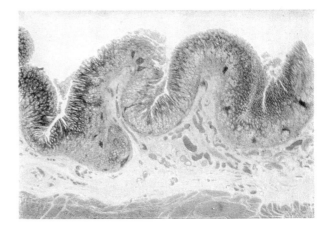

Fig. 151. Chronic hypertrophic gastritis;
H & E, 11 ×.

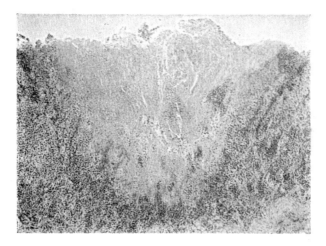

Fig. 152. Hemorrhagic infarct of the gastric mucosa; H & E, 72 ×.

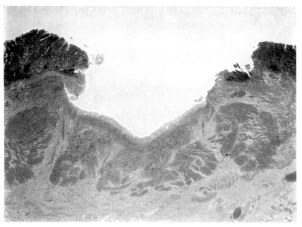

Fig. 153. Fresh gastric ulcer; H & E, 14×.

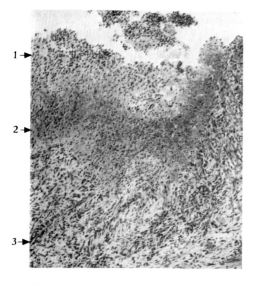

Fig. 154. Base of a gastric ulcer; H & E, 102×.

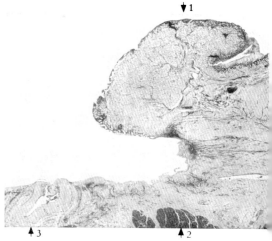

Fig. 155. Chronic penetrating gastric ulcer; H & E, 6×.

Gastric Ulcer

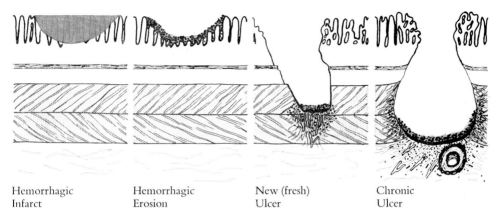

| Hemorrhagic | Hemorrhagic | New (fresh) | Chronic |
| Infarct | Erosion | Ulcer | Ulcer |

Fig. 156. Probable pathogenesis of a gastric ulcer.

Fig. 156 shows the **histogenesis of a gastric ulcer.**

First stage: *hemorrhagic infarction of the mucosa* (see Fig. 152). The necrotic material is being excavated into the lumen *(hemorrhagic erosion)*. The erosion can either heal or progress to ulceration. A *new ulcer* (Fig. 153) frequently is step-like on the oral edge, while on the aboral edge it rises steeply. A *chronic ulcer* (Fig. 155), in contrast, is flask shaped with a margin of dense scar tissue.

Hemorrhagic infarct (Fig. 152). A wedge-shaped red area lacking stained nuclei is seen in the mucosa. Medium magnification shows erythrocytes lying in acellular necrotic tissue, the greater part of which stains only faintly. The villi of the surface mucosa have disappeared (slight erosion).

Macroscopic: Irregularly shaped black foci with shallow mucosal defects.

Fresh gastric ulcer (Fig. 153). Under low magnification, the defect in the wall can be seen extending to the muscularis and showing the usual mucosal overhang (on the aboral edge to the left of the illustration). In the base of the ulcer, there is a pale grayish red zone (fibrin) and a darker zone (necrosis and granulation tissue). Under higher magnification, it is easier to analyze these layers. **Base of a gastric ulcer** (Fig. 154). At the top, there is a loose layer of fibrin and polymorphonuclear leukocytes ($\rightarrow$ 1) lying on an intensely eosinophilic band-like zone of fibrinoid necrosis ($\rightarrow$ 2) (necrotic material composed of fibrin and nuclear fragments). Granulation tissue ($\rightarrow$ 3) surrounds the necrotic layer and invades it. The capillaries in the granulation tissue run perpendicularly to the surface. Lymphocytes, histiocytes and mature connective tissue make up the lower third of this zone.

Macroscopic: A step-like or flat, round or oval defect in the wall. The base is gray.

Chronic penetrating ulcer (Fig. 155). In this figure, the mucous membrane has been elevated ($\rightarrow$ 1) and contains hyperplastic pyloric glands. In the neighborhood of the ulcer, there is an increased amount of connective tissue. The defect in this instance extends to the pancreas ($\rightarrow$ 2). The necrosis has eroded a large artery $\rightarrow$ 3 (clinically: fatal hemorrhage).

Macroscopic: A round defect with firm margins and a smooth base. Pancreatic lobules can often be seen in the base of the ulcer.

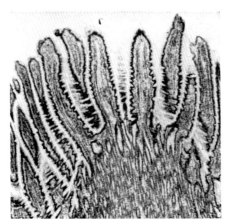

Fig. 157. Normal jejunum (dog);
H & E, 40×.

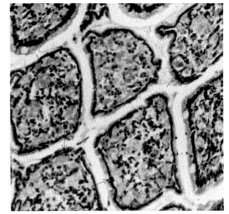

Fig. 158. Hyperemia of villi (cross section);
H & E, 170×.

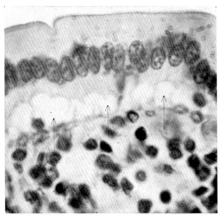

Fig. 159. Serous exudation with lifting of
surface cells;
H & E, 700×.

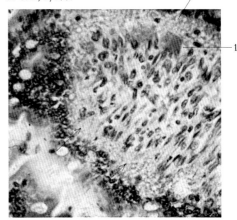

Fig. 160. Marked protein exudation in the
subepithelial space;
H & E, 400×.

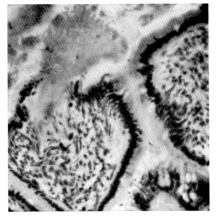

Fig. 161. Beginning necrosis of the tip of a
villus; H & E, 180×.

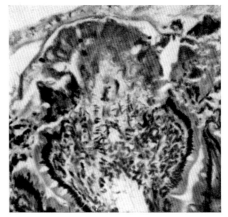

Fig. 162. Complete necrosis of the tip of a
villus; H & E, 190×.

106

Enterocolitis

All the infectious agents (e. g., pneumococci, streptococci, viruses, dysenteric organisms, cholera) or their toxins, as well as non-infectious toxic agents (e. g., allergy, uremia) cause a similar series of tissue reactions in the intestinal mucosa, which succeed one another in an orderly progression and have as a common basis changes in the terminal vascular system. The early stages cannot be as well seen in humans as in experimental animals because of the rapid onset of autolysis. The photographs on page 106 illustrate such a series of experiments in dogs given dysentery toxin intravenously (Croneberg and Sandritter, 1952).

The dysentery toxin first causes shock, with a fall in blood pressure, then an increase in peripheral resistance due to contraction of the arterioles. Following this, a disturbance of the microcirculation develops, resulting in aggregation of erythrocytes (sludge phenomenon) and of platelets (Fig. 97) which cause reduced venous return to the heart. In the terminal phase, hyalin thrombi form in the arterioles and venules and cause necrosis and hemorrhage. The central feature of this sort of shock is an alteration of blood coagulation in which consumption of coagulation factors and blockade of the reticuloendothelial system (Fig. 16) play an essential part (for *consumption of coagulation factors,* see Lasch, 1963, 1964; for morphology, see Sandritter and Lasch, 1966). In the dog, the intestine must be regarded as a shock organ. The alteration in the microcirculation first becomes apparent as hyperemia (Fig. 158 → hyperemic capillaries) of the villi of the small intestine (compare them with the slender villi of normal *jejunum* in Fig. 157). Simultaneously with the hyperemia, there is exudation into the stroma of the villi.

The exudate lifts the epithelium. The result is the formation of a *subepithelial space* (→ in Fig. 159). With increasing capillary circulatory disturbance (hyalin thrombi), more fluid accumulates in the subepithelial space (→ in Fig. 160), so that the entire epithelium is elevated. Figure 160 shows the **granular protein masses** (formed from the fluid during fixation) under the epithelium (→). The stasis has led to circumscribed *necrosis of the tips of the villi* (Fig. 161), characterized by a homogeneous mass of epithelium, villus stroma and fibrin. Finally, the entire upper third of the villi becomes necrotic (**complete necrosis of the tips of the villi,** Fig. 162). In the end stage, one sees a broad necrotic zone with nuclear fragmentation, exudate and leukocytes.

The experimental observations just described can serve as a model for the development of the morphological consequences of shock (e. g., renal cortical necrosis, hemorrhagic necrosis of the adrenal or Waterhouse-Friderichsen syndrome, etc.) and for enteritis in man.

In the subacute and chronic stages, the necrotic material is cleared away (by mechanical means or leukocytic ingestion). Ulcers develop which may extend deeply and so lay bare the muscularis (*ulcerative colitis,* Fig. 165). In chronic cases, secondary proliferation of the mucosa occurs at the edges of the ulcers (so-called pseudopolyposis, Fig. 165).

In many cases, a fibrinous exudate predominates, with more or less marked necrosis of the tips of the villi (pseudomembranous colitis, e. g., in uremia). Figure 163 (**superficial fibrinous and necrotizing colitis**) shows such an inflammation with a broad layer of fibrin and leukocytes (→ 1) and beginning necrosis of the tips of villi. The mucosa is markedly hyperemic and the submucosa is thickened by edema (→ 2: muscularis mucosae).

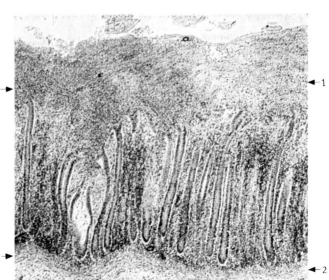

Fig. 163. Superficial fibrinous and necrotizing colitis;
H & E, 46×.

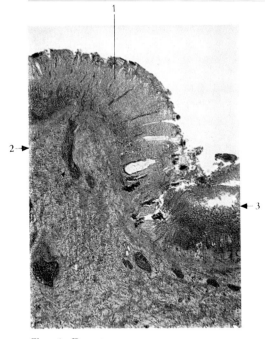

Fig. 164. Dysentery;
H & E, 28×.

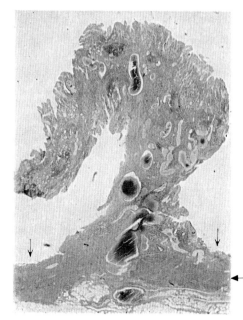

Fig. 165. Chronic ulcerative colitis;
H & E, 11×.

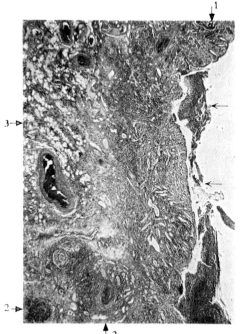

Fig. 166. Regional ileitis;
H & E, 20×.

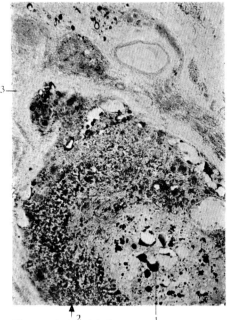

Fig. 167. Whipple's disease;
Sudan–hematoxylin, 64×.

Dysentery (Fig. 164). *Intestinal infestation by Shigella organisms or amebae. The colon is most frequently affected, and less frequently the distal ileum. In the early stages, there is edema and hyperemia of the mucosa, which is followed by hemorrhagic inflammation, necrosis, and a fibrinous exudate on the surface of the mucosa (pseudomembranous, necrotizing inflammation). The terminal stages show ulceration.* Figure 164 shows an area of expanding necrosis of the colonic mucosa (→ 1) and considerable edematous loosening of the submucosa (→ 2). The blood vessels are widely dilated and partly filled with erythrocytes and fibrin thrombi (→). There is a longitudinal pseudomembranous layer of fibrin (→ 3).

Macroscopic: Redness and edema of the intestinal wall. Mucosal necrosis forming a dirty, yellowish brown, clay-like covering. Sharply circumscribed ulcers with undermined margins. The colon contains bloody mucus.

Ulcerative colitis (Fig. 165). *This is a chronic inflammation of the mucosa of the colon, characterized by a long course and ulceration. It is not related to chemotherapy* (MOHR, 1963), *but is probably due to the development of autoantibodies* (BROBERGER et al., 1959, 1962). In the fully developed disease, there are extensive ulcers (→) extending to the muscularis propria (→ 1), together with islands of preserved colonic mucosa. These islands of colonic mucosa are polypoid and have stalks containing connective tissue (the elevation of the mucosa to the left in the illustration is an artifact).

Macroscopic: Extensive, irregular, longitudinal mucosal defects with polypoid overgrowth of mucosal islands. The wall is stiff and the lumen narrowed. The muscularis shows cross rippling.

Regional ileitis (regional enteritis, Crohn's disease, Fig. 166). *This is a chronic, recurrent disease of unknown etiology, but with a familial frequency. In 95% of cases, the terminal portion of the ileum is affected.* After the edema, hyperemia and hemorrhage of the acute stage, the chronic stage is characterized by extensive ulceration (→) with thickened mucosa (→ 1) and accompanied by a chronic inflammatory infiltrate and epithelioid cell granulomas (→ 2) with Langhans type giant cells (this is not tuberculosis, but rather a non-specific granuloma). In Figure 166, the ulcer extends to the subserosa (→ 3). Beneath this, there is an increased amount of collagenous connective tissue (scarring) and hypertrophy of the muscularis.

Macroscopic: In the chronic stage, the intestinal wall is thick and rigid, the surrounding tissues are adherent and there are irregular mucosal defects.

Complications: Perforation, hemorrhage and stenosis.

Whipple's disease (intestinal lipodystrophy, Fig. 167). *This is a progressive disease of the small intestine and mesenteric lymph nodes in which there is stasis of chyle, fat storage and granulomatous inflammation. It is probably caused by a bacterial infection (Cornybacteria?, Hemophilis?,* CHEARS and ASHWORTH, 1961; WHIPPLE, 1907). Histologically, the intestinal lymph vessels are dilated and filled with fat. The sinuses of enlarged mesenteric lymph nodes are also dilated, cystic and crammed with phagocytosed fat (partially dissolved during fixation → 1). Histiocytic granulation tissue is present throughout (→ 2) with large foam cells containing lipid droplets (also glycoproteins). It is in these cells that the above-mentioned bacteria have been demonstrated. In the later stages, scarring may result from the chronic inflammation (→ 3).

Macroscopic: Chylous ascites, dilated, yellow lymphatic channels in the intestinal serosa, enlarged cystic lymph nodes with yellow contents.
Pathogenesis: Obstruction of the thoracic duct (stasis?). Primary metabolic disorder? Bacterial infection?
Clinical: Chiefly rheumatic complaints, endocarditis, steatorrhea, anemia, cachexia.

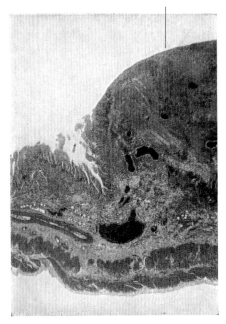

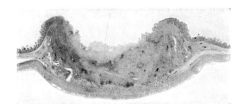

Fig. 169. Typhoid fever: ulceration and scab formation; H & E, 6 ×.

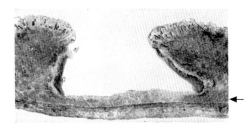

Fig. 168. Typhoid fever: marked inflammatory swelling; H & E, 26×.

Fig. 170. Typhoid fever: ulcer; H & E, 8 ×.

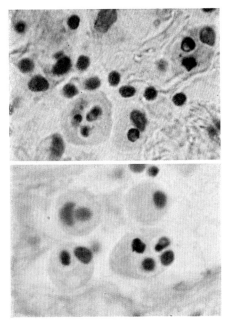

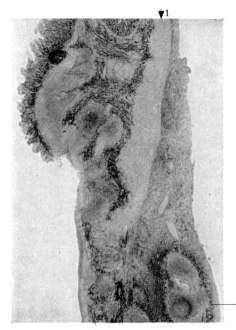

Fig. 171. Typhoid fever: large macrophages; H & E, 640×.

Fig. 172. Tuberculous ulcer of intestine; van Gieson stain, 12 ×.

Typhoid Fever

The typhoid bacillis (Salmonella typhosa) causes a characteristic inflammatory disease of the lower ileum that runs a limited course. The inflammation starts in the region of Peyer's patches and progresses to necrosis and ulceration. Four stages are recognized, each lasting approximately one week. Both the intensity of the inflammation and the duration of the disease vary greatly.

1st stage (1 week); **marked inflammatory swelling** (Fig. 168), with either diffuse or focal enlargement of the lymphoid follicles (typhoid nodules. see also Fig. 195, p. 122) which is characterized by infiltration of swollen reticuloendothelial cells and palely stained lymphocytes. Figure 168 shows the dense cellular infiltration of a swollen follicle (bluish red), with beginning necrosis of the surface mucosa (→). **Higher magnification** (Fig. 171) reveals an increased number of round reticulum cells (phagocytes, histiocytes) with abundant cytoplasm and pyknotic nuclei. Nuclear fragments and erythrocytes are also present.

Macroscopic: Pea-sized, grayish red nodules or gray plaques.

2nd stage (2 weeks); a **scab** (Fig. 169) can be seen in the necrotic portion of the markedly swollen and superficially ulcerated tissue (area devoid of nuclei). The necrotic area is surrounded by leukocytes.

Macroscopic: Yellowish green necrosis.

In the third week the necrotic tissue sloughs, and this results in the *3rd stage: ulceration* (Fig. 170). The ulcer extends to the muscularis (→). A narrow strip of necrotic tissue can still be recognized in the edges at each side.

In the *4th stage* (4 weeks) *the ulcer is cleaned up finally* by granulation tissue, which is then converted to a *scar* and finally epithelialized from the adjacent mucosa. The scars are smooth and thin because of the absence of lymph follicles. After about four months, only a thin zone in the intestinal wall marks the previously diseased area. Typhoid scars never cause stenosis.

Complications: Perforation with peritonitis in the ulcer stage (3–4 weeks), fatal intestinal hemorrhage, typhoid pneumonia, waxy hyalin degeneration of the abdominal muscles (see Fig. 331, p. 203).

Intestinal tuberculosis (Fig. 172). *Tubercle bacilli may colonize the lymph follicles of Peyer's patches and cause caseous tuberculosis.* Under very low magnification, a defect is seen which extends to the muscularis (→ 1). The base is formed by a narrow zone of necrosis (caseation) containing many polymorphonuclear leukocytes (secondary infection). At the margins, there are round nodules that can be identified as typical tubercles under higher magnification. The tubercles extend through the entire wall at the base of the ulcer and into the serosa (→ 2). There is an increase in connective tissue.

Macroscopic: Flat ulcers with tattered margins, often surrounded by a circle of small white nodules on the serosa. Tuberculous lymphangiitis develops. The nearest lymph nodes draining the area are also always involved. Intestinal tuberculosis appears either as a result of ingestion of tubercle bacilli (primary intestinal tuberculosis with a primary complex) or, more frequently, as a secondary tuberculous process in association with active pulmonary tuberculosis.
Complications: Scarring of the ulcers with resultant intestinal stenosis, rarely perforation into the peritoneal cavity or into neighboring hollow organs. Bleeding may occur from a tuberculous ulcer, or generalized tuberculous peritonitis may develop.

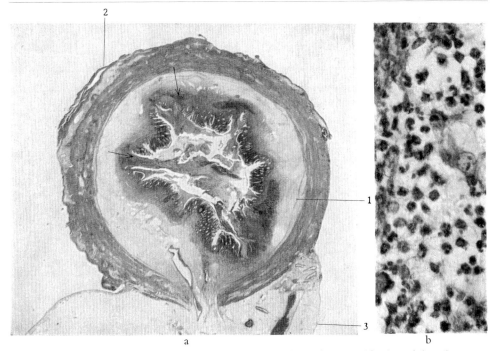

a   b

Fig. 173 a. Phlegmonous appendicitis; H & E, 10×. Fig. 173 b. Higher magnification of the submucosa, 600×.

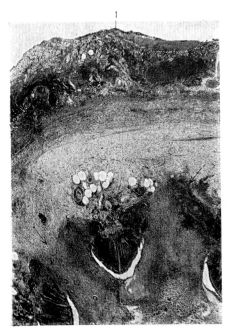

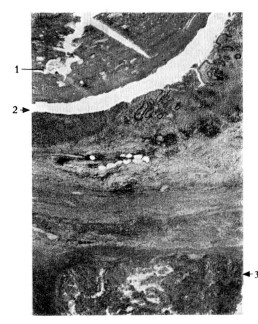

Fig. 174. Acute appendicitis with a so-called focus of primary infection; H & E, 23×.

Fig. 175. Appendicitis with a fecolith; H & E, 41×.

Appendicitis

Inflammation of the vermiform appendix usually has an intestinal origin (invasion of obstructed glands by intestinal bacterial flora or streptococci: or obstruction from a fecolith). Only rarely is appendicitis hematogenous, although it may follow an acute viral infection such as influenza, chicken pox or measles.

The *inflammation* starts in a small focus in the mucosa (*primary infection* of ASCHOFF, 1908) and then spreads like a *phlegmon* through all coats of the wall. Intramural abscesses, secondary ulceration, empyema, necrosis and gangrene of the wall frequently occur as a result of the development of arteritis and hemorrhagic infarction. *Chronic inflammation* leads to fibrosis and partial or complete obliteration of the lumen (Fig. 176), sometimes with retention of secretions (hydrops or mucocele).

Figure 173a shows an example of **acute phlegmonous appendicitis** at very low magnification. Fibrin and leukocytes fill the lumen. Several primary sites of infection are seen with mucosal necrosis covered with fibrin and leukocytes. The markedly increased thickness of the submucosa (edema → 1) and sparsity of leukocytic infiltration are remarkable (higher magnification Fig. 173b). Fibrin covers the peritoneum (→ 2). The inflammation also commonly extends into the mesentery (→ 3).

In Figure 174, two **primary foci of infection** can be seen under higher magnification (2 arrows in the picture). The inflammation has originated in a crypt and the leukocytic exudation has involved the tunica propria. Following this, the epithelium is breached and the mucosa destroyed by focal inflammatory exudation of fibrin and leukocytes. In Figure 174, the whole wall is infiltrated with leukocytes (→ 1: peritoneum covered with fibrin and leukocytes).

Fecal stasis (Fig. 175) in the appendix (inadequate peristalsis?) can lead to the development of a fecolith (from deposition of calcium and magnesium). Undigested food particles (→ 1: fragment of vegetable matter) are frequently seen in fecoliths. *Mucosal ulceration* (→ 2) may develop from the trauma of the pressure of such particles and result in *phlegmonous inflammation* involving all the intestinal coats. Figure 175 shows also *an intramural abscess* (→ 3) in the muscularis.

Acute appendicitis is usually a rapidly progressive illness that requires prompt surgical intervention. The urgency of the intervention becomes clear when the number of serious complications of untreated appendicitis are compared with the rapidity of recovery after appendectomy.

Chronic appendicitis (Fig. 176) results in disappearance of the mucosa and usually obliteration of the lumen. In Figure 176, the lumen is closed by connective tissue. Occasional lymph follicles remain. The submucosa is greatly thickened by fibrosis (→) and contains nodules of fat tissue (→ 1).

Complications of appendicitis: Perforation, peritonitis, pericecal abscess (typhlitis), spreading retroperitoneal inflammation (phlegmonous), subphrenic abscess, pyelophlebitic liver abscess, chiefly in the left lobe, hydrops, mucocele.

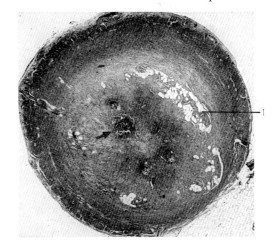

Fig. 176. Chronic obliterative appendicitis; H & E, 15 ×.

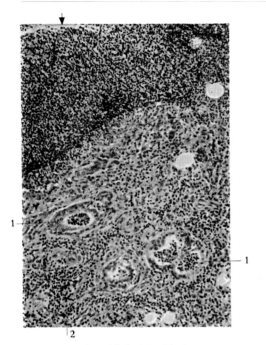

Fig. 177. Purulent sialadenitis with abscess formation; H & E, 120×.

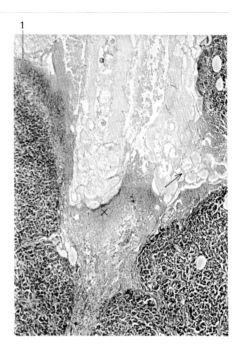

Fig. 178. Parenchymatous and fat necrosis of the pancreas; H & E, 43×.

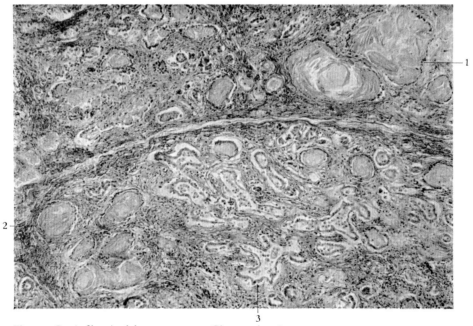

Fig. 179. Cystic fibrosis of the pancreas; van Gieson stain, 78×.

Purulent sialadenitis with abscess formation (Fig. 177). *Inflammation of the salivary glands may be due to a primary viral infection, for example, mumps parotitis (lymphocytic exudate), or it may be due to secondary infection, for example, a staphylococcal infection in general debilitation (cachexia). The condition usually arises as an ascending infection (e. g., following stones in a salivary duct), but occasionally it is hematogenous in origin. Chronic recurring inflammation with plasma cells and marked fibrous induration may develop when the salivary ducts are obstructed (so-called inflammatory tumor usually seen in 30–40 year old men. In 50% of cases, there are salivary stones). In Sjögren's syndrome (chiefly occurring in menopausal women) there is also a chronic recurrent form of inflammation which eventually results in atrophy of the parotid and the neighboring salivary and tear glands.* Histologically, purulent sialadenitis shows leukocytes in dilated ducts (→ 1) as well as in the interstitial tissues. The glands are widely separated because of the inflammatory edema and infiltration with polymorphonuclear leukocytes and lymphocytes (→ 2). Tissue destruction with abscess formation is common (→).

Fat necrosis of the pancreas (Fig. 178). *Necrosis of the parenchyma and fat tissue of the pancreas is initiated by autodigestion (trypsin, lipase) resulting from previous disturbance of the local circulation. The pathogenesis of this very complex process is still under dispute.* Microscopically, there is necrosis of the parenchyma and islands of fat tissue in the pancreas, frequently accompanied by hemorrhage *(hemorrhagic pancreatic necrosis)*. Under low magnification, the ghost-like outlines of the fat cells can be recognized in many of the necrotic areas (→). In other areas, the fat is replaced by homogeneous, pale pink or blue material. Often, crystals of fatty acids are precipitated. In Figure 178, hematoidin is deposited at the edge of the area of fat necrosis (×). The necrosis also extends into the parenchyma (→ 1), which appears eosinophilic and shows loss of nuclei. In the acute stages of the necrosis, leukocytes accumulate at the margins, while in later stages a collar of granulation tissue or mature connective tissue containing foam cells may be found. Fat necrosis developing after death lacks any evidence of tissue reaction such as exudation of leukocytes.

Macroscopic: In the initial stages, there is edema and focal parenchymatous necrosis (large, dirty-gray pancreas): in hemorrhagic necrosis, the pancreas is dark red and bloody; secondary liquefaction with cyst formation may develop. Fat necrosis appears as chalky white, freckle-sized nodules.

Cystic fibrosis of the pancreas (Fig. 179). *Not only is the pancreas involved in this disease but also the mucous glands of the intestine, bile ducts, lungs and salivary glands (mucoviscidosis, Anderson, 1962). It affects chiefly children who have meconium ileus. Marked inflammatory changes are present in the lungs of these children (bronchiectasis) and, finally, chronic deficiency of pancreatic enzymes leads to the development of celiac disease. The basic disease process is a "dyscholasia", that is, the development of stasis and a secretion of high viscosity.* Microscopically, the normal lobular structures are surrounded by strands of connective tissue. Both the ducts (→ 1) and acini (→ 2, 3) are widely dilated and cystic. The contents of the cysts consist of homogeneous or laminated secretions. An increased amount of interstitial tissue is distributed randomly through the lobules (red connective tissue in van Gieson stain). In addition, there is scanty infiltration of leukocytes and plasma cells. In general, the organ is reconstructed in a way similar to hepatic cirrhosis.

Macroscopic: The pancreas is firm and grayish white. In the late stages, there are numerous small cysts and the surface is granular.

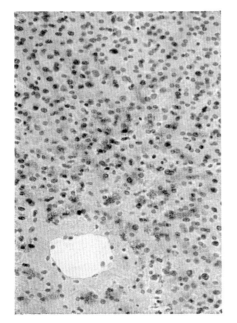

Fig. 180. Brown atrophy of the liver;
111×.

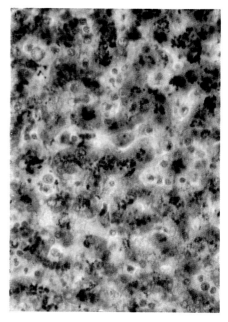

Fig. 181. Siderosis of the liver;
Berlin blue reaction, 456×.

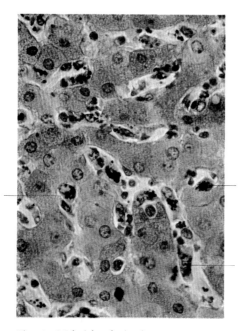

Fig. 182. Malarial melanin pigment;
H & E, 480×.

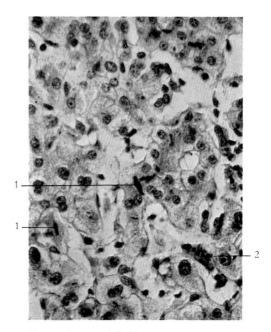

Fig. 183. Icterus of the liver;
H & E, 310×.

Liver

Familiarity with the normal microscopic anatomy of the liver is an essential prerequisite for interpretation of the microscopic appearances of abnormal liver. For purposes of orientation, the *periportal field* will serve as a good starting point [Glisson's triad of bile ducts (cylindrical epithelium), artery (heavy muscular wall) and branches of the portal vein]. The periportal field is enveloped by a sheath of liver cells, known as the *limiting plate* (POPPER and SCHAFFNER). Cords of liver cells accompanied by sinusoids course toward the central vein. When trying to understand pathological changes in the liver lobules, it should be borne in mind that different parts of the liver lobule can be affected separately (e. g., either the central or peripheral zones). This depends upon peculiarities of the circulation and of the cellular complement of enzymes. Concepts about the fundamental functional unit of the liver are still not well established. For example, instead of the "classic" liver lobule centered around the central vein *(central vein unit)*, a so-called *portal vein unit* has been proposed (see RAPPAPORT, 1954). In this scheme, the periportal zone lies at the center and the central vein marks the peripheral boundary of the liver lobule. Many pathological alterations can be well correlated with the functional findings with this concept (e. g., the pattern of stasis). *Attention should be paid to the following features in pathological material:* The cell constituents of the periportal field, the integrity of the liver cell cords, and of the liver cells themselves, particularly in the limiting plate, Kupffer cells and any deposits of pigments or other substances (e. g., fat, amyloid).

Brown atrophy of the liver (Fig. 180). *In brown atrophy, which may affect any internal organ and especially the heart and liver, there is an increase in lipofuscin.* The pigment is best seen in histological sections stained with hemotoxylin without a counterstain. Low magnification shows a prominent brownish cast in the region of the central portion of the lobule. Under higher magnification, brown cytoplasmic granules can be seen. Figure 180 shows the central vein and surrounding cords of liver cells, which contain less and less pigment the farther they are situated from the center of the lobule. In addition, the liver cells are also atrophic and have compactly arranged nuclei.

Macroscopic: Brown, shrunken organ with a wrinkled capsule.

Siderosis of the liver (Fig. 181). *In this condition, iron-containing pigment, usually derived from hemoglobin, is deposited in the cytoplasm of both the liver and the Kupffer cells.* In contrast to lipofuscin pigment, siderosis is found chiefly in the periphery of the liver lobule, especially in the cytoplasm of cells lying next to bile ductules (see also Figs. 13, 369). In this way, the midline between two rows of cells becomes intensified. The pigment appears yellowish brown in sections stained with hematoxylin and eosin, but the Berlin blue reaction colors the pigment a deep blue. The stellate-shaped Kupffer cells also contain deposits of iron pigment.

Macroscopic: A brown liver of normal size, often associated with siderosis of other organs (pancreas, spleen, salivary glands), especially in hemochromatosis (see Fig. 206).

Malarial melanin pigment (Fig. 182). *Brownish black pigment originating from destruction of blood cells in malaria is deposited in the reticuloendothelial cells.* Accordingly, it is found in the Kupffer cells of the liver. Figure 182 shows the black granules in the swollen Kupffer cells (→), and is a good demonstration of the phagocytic capacities of these lining cells of the sinusoids (see Fig. 16).

Macroscopic: Smoky gray discoloration of liver and spleen.

Icterus of the liver (Fig. 183). *In jaundice, granules of bile pigment appear in the cytoplasm of the liver cells and bile casts form in the ductules or larger bile ducts.* Under low magnification, greenish, sausage-shaped secretions (bile casts, incorrectly called bile thrombi → 1, see also Figs. 215, 216) can be seen. Isolated, fine droplets of bile are also seen in the cytoplasm of the liver cells. In obstructive jaundice and extrahepatic jaundice, the central zone of the liver lobule is particularly affected, whereas in hepatocellular jaundice all parts of the lobule are involved. The Kupffer cells may also contain bile pigment (→ 2) or phagocytosed necrotic liver cells.

Macroscopic: The liver has either a green (biliverdin) or a golden brown color (bilirubin).

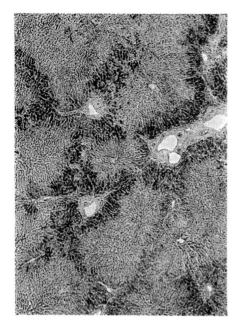

Fig. 184. Peripheral fatty degeneration
of the liver;
Sudan stain, 22×.

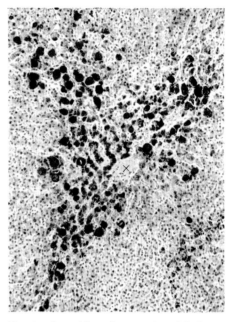

Fig. 185. Central fatty degeneration of the liver;
Sudan stain, 84×.

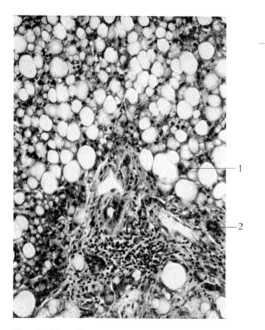

Fig. 186. Fatty liver;
H & E, 170×.

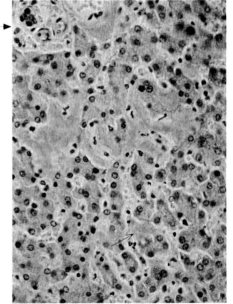

Fig. 187. Amyloidosis of the liver;
Congo red stain, 155×.

Fatty Degeneration of the Liver

The lipids of the liver cells are bound to the cell components and are not normally seen. When fat appears in the form of droplets in the cytoplasm of the liver cells, the condition is known as *fatty degeneration* (fatty metamorphosis). Three forms of fatty degeneration occur in the liver: *peripheral fatty degeneration* (e. g., alimentary fatty degeneration), *central fatty degeneration* (e. g., metabolic or toxic) and *diffuse fatty degeneration* (see p. 7).

Peripheral fatty degeneration (Fig. 184) is manifested by the occurrence of large droplets of fat in the cytoplasm of liver cells at the periphery of the lobules. Low-power examination of preparations stained with Sudan shows a red ring surrounding the pale central zone. Higher magnification shows that the liver cells are filled with large droplets of fat; frequently, these are large round globules. The nucleus is displaced to the periphery of the cells.

Macroscopic: Yellow ring-shaped network with brownish red centers.

Central fatty degeneration (Fig. 185) shows the reverse picture. With the scanning lens, the central zones of the lobule appear as red areas surrounded by a blue halo. Low magnification reveals the position of the fat deposits. The central vein ($\times$) lies in the middle of the fatty area. A further point of distinction from peripheral fatty degeneration is the fact that most of the fat droplets are very fine and distributed diffusely through the cytoplasm.

Macroscopic: Small yellow point-like lesions scattered on a brown background.

Fatty liver (Fig. 186). In this condition, almost all the liver cells are filled with large droplets of fat, without preferential localization. Several cells may fuse and form so-called fat cysts ($\rightarrow$ 1). The periportal connective tissue contains proliferated bile ducts ($\rightarrow$ 2), inflammatory exudate and an increased amount of connective tissue. As a result, the picture of portal cirrhosis develops (*fatty cirrhosis*, see Fig. 205). In Figure 186 (a paraffin section), only the empty spaces are seen from which the fat has been dissolved.

Macroscopic: Large, soft organ of doughy consistency and with yellow dull cut surfaces instead of the normal glistening ones. Fat droplets coat the knife.

Amyloidosis of the liver (Fig. 187). The amyloid, which is a pathological protein, is deposited in the space between the walls of the sinusoids and the liver cells (Dissé's space). At first only a narrow strip of homogeneous red material (positive for Congo red) is seen next to the capillaries ($\rightarrow$ inside picture). The lumens of the sinusoids may be greatly reduced as a consequence of the infiltration. Amyloid stains with either Congo red or methyl violet (red metachromasia, see pp. 10, 171). Amyloid stained with Congo red is doubly refractive and shows an abnormal green color when viewed with polarized light.

Macroscopic: Large, firm organ having a wooden consistency and glassy cut surfaces. Suspected cases of amyloidosis may sometimes be confirmed by either a needle biopsy of the liver or a punch biopsy of the rectum.

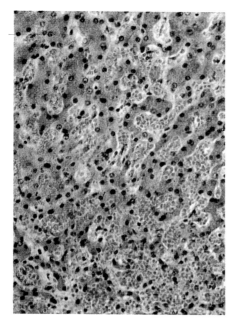

Fig. 188. Mild congestion (stasis) of liver;
H & E, 250×.

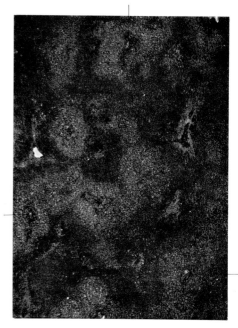

Fig. 189. Marked congestion of liver;
H & E, 29×.

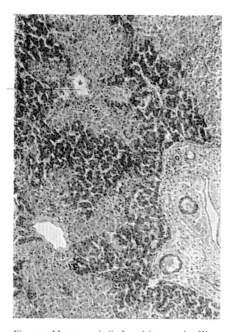

Fig. 190. Hypoxemic (ischemic) necrosis of liver;
H & E, 60×.

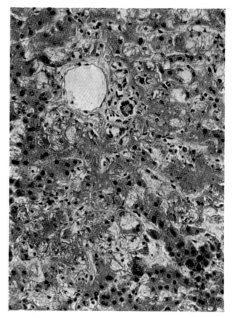

Fig. 191. Liver necrosis in eclampsia;
H & E, 200×.

Congestion of the liver (Fig. 188). Stasis due to obstruction of the venous return to the right heart manifests itself first in the *central zones of the liver lobules*. At a later stage, lake-like vascular channels develop by fusion of the congested central zones of adjacent liver lobules. In the early stages, low-power magnification reveals red zones in the center of the lobules; higher magnification discloses the greatly dilated sinusoids. Figure 188 shows a section of the central zone (the central vein lies below and outside the picture), with the sinusoids greatly distended by numerous erythrocytes. If the liver cells in the uncongested upper portion of the illustration are compared with those in the congested areas, it can be clearly seen that the liver cells in the latter are atrophic because of compression by dilated sinuses. This often leads to deficient oxygenation of the cells so that they also show fatty degeneration (→: unaltered Kupffer cell).

Macroscopic: Enlarged, firm liver. The cut surfaces show dark red central areas surrounded by pale brown peripheral zones. Often, fatty degeneration is also present and imparts a yellow appearance.

Marked congestion of the liver (Fig. 189). When congestion has been present for a long time, it involves not only the intermediate and peripheral zones of the lobule, but also the adjacent lobule. In this manner, congested channels are formed which connect one liver lobule with another and lead to a *reversal of the normal liver pattern* so that the periportal field (→) is in the middle of a red ring of hyperemia (see notes on histology on p. 117). The red ring and the broad channels can be seen even with the scanning lens. With low-power magnification, the periportal field is seen to be at the center. Higher magnification of the congested area shows the greatly dilated sinusoids. In these areas, the liver cells have disappeared. Frequently, the walls of the sinusoids cannot be recognized. A great lake of blood has formed. Most of the intact parenchyma shows fatty degeneration.

Macroscopic: The liver is large and dark red. The cut surfaces show a dark red network on a yellow background (fatty degeneration), the so-called nutmeg liver.

Hypoxic (Ischemic) **liver necrosis** (Fig. 190). *Necrosis of the liver can affect either single cells (see hepatitis, p. 126) or groups of cells in either the intermediate zone of the lobules or without any particular localization.* Focal necrosis can be caused by *toxins* (e. g., diphtheria) or it may be dependent upon *acute oxygen lack.* Figure 190 shows geographical areas of necrosis in the centers of the liver lobules (→: central vein). The areas of necrotic liver cells are apparent from the pale red stain. Nuclei are decreased in number. Kupffer cells, for the most part, are preserved.

Liver necrosis in eclampsia (Fig. 191). *Eclampsia usually develops toward the end of pregnancy but before labor has occurred. The pathogenesis is now considered to be the result either of direct toxic action on the parenchymatous cells or a secondary outcome of a disturbance of the circulation. Liver, kidney and brain are preferentially affected.* In contrast to hypoxic liver necrosis, which develops in the area of greatest oxygen deficiency, the necrosis of eclampsia is distributed at random throughout the lobule. Examination with a scanning lens discloses irregularly scattered, eosinophilic, map-like lesions. Low-power magnification shows that the liver cell cords and sinusoids in the homogeneous red areas are no longer arranged next to one another. Cell nuclei have disappeared. The cytoplasm of the liver cells has become homogeneous and structureless. The blood in the sinusoids is coagulated into solid masses (→) as a result of stasis or the formation of fibrin and platelet thrombi (hyalin thrombi).

Macroscopic: Gray or grayish yellow, map-like lesions.

121

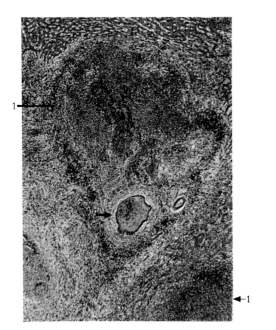

Fig. 192. Ascending suppurative cholangitis;
H & E, 50×.

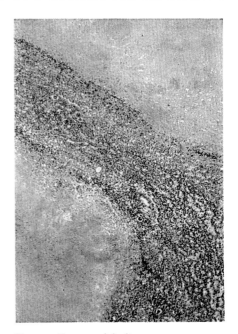

Fig. 193. Gumma of the liver;
van Gieson stain, 56×.

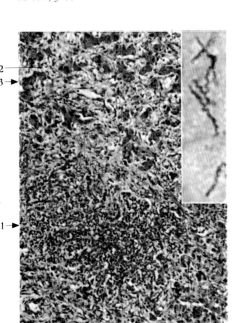

Fig. 194. Congenital syphilis of the liver;
H & E, 120×.
Inset: spirochetes;
Levaditi stain, 2,350×.

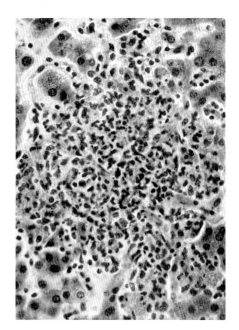

Fig. 195. Typhoid nodule in the liver;
H & E, 330×.

Ascending suppurative cholangitis (Fig. 192). *This is caused by ascending bacterial infection (mostly Escherichia coli) of the bile ducts and is often associated with bile stasis (stones, tumors).* The bile ducts in the periportal spaces are dilated and contain exudate rich in polymorphonuclear leukocytes (→). The entire periportal field is infiltrated with polymorphonuclear leukocytes, which also are found in the adjacent parenchyma where there is tissue necrosis (*cholangiolytic abscess* → 1). In Figure 192 there is an increase in the periportal fibrous tissue which forms a concentric, collar-like arrangement around the bile ducts. This is often an indication of previous cholangitic disease.

Macroscopic: The liver is bile-stained, with widening and proliferation of the periportal fields and foci of greenish necrosis.

Gumma of the liver (Fig. 193). *In the third stage of syphilis, granulomas (gummas) with a rubbery consistency appear in affected organs.* These are sharply demarcated, round or map-like foci of necrosis which, as can be easily seen with elastica and van Gieson stains, contain connective tissue or elastic fibers which arise in the surrounding tissues and penetrate the necrotic area. Figure 193 shows the necrotic center (yellow with van Gieson stain and lacking nuclei) surrounded by a narrow band of granulation tissue. Epithelioid cells resembling those of tuberculosis (Fig. 141, p. 98) are seen in the granulation tissue. These, however, are present in smaller numbers than in tuberculosis. Next to this there is a layer of connective tissue vascularized with capillaries and containing fibroblasts and lymphocytes. In the outermost zone, scar tissue has formed (red in van Gieson's stain). As in tuberculosis, there are also Langhans type giant cells. However, in contrast to tuberculosis, numbers of plasma cells are present in the granulation tissue of a gumma and the neighboring blood vessels show endarteritis.

Macroscopic: Yellow, map-like areas of necrosis having a rubbery consistency.

Congenital syphilis of the liver (Fig. 194). Under low magnification, the normal architecture of the liver can be scarcely recognized. There are small, richly cellular, blue-staining focal lesions (*syphilomas*). The liver cords are widely separated by an interstitial cellular infiltrate, and individual groups of liver cells have been destroyed. Medium magnification reveals miliary granulomas (→ 1) showing areas of fresh necrosis, nuclear fragments, polymorphonuclear leukocytes and lymphocytes. In these areas, the liver cells are completely destroyed. In the surrounding tissue, a chronic interstitial hepatitis has developed in which the interstitial tissue is markedly distended with histiocytes (→ 2), fibroblasts, lymphocytes and fibrous tissue. Remnants of liver cords lie in between (→ 3). Numerous *spirochetes* can be demonstrated with special stains (Levaditi silver stain, inset, Fig. 194).

Macroscopic: The liver is of firm consistency and the cut surfaces show grayish brown flecks.

Congenital syphilis localizes principally in the skeletal system (*syphilitic osteochondritis*, p. 209, *syphilitic saddle nose, syphilitic periosteitis*), in the skin (*syphilitic pemphigus*), lungs (*pneumonia alba*) and brain. In addition, the victims may show the so-called *Hutchinson triad* (keratitis, inner ear deafness and malformed teeth).

Typhoid nodule of the liver (Fig. 195). The granuloma of typhoid fever has been chosen as an example of a nodular, granulomatous inflammation of the liver. There is nodular proliferation of the local cells of the reticuloendothelial system (i. e., the Kupffer cells) which come to resemble epithelioid cells. In addition, a few lymphocytes and an occasional solitary polymorphonuclear leukocytes are to be seen. The liver cells in the area have been destroyed (see typhoid fever on p. 110).

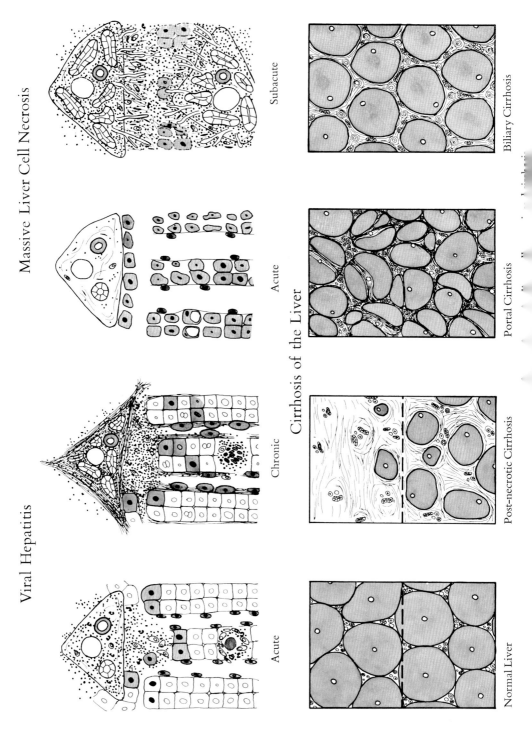

Massive Liver Cell Necrosis

Subacute

Acute

Viral Hepatitis

Chronic

Acute

Cirrhosis of the Liver

Biliary Cirrhosis

Portal Cirrhosis

Post-necrotic Cirrhosis

Normal Liver

Viral Hepatitis – Massive Liver Cell Necrosis – Cirrhosis

Figure 196 shows in schematic form the histological appearances of these three diseases, which will be considered together because of certain similarities. *In essence, all three show destruction of liver cells (necrosis) accompanied by a secondary mesenchymal reaction that takes the form of granulation tissue. There is, in addition, reorganization of the structure of the liver and parenchymal regeneration.* In many cases of cirrhosis, *primary proliferation of granulation tissue (inflammation) with simultaneous or subsequent destruction of parenchyma* occupy a prominent place.

Viral hepatitis (see also pp. 126, 127) is initiated by *necrosis of single cells* (acidophilic necrotic cytoplasm). These are resorbed by histiocytes. The periportal zones show an infiltrate of lymphocytes and histiocytes which destroy the limiting plate and extend farther into the parenchyma. In *subacute* and *chronic stages*, the foci of resorption may persist for a long time as *residual nodules*. The Kupffer cells are enlarged and increased in number. Collagen is deposited in the walls of the sinusoids, and the periportal spaces contain increased amounts of fibrous tissue and a dense inflammatory exudate.

In massive liver cell necrosis (see also pp. 128, 129), the necrosis involves either the entire liver or a part of it. In the majority of cases, it is now thought to be a *fulminant form of viral hepatitis*. The acute stage *(massive cytolytic necrosis,* formerly *acute yellow atrophy)* is manifested by dissociation of the liver cell cords, necrosis of cells and pyknosis of nuclei. In the *subacute stages*, a large part of the parenchyma is demolished and the periportal zones collapse and are infiltrated with chronic inflammatory cells.

Cirrhosis of the liver (see also pp. 130, 131) is a disease in which there is *destruction of parenchyma* with *progressive reconstruction* of the entire liver and formation of *pseudolobules*.
Three essentially different types of cirrhosis are recognized: 1. *postnecrotic cirrhosis*, 2. *portal cirrhosis*, 3. *biliary cirrhosis*.

The theoretical origin of **postnecrotic cirrhosis** is clearly shown in the first two diagrams in the lower row of Figure 196: a portion of the liver parenchyma is destroyed (portion above the broken line in the figure) and a large scar results in which only a few clusters of parenchymatous cells remain. The periportal zones are compressed and lie closer together. The lower portion of the diagram shows a less marked degree of the same process with various sized pseudolobules. Frequently, a whole lobe of the liver or a large part of it is destroyed (see also Fig. 203).

In **portal cirrhosis** (see also Fig. 204), the architecture of the liver lobules is considerably altered by bands of fibrous tissue arising from the periportal zones and coursing through the lobules in irregular fashion to form pseudolobules. In the residual areas of parenchyma, the central veins no longer lie at the center. The *etiology* is either a virus infection (hepatitis) or a toxic injury of the liver (e. g., alcohol or an ingested poison, etc.).

Biliary cirrhosis results from a combination of bile obstruction and ascending inflammation. The inflammation and reorganization of the parenchyma originate in the periportal zones, encroach upon the parenchyma and extend to the periphery of the liver lobules. This results in a portal type of cirrhosis, but it differs in being more uniform. A similar appearance develops in fatty cirrhosis and pigment cirrhosis (see Figs. 205, 206).

125

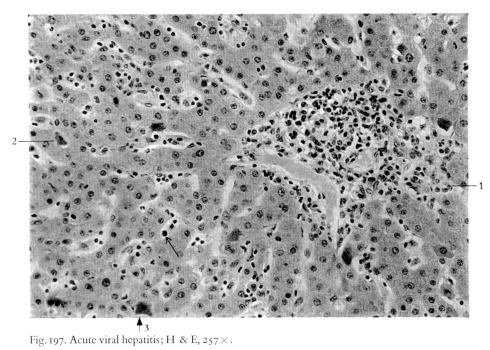

Fig. 197. Acute viral hepatitis; H & E, 257×.

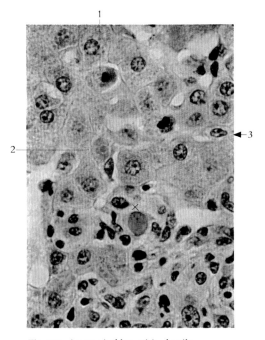

Fig. 198. Acute viral hepatitis, detail;
H & E, 512×.

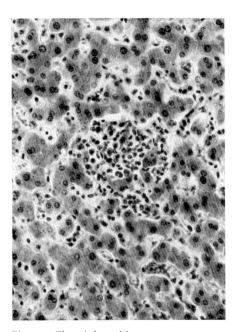

Fig. 199: Chronic hepatitis;
H & E, 225×.

Viral Hepatitis

Viral hepatitis shows a *characteristic histological picture* so that, in most cases, *an etiological diagnosis can be made from the microscopic examination.* Study of needle biopsy specimens has aided in unraveling the course of the disease.

Acute viral hepatitis (Figs. 197, 198). Low magnification reveals widening and cellular infiltration of the periportal fields, but with preservation of architecture and scanty cellular infiltration of the parenchyma. Somewhat higher magnification (Fig. 197) shows the periportal infiltrate to consist of lymphocytes and a few polymorphonuclear leukocytes which have breached the limiting plate of the lobule and invaded the parenchyma ($\rightarrow$ 1). Between the liver cell cords there are *swollen Kupffer cells* (stellate shaped) and round, mobilized reticuloendothelial cells (histiocytes, $\rightarrow$ in the picture). In addition, individual liver cells are small and shrunken, with striking angular cytoplasm and pyknotic nuclei ($\rightarrow$ 2, $\rightarrow$ 3).

High magnification, Figure 198, **acute viral hepatitis** (detail, see also Figs. 219, 220), shows necrosis of individual cells and the reaction in the liver. At $\rightarrow$ 1, a necrotic cell with nuclear pyknosis is seen. At $\rightarrow$ 2 (also $\times$), there is the ghost of an anuclear cell forming a typical eosinophilic body (so-called hyalin or Councilman body, see also Fig. 219). These "hyalin bodies" are not specific for hepatitis, as they are also observed in other conditions. The individual necrotic cells are surrounded by lymphocytes and histiocytes with plump, oval or slightly indented nuclei (see Fig. 219). At $\rightarrow$ 3, there is a swollen Kupffer cell. In the acute stages there are, in addition, bile pigmentation of liver cells and bile casts in the central zones (see Figs. 215, 216). Mitoses and multinucleated giant cells indicate the onset of liver cell regeneration.

Macroscopic: The liver is enlarged, with rounded edges and spotted, yellow, reddish brown external and cut surfaces.

Chronic hepatitis (Fig. 199). The microscopic picture consists only of cellular infiltration in the periportal zone which, however, may persist for a long time after the clinical signs have subsided. The Kupffer cells are usually also swollen and increased in number, and foci of lymphocytes and proliferated reticulum cells (granulomas) may be present in the parenchyma. Removal of the individual necrotic cells seen in the acute stages is now complete. The cell nuclei vary in size. In van Gieson preparations, the deposition of collagen in the walls of the sinusoids can be seen as well as frequent small, sparsely cellular scars.

Two different courses may be recognized, both morphologically and clinically:

1. *Chronic active hepatitis with transition to cirrhosis* in which the chronic inflammatory infiltrate of the periportal fields encroaches on the parenchyma.

2. *Persistent hepatitis* with a prolonged anicteric course which may last for years and without extension of the periportal inflammation.

Giant cell hepatitis is considered on p. 132.

Macroscopic: The liver is of normal size, firm and brown. Eventually, it may become slightly nodular. *Clinical:* Jaundice of some duration is common, but an anicteric form also occurs. The disease can appear in epidemics, which are particularly common during wars and immediately thereafter. Transmission is either peroral (Virus A, epidemic hepatitis in the true sense of the term with an incubation period of 2–4 weeks) or parenteral. In the latter, the causative agent (Virus B) is introduced by a blood transfusion or by an injection of some sort. The incubation period varies between 45 and 160 days.

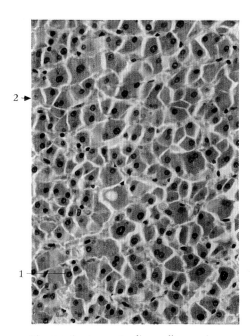

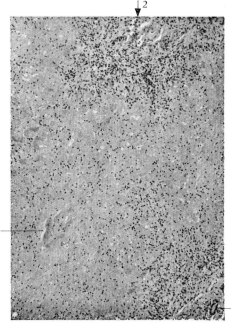

Fig. 200. Acute massive liver cell necrosis showing disorganization of the liver cell cords; H & E, 270×.

Fig. 201. Acute massive liver cell necrosis (4–6 days old); H & E, 110×.

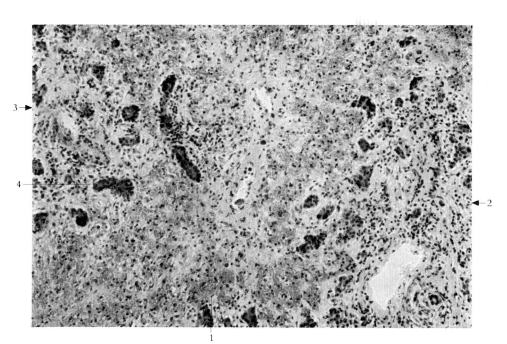

Fig. 202. Subacute massive liver cell necrosis; H & E, 165×.

Massive Liver Cell Necrosis

In **acute massive liver cell necrosis** (Figs. 200, 201), the whole organ is necrotic. It may be caused by various etiological agents and may lead to death within a few days. Among causative agents are: 1. *Potent poisons* (e. g., phosphorus, poisonous fungi, arsenic and others: these cause so-called toxic liver necrosis). In toxic liver injury, a marked degree of fatty degeneration of liver cells is seen at the beginning of the illness. Necrosis develops secondarily and affects the peripheral zones of the lobules preferentially. 2. *Metabolic disturbances* (usually protein). 3. *Viral infection*. This causes a *fulminant* or *malignant form of viral hepatitis* and has increased greatly in incidence during the past 20 years.

The microscopic picture of acute massive liver cell necrosis varies with the age of the illness and with the time that has elapsed between death and performance of the autopsy. In fresh cases (6–8 hours after death), there is disorganization of the liver cell cords, that is, the individual liver cells have become unattached and appear as separated cellular elements. The cells vary in size, and some are already shrunken ($\rightarrow$ 1, Fig. 200). The cytoplasm is homogeneous and stains more blue than normal (decrease in glycogen content). The nuclei are small and frequently either pyknotic ($\rightarrow$) or more faintly stained than normal (karyolysis $\rightarrow$ 2).

Figure 200 shows the liver of a patient who was ill of a clinically obscure "upper abdominal syndrome". At laparotomy, the liver was yellow and slightly reduced in size. An incisional biopsy was taken (see Fig. 200). Nineteen hours later, the patient died and at autopsy showed the typical picture of massive liver cell necrosis. Histologically, at autopsy the liver cells were without nuclei and the cytoplasm was faded and finely granular. There was no inflammatory infiltrate.

Acute massive liver cell necrosis, 4-6 days old (Fig. 201). If a patient with acute massive liver cell necrosis survives for a few days and then dies, almost complete dissolution of the liver cells occurs. Only homogeneous, eosinophilic material now remains. Intact individual Kupffer cells, however, are still present. The band-like areas of strongly eosinophilic material ($\rightarrow$ 1) still contain anuclear remnants of liver cell cords. The periportal fields ($\rightarrow$ 2) are infiltrated with inflammatory cells (lymphocytes), and show occasional proliferated bile ducts ($\rightarrow$ 3).

Macroscopic: The liver is small and flaccid and the capsule is wrinkled. The cut surfaces are yellow, yellowish green or ocher yellow. The liver may weigh as little as 500 Gm. (normal weight is 1,500 Gm.). Frequently, crystals of leucine and tyrosine can be seen on the cut surfaces or on the surface of the capsule (*microscopically:* round granules or crystalline tufts).

Subacute massive liver cell necrosis (Fig. 202). When only a part of the liver is affected by the necrosis (e. g., a lobe or a part of a lobe), or if the disease runs a slow course, subacute red atrophy ensues in which cell detritus, the remnants of liver cells, can be seen between the dilated sinusoids ($\rightarrow$ 1). Resorption of the necrotic tissue is far advanced and, as a result, the supporting hepatic framework has collapsed and the periportal spaces lie closer to one another ($\rightarrow$ 2 and $\rightarrow$ 3 indicate respectively two portal fields). There are numerous proliferated bile ducts ($\rightarrow$ 4) in addition to lymphocytic infiltration. Two central veins can be seen in the middle of the picture between the portal fields. At very low magnification, the increased width of the periportal fields and the proliferation of bile ducts are plainly visible.

Macroscopic: The liver is reduced in size, tough in consistency and has red and yellow, marble-like cut surfaces. The red color is due to hyperemia and pooling of blood. Islands of fatty parenchymous tissue are yellow.

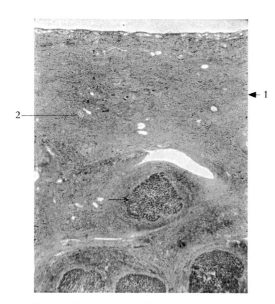

Fig. 203. Postnecrotic cirrhosis;
H & E, 14×.

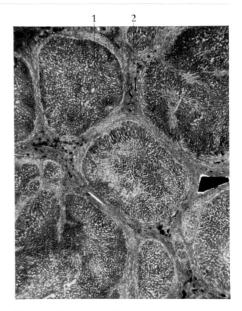

Fig. 204. Portal cirrhosis;
H & E, 30×.

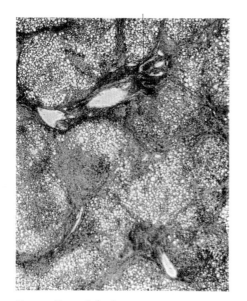

Fig. 205. Fatty cirrhosis;
van Gieson stain, 40×.

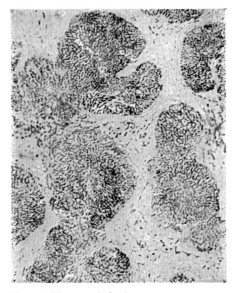

Fig. 206. Pigment cirrhosis;
Berlin-blue reaction, 30×.

Hepatic Cirrhosis

Postnecrotic cirrhosis (Fig. 203). The results of patchy parenchymatous necrosis are clearly seen in the picture. There is a large area of subcapsular tissue destruction ($\rightarrow$ 1), the lobular pattern has disappeared and the periportal zones are collapsed and compressed on one another. This has resulted in large scars that are rich in collagenous tissue and infiltrated with chronic inflammatory cells. The periportal zones also are infiltrated with lymphocytes and, in addition, show bile duct proliferation ($\rightarrow$ 2). Islands of remaining parenchyma ($\rightarrow$) can still be seen in the scarred tissue. Some of these show central veins or periportal zones, but they no longer have an orderly arrangement, since the necrosis of the lobules has been irregular. The central vein, for example, may lie at the edge of the lobule or the periportal zone lie in the middle of it *(pseudolobules)*. Other masses of regenerating liver cells have formed nodules with an abnormal architectural arrangement of the liver cell cords *(regeneration adenomas)*.

Macroscopic: The liver is irregularly nodular with depressed large and small scars and coarse nodules (regenerating parenchymal remnants).

Portal cirrhosis (Fig. 204). Examination with the scanning lens discloses various sized foci of red parenchymatous tissue traversed by bluish red septa of scar tissue. With low-power magnification, the pseudolobules and connective tissue septa connecting the periportal zones can be seen more clearly. Various sized islands of liver tissue with abnormally situated central veins have been formed in this way ($\rightarrow$ 1). The connective tissue ($\rightarrow$ 2) is infiltrated with cells (lymphocytes, histiocytes and a few polymorphonuclear leukocytes) and contains proliferated bile ducts. The progress of the cirrhosis is indicated by the degree of involvement of the parenchyma by cellular exudate.

Macroscopic: The liver shows fine, fairly regular nodularity (so-called hobnail liver).

In the final stages, the various forms of cirrhosis often become indistinguishable from one another. In this case, it is best to use the designation *Laennec's cirrhosis*.

Fatty cirrhosis (Fig. 205). In this condition, the alteration of architecture develops in a regular fashion from the periportal zones just as in biliary cirrhosis. With the scanning lens, it is scarcely possible to recognize the tissue as liver. In van Gieson preparations, red connective tissue septa can be seen, while the tissue between has a vacuolated appearance. Low magnification shows lymphocytic infiltration of the periportal fields and bile duct proliferation ($\rightarrow$). The liver cells contain round, optically empty droplets (the fat has been dissolved out in the process of preparation). In some places, larger fat cysts have formed (from fusion of fatty cells) (see also Fig. 186).

Macroscopic: Large, yellow, finely granular, firm liver.

Pigment cirrhosis (Fig. 206). *This occurs mostly as a part of hemochromatosis (bronze diabetes), an illness in which siderin pigment is deposited in the pancreas, spleen, lymph nodes, salivary glands and many other organs.* Very low magnification of sections treated with Berlin-blue shows irregular, blue-stained masses of parenchyma traversed by red-stained connective tissue septa of various widths. Higher magnification shows granules of blue pigment in the cytoplasm of the liver and Kupffer cells and in the lining cells of proliferated bile ducts.

Macroscopic: The liver is small, firm and brown and shows either fine or coarse granularity.

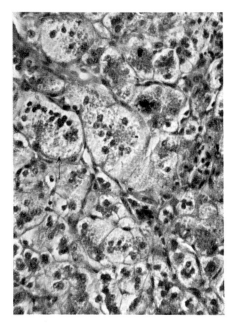

Fig. 207. Giant cell hepatitis;
H & E, 300×.

Fig. 208. Myeloid leukemia involving the liver;
H & E, 108×.

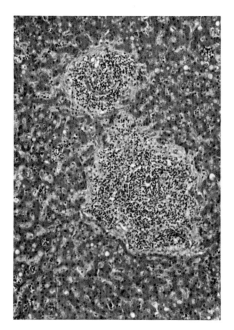

Fig. 209. Lymphatic leukemia involving
the liver; H & E, 108×.

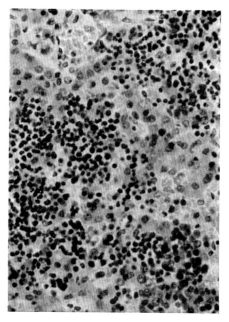

Fig. 210. Erythroblastosis of the liver;
H & E, 388×.

Giant cell hepatitis (Fig. 207).
Giant cell hepatitis of the newborn or infant is the expression of a particular reaction by the infant liver to various noxious stimuli (mainly viral hepatitis, although other causes are possible). The symptoms which are most prominent clinically are those resulting from obstructive jaundice. Microscopically (Fig. 207), the normal cords of liver cells are replaced by numerous, bizarre multinucleated giant cells (→). They frequently are the width of two or more liver cords. The cytoplasm of these giant cells is vacuolated and often filled with bile pigment (→ in the picture). These giant cells are an expression of faulty regeneration following liver cell damage. Proliferation of connective tissue cells (stellate cells, cells in the periportal fields) is not very prominent in this phase of the disease.

Macroscopic: Enlarged liver, with a marked green discoloration.

Myeloid leukemia involving the liver (Fig. 208). *In this form of leukemia, there is an unregulated increase in immature early forms of granulocytes in the bone marrow with spillover into the blood. It usually leads to infiltration of the spleen and lymph nodes and to accumulation and increase of myeloblasts, promyelocytes and myelocytes in the sinusoids of the liver* (see also Figs. 290, 291). The scanning lens reveals preservation of the architecture. Low magnification shows the markedly increased cell content of the sinusoids, most of which are distended and plugged with large, nucleated blood cells (myelocytes with round, vesiculated nuclei and, when more mature, granular cytoplasm; myeloblasts with oval or bean-shaped nuclei, see Fig. 290). The portal fields are, for the most part, either not involved or only slightly infiltrated with leukemic cells. The liver cells may undergo pressure atrophy and show degenerative changes.

Macroscopic: The liver is enlarged, grayish red and the lobules are indistinct. In paramyeloblastic leukemia, the periportal zones are especially affected.

Lymphatic leukemia involving liver (Fig. 209, also Fig. 289). In contrast to myeloid leukemia, the *periportal zones* in chronic lymphatic leukemia are permeated with immature cells (lymphoblasts, lymphocytes), whereas the sinusoids contain only small numbers of nucleated cells. Under low magnification, the markedly increased, blue appearing, spherical periportal zones are at once apparent. Higher magnification shows infiltration of the periportal connective tissue by lymphatic cells, with dense or vesiculated nuclei and scanty cytoplasm.

Macroscopic: The liver is enlarged. The periportal spaces are often visible on the cut surfaces as small, white nodules.

Erythroblastosis of the liver (Fig. 210). *In this condition, the fetus or newborn infant develops hemolytic anemia as a result of immunization of the mother during pregnancy by the father's blood factors. (Most commonly this is Rh incompatibility and less commonly incompatibility of ABO or some other factor.) The anemia results in a marked reactive increase in blood formation in the bone marrow and other hematopoietic tissues, including the liver (this occurs normally in newborns).* Nodules of cellular infiltration are seen in the liver. Under high magnification, these can be identified as foci of intrasinusoidal hematopoiesis. The cells are chiefly erythropoietic (in particular, erythroblasts and normoblasts), with a few from the white cell series and some megakaryocytes. In addition, there is hepatocellular jaundice, since, in most cases, the liver cells are unable to produce indirect reacting bilirubin. Bile casts and siderosis may also be seen.

Macroscopic: A large, red liver. In late stages, there may be generalized edema *(congenital hydrops)*, anemia and *severe jaundice* (icterus gravis, often associated with kernicterus).

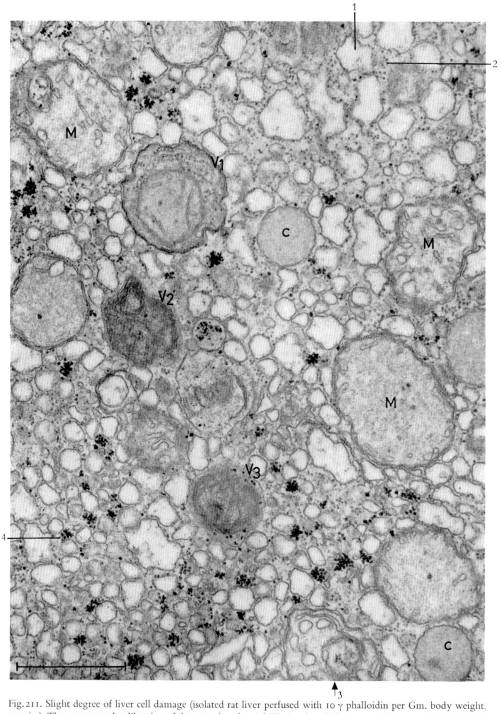

Fig. 211. Slight degree of liver cell damage (isolated rat liver perfused with 10 γ phalloidin per Gm. body weight, 30 min.). There are vacuolar dilatation of the smooth and rough ER (→ 1) and ribosomes without membranes (→ 2). There are also numbers of autolysosomes (autophagocytotic vacuoles) with accumulated mitochondria (V₁; also see Fig. 212), and myelin figures (V₂ and V₃) which are presumably a manifestation of the digestion of membranes in these lysosomes. → 3 Golgi apparatus, M = mitochondria, C = cytosome, → 4 glycogen. 32,000 × (Dr. MILLER).

Electron Microscopy of Lifer Injury

The electron microscopic changes of the liver cell organelles are rather uniform and, for the most part, nonspecific. Theoretically, all the changes described in Table 4 may occur. In acute toxic injury (alcohol, carbon tetrachloride, partial hepatectomy, see Fig. 213, or anoxia), the mitochondria are swollen (cloudy swelling) and the endoplasmic reticulum or ground substance becomes vacuolated (hydropic degeneration, Fig. 217). Glycogen stores disappear, the rough endoplasmic reticulum becomes disorganized and frequently loses its ribosomes (reduction of protein synthesis) and, finally, the cell membranes become fragmented, vacuolated and are destroyed (Figs. 214, 217). The lysosomes contain parts of the cellular organelles (Fig. 212). Similar pictures are seen in acute viral hepatitis, in which hyalin bodies, also called Councilman bodies (Fig. 219), appear, i.e., necrotic, shrunken liver cells. Proof of virus particles has not been substantiated in the human. Chronic liver damage entails primarily focal or diffuse prolif-eration of the endoplasmic reticulum (Fig. 218, intensification of the detoxification process) and, as a result, glycogen disappears. In chronic *alcoholic intoxication*, focal filamentous masses may be seen which are interpreted to be altered ergastoplasm (*Mallory bodies*, alcoholic hyalin, Fig. 221). Terminally, the ER may be entirely disrupted. The smooth endoplasmic reticulum may also appear to form myelin-like whorls (fingerprints, Fig. 218). Fat droplets may be seen either in acute or chronic liver damage. In chronic hepatitis, there is also proliferation of collagen fibers in the space of Dissé, and a basement membrane may form. In intra- (hepatitis, toxic) and extrahepatic cholestasis the bile canaliculi are dilated, the microvilli are swollen at first, then disappear (Fig. 215), and the pericanalicular cytoplasm has a denser appearance. Lysosomes and cytosomes (pericanalicular dense bodies), increase in number and are spread throughout the cytoplasm (activation of acid phosphatase). In addition, bile droplets can be seen in the cytoplasm (Fig. 216). Determination of the path of bile into the blood stream (whether between or through hepatic cells) has not been successful even with the electron microscope. In hepatic cirrhosis, nonspecific changes again are seen (enlargement and clumping of mitochondria, myelin-like degeneration, vacuoles in the ER, proliferation of collagen fibers around the liver cells, autophagolysosomes, localized cell destruction, fat deposition, localized glycogen aggregation, pigmentation, bile tubule proliferation and hemosiderin).

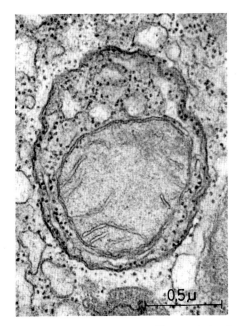

Fig. 212. *Autophagolysosome*, "focus of local degradation" in a liver cell of a rat. Treatment as in Figure 211. Within the surrounding membrane there is a well-preserved mitochon-drion and parts of rough endoplasmic reticulum (ribosomes, membranes). 45,000 × (Dr. MILLER).

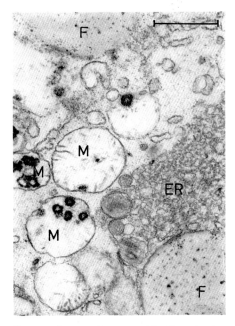

Fig. 213. Acute carbon tetrachloride poisoning (after 24 hours, liver, mouse). Focal prolifera-tion of the smooth endoplasmic reticulum (ER), fat droplets (F) as well as swollen mitochondria (matrix type) with round, black-appearing matrix aggregates (calcium deposits, REYNOLDS, 1963). 35,000 × (Dr. HÜBNER).

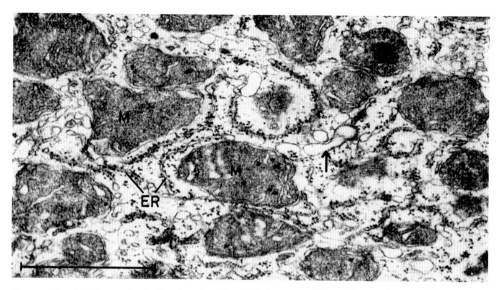

Fig. 214. *Chronic toxic necrosis of a liver* (rat, 8 weeks of N-nitrosomorphilin = liver carcinogen). Disorganization of the rough endoplasmic reticulum (ER) may be seen, which no longer shows parallel-layered membrane systems as in the normal, but lies isolated between mitochondria. The ribosomal mass is partly reduced or has irregular borders. M = mitochondria with dense matrix and some matrix aggregates. Isolated cisternae in the smooth ER are dilated (→). 37,000 × (Dr. BANNASCH).

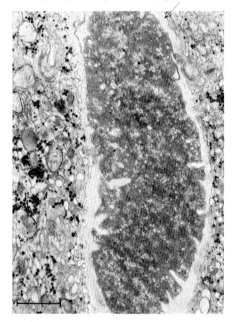

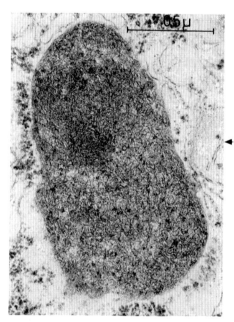

Fig. 215. *Bile cast* in a canaliculus (human, viral hepatitis). There are no microvilli (Fig. 11), the lumen is filled with bile pigment as well as with markedly fragmented smooth membranes (finely fibrillar material). Notice the ground substance surrounding the canaliculus (→). 12,000 × (Dr. BIAVA, 1964, p. 1099).

Fig. 216. *Bile droplet in the cytoplasm* (viral hepatitis) delineated by a membrane and containing very closely layered smooth membranes (interpreted as focal cytoplasmic degradation). In the vicinity there is glycogen. → part of a mitochondrion. 50,000 × (Dr. BIAVA, 1964, p. 1099).

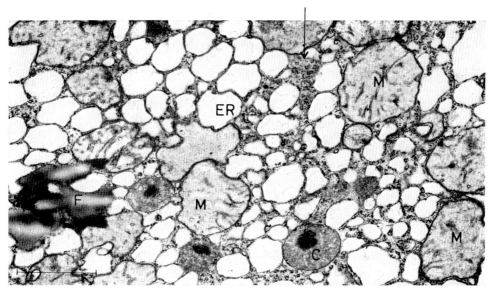

Fig. 217. *Hydropic degeneration* of a liver cell after partial hepatectomy (rat, after 24 hours). The rough endoplasmic reticulum is very much dilated (ER) with many loose ribosomes (→). The mitochondria (M) are swollen (matrix type). In addition, there are cytosomes (C) and fat droplets (F). 22,000× (Dr. BAN-NASCH).

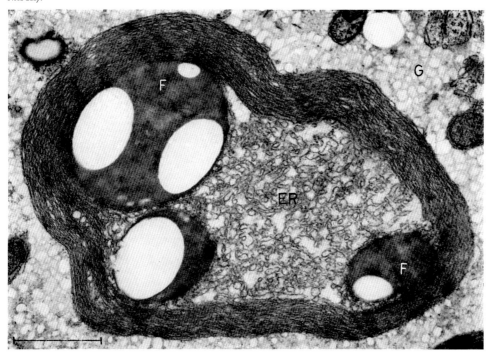

Fig. 218. Concentrically layered membrane complexes of the smooth endoplasmic reticulum (fingerprints, myelin figures) with enclosed fat droplets (F) and a network of smooth endoplasmic reticulum (ER). Plentiful glycogen (G) is in the vicinity (here appearing light, since it is not stained with lead). Same experiment as in Figure 214. 24,000× (Dr. BANNASCH).

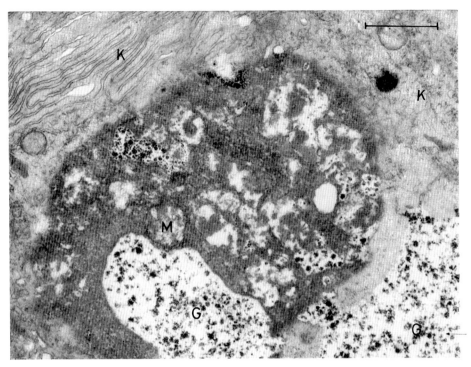

Fig. 219. *Hyalin (acidophil) body*, also called *Councilman body*, in viral hepatitis (compare with Fig. 198). A necrotic, rounded and shrunken liver cell with dense endoplasmic reticulum (M = remnants of mitochondria, G = glycogen, partly in the cells, partly in the sinus →) is surrounded by a Kupffer cell (K) (above, smooth endoplasmic reticulum of the Kupffer cell). 20,000 × (BIAVA et al., 1965).

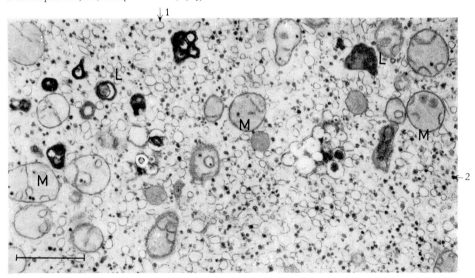

Fig. 220. *Liver cell in viral hepatitis*. The endoplasmic reticulum is vacuolated and lacks ribosomes (→ 1 and L = lyso-somes, which contain membrane components, perhaps also bile pigment). In addition, there are mitochondria (M) with serpentine cristae (more frequently found in cholestasis). → 2 glycogen, diffusely distributed. 12,000 × (SCHAFF-NER, POPPER, 1966).

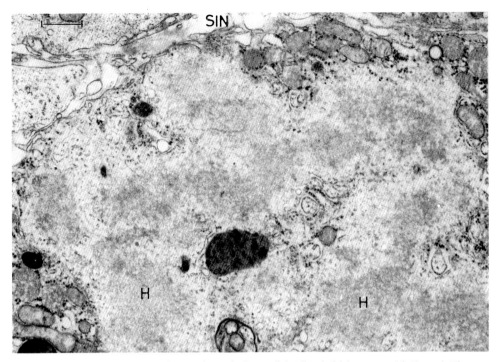

Fig. 221. *Alcoholic hyalin* (human) in the cytoplasm of a liver cell *(Mallory body)* (compare with Fig. 223). There are confluent finely filamentous and granular masses (H = hyalin, compare with Fig. 222), which are not limited by a membrane. According to BIAVA, 1964 (p. 301), the granular masses represent fragmented rough endoplasmic reticulum and ribosomes. In the vicinity of the hyalin, there are light-appearing cytoplasmic portions (empty-appearing portions under the light microscope. Fig. 223) and at the periphery plentiful free ribosomes. SIN = Sinus. 10,000 × (BIAVA, 1964, p. 301).

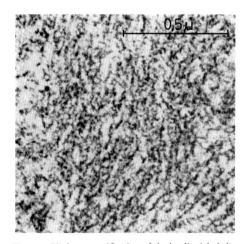

Fig. 222. Higher magnification of the hyalin *(alcoholic hyalin, Mallory bodies)*. There are parallel-stacked fragmented portions of endoplasmic reticulum and some granular material. Ribosome-like bodies may be seen. 60,000 × (BIAVA, 1964, p. 301).

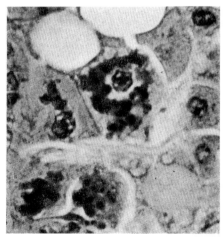

Fig. 223. Mallory bodies in liver cells. They appear as dark red, irregularly shaped cytoplasmic condensations that are in part branching and in part droplet forms. Modified Azan stain, 700 ×.

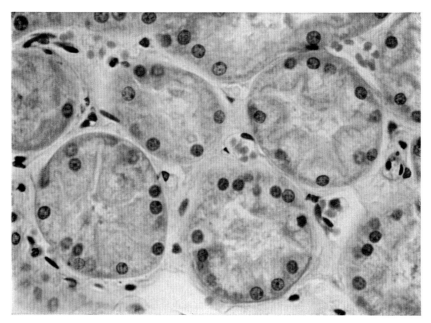

Fig. 224. Cloudy swelling of proximal tubules of the kidney; H & E, 600 ×.

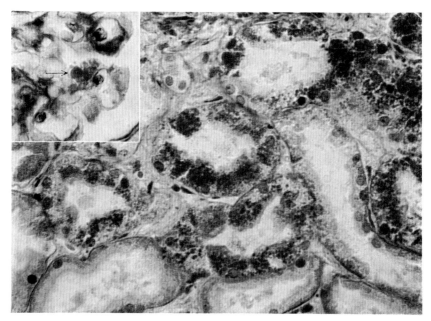

Fig. 225. Hyalin droplet degeneration; Azan stain, 456×. Inset: Hyalin degeneration in the investing epithelium of a glomerulus (rat); experimental glomerulonephritis; PAS, ca. 500×.

Kidney

Histologic examination of kidney sections should proceed according to the following guide lines. Evaluation of the *thickness of cortex and medulla* in the specimen. *Alterations of vessels:* especially at the corticomedullary junction and in the afferent arterioles. *Glomeruli:* cellularity, the condition of the basement membrane, capsular lining epithelium, focal or diffuse necrosis of the glomerulus. *Tubules:* size of lumen, size of cells, cytoplasmic deposits, segments affected. *Interstitium:* cellular and fibrous content.

Cloudy swelling (Fig. 224). *This is a disturbance of the ionic milieu of the cell that entails retention of water and sodium with concomitant loss of potassium from the cells, which then begin to swell.* The swelling affects mitochondria particularly (see p. 146f.). The resulting increase in the size of particulate matter leads to increased dispersion of light and, thereby, to a Tyndall effect, i. e., to cloudiness. Figure 224 shows proximal tubular epithelium, the cytoplasm of which is filled with fine, pale droplets (swollen mitochondria), giving rise to a finely granular appearance. Fine, granular, coagulated protein material is also seen in the narrowed lumens of the tubules. The same changes occur also in postmortem specimens and are differentiated only with difficulty from antemortem cloudy swelling. If the tissue sections are treated with dilute acetic acid, the contents of the mitochondria precipitate on the mitochondrial membrane, and the cytoplasm again becomes clear.

Macroscopic: Enlarged, soft organ with dull cut surfaces. The parenchyma bulges above the cut surface. Cloudy swelling occurs, especially with toxic injury (e. g., diphtheria).

In *hydropic degeneration* (Fig. 231), the process is identical – free water accumulates in the cell and forms vacuoles (mitochondria, endoplasmic reticulum and ground substance). Microscopically, the cytoplasm is filled with large and small optically empty vacuoles. In some instances, perinuclear halos also appear (similar to Fig. 228). Hydropic degeneration is seen particularly in cases of acute anoxia, toxic inhibition of glycolysis (e. g., cyanide poisoning), substrate depletion or inhibition of oxidative phosphorylation (e. g., barbiturate poisoning, see p. 146).

Hyalin droplet degeneration (Fig. 225 and p. 148). *Proteinaceous droplets appear in the cytoplasm of the proximal tubular epithelium due to tubular reabsorption, e. g., in glomerulonephritis.* Histologically, medium magnification reveals swelling of the proximal tubular cells due to infiltration of deep red-staining and somewhat refractile protein droplets. The lumen contains hyalin casts or granular precipitates of protein. At this stage, single epithelial cells, filled with proteinaceous droplets, are also found in the lumen.

In rare cases, hyalin droplet degeneration also involves the epithelial cells of glomerular loops, which are, of course, related morphologically to the tubular epithelium. The inset in Figure 225 shows experimental glomerulonephritis in a rat in which there is marked thickening of the basement membrane and proliferation of epithelial and endothelial cells. The arrow points to an epithelial cell with round, hyalin droplets in the cytoplasm (see also Fig. 252b).

Macroscopic: Enlarged, pale grayish white kidneys (large, white kidney), e. g., in amyloidosis or myeloma (myeloma nephrosis).

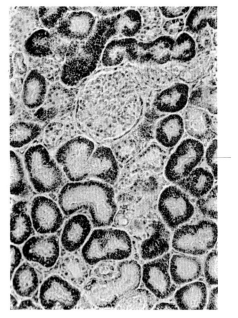

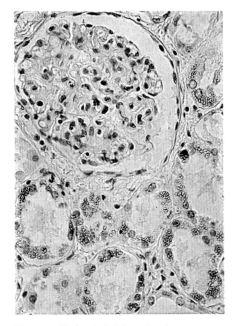

Fig. 226. Fatty degeneration of the proximal tubules of the cortex. Sudan-hematoxylin stain; 160×.

Fig. 227. Cholemic (bile) nephrosis. Hematoxylin; 459×.

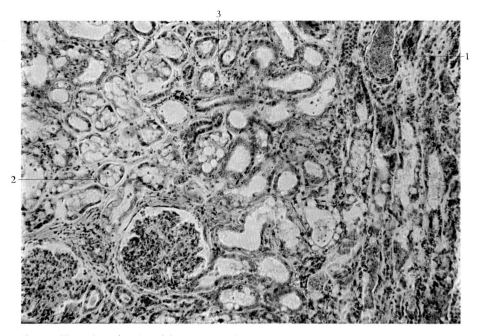

Fig. 228. Hypoxic nephrosis with hypopotassemia; H & E, 111×.

Nephrosis

By the term nephrosis is meant noninflammatory renal disease characterized morphologically by degenerative tubular changes.

Fatty degeneration of proximal tubules of the cortex (Fig. 226). *Deposition of neutral fats and lipids in the tubular epithelial cells can result either from reabsorption by the tubular cells (e. g., lipoid nephrosis associated with diabetes), from hypoxia or from toxic injury.* The figure shows fatty changes resulting from the hypoxia of anemia. Scanning the section at low magnification reveals accumulation of the Sudan stain in the cortex. The medullary border is sharply delineated, and with medium high magnification (Fig. 226) the loops of Henle are seen to be mostly spared. Fine lipid droplets are deposited in the epithelial cells of the proximal convoluted tubules of the cortex. The lipid droplets either lie in the basal portion of the cell or completely fill it. The cells are swollen. The tubular lumen is narrowed. The portions of the distal tubules next to the glomeruli (→) are not involved.

Lipoid nephrosis, when it occurs as an independent disease, is also characterized by marked fatty changes of the tubular system with deposition of neutral fats and lipids (doubly refractile). In addition, fatty deposits are found in the interstitium. There is evidence, furthermore, of injury to the basement membrane of the glomeruli, as shown by splitting, swelling and thickening. Most authors now consider the condition as membranous glomerulonephritis (see p. 159) rather than glomerulonephrosis.

Macroscopic: The kidney is slightly enlarged and the cortex is yellow.

Bile or cholemic nephrosis (Fig. 227) *signifies degenerative changes and deposition of bile pigments in the proximal tubular epithelial cells during the course of jaundice (reabsorption, see p. 148).* Hematoxylin stain brings out very well the yellow-to-green color of the bile pigment. Medium magnification reveals granular deposits of bile pigment in the cytoplasm of the proximal tubular epithelium. In addition, there are degenerative changes such as cloudy swelling and slight fatty changes. Occasional shed cells can also be found in the lumens of the tubules. Bile-stained hyalin casts are present in the collecting ducts. For the most part, the glomeruli are not affected. In Figure 227, however, there is slight edematous swelling of the basement membrane.

Macroscopic: Slightly enlarged kidney, green-to-yellowish brown cortex and medulla.

Hypoxic nephrosis with hypokalemia (Fig. 228). *(Synonyms: hemoglobinuric nephrosis, myoglobinuric nephrosis, crush kidney, shock kidney, lower nephron nephrosis.)*
This is an acute process that may be caused by various injurious agents (trauma, poisons) and is characterized by the onset of severe shock, hemolysis or myolysis and degeneration and necrosis of renal tubules. The term vascular-tubular syndrome describes the two essential components: vascular collapse (disturbance of perfusion) and toxic tubular degeneration. Microscopically, the most striking finding is the presence of proteinaceous casts containing hemoglobin or myoglobin (brown casts in the collecting ducts, → 1) in the distal tubules, Henle's loops and collecting ducts. Proximal convoluted tubules may show focal necrosis. In addition, degenerative changes of the tubular epithelium may be seen (cloudy swelling, fatty degeneration). There is an accompanying hypokalemia (polyuric phase of the shock kidney) causing cystic dilatation of the base of the tubular epithelial cells (proximal), which microscopically gives the impression of vacuolar degeneration (→ 2). Later, tubular rhexis develops (rupture of kidney tubules). The epithelium of the proximal tubules in Figure 228 is for the most part, flattened (a sign of insufficiency). The interstitial tissues are swollen by edema (→ 3). The glomeruli are hyperemic and have wide basement membranes.

Macroscopic: Enlarged kidneys; dirty grayish brown color.

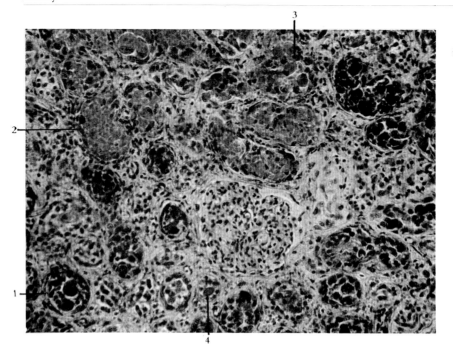

Fig. 229. Mercuric bichloride nephrosis; H & E, 200 ×.

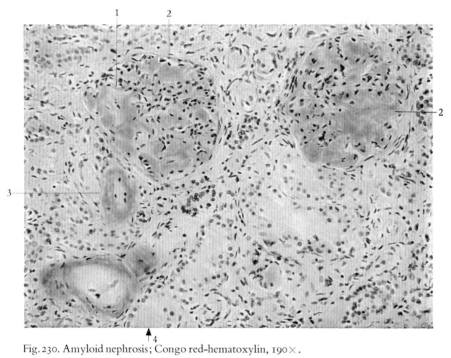

Fig. 230. Amyloid nephrosis; Congo red–hematoxylin, 190×.

Mercuric bichloride nephrosis (Fig. 229). *Corrosive mercuric bichloride produces a marked, necrotizing nephrosis, with secondary calcification of necrotic tubular cells.* It involves particularly the proximal convoluted tubules. There is considerable controversy concerning the pathogenesis and site of action of the mercury, but, if death occurs during the acute phase, necrosis of the proximal convoluted tubules is seen. Within a few days, deposits of calcium can be found in the necrotic areas (see Fig. 234, matrix aggregates). Regeneration of tubules follows survival of the acute phase, as evidenced by the marked proliferation of flat epithelial cells which may be the predominant feature of the microscopic picture.

Microscopic examination of the cortex in the acute and subacute stages reveals necrotic red-staining tubules and dark blue-staining deposits of calcium. Medium magnification (Fig. 229) shows irregular blue calcium deposits of varying size as well as calcified epithelial cells that have been partly shed into the lumen ($\rightarrow$ 1), with the result that cross sections of the tubule may appear completely filled. In other areas, tubules are filled with granular, eosinophilic masses ($\rightarrow$ 2). Here, the epithelium is necrotic and, together with the shed epithelial cells ($\rightarrow$ 3) and protein casts, forms a homogeneous concrement. Other segments of the tubules also contain casts (distal tubule, $\rightarrow$ 4). The interstitium is edematous. The glomeruli are avascular, normally cellular and have delicate basement membranes (see also Figs. 231–234).

Macroscopic: Enlarged, soft kidney with dull red or grayish white external and cut surfaces.

Amyloid nephrosis (Fig. 230). *This is due to secondary amyloidosis (spleen, liver, adrenal and intestine, etc., are also involved) and is manifested by deposition of abnormal protein, amyloid, in the glomeruli and afferent arterioles.*

Examination of an H & E section with a scanning lens reveals large, homogeneous, eosinophilic, hyalinized cortical glomeruli. Medium magnification shows arterioles with homogeneous, hyalinized walls. The hyalinized protein material stains readily with Congo red or methyl violet (amyloid stains red, surrounding tissue pale blue): the red stain is specific for amyloid. The amyloid accumulation appears first as a fine red streak lying between the basement membrane and the endothelium of the glomeruli ($\rightarrow$ 1, see also Fig. 253). With increasing deposition, the glomerular loop thickens and the lumen is narrowed. As a result, the loops take on a homogeneous, anuclear appearance. Adjacent affected glomeruli may merge to produce a uniformly red area ($\rightarrow$ 2). The and stage is an obliterated glomerulus. The same process occurs in the media of the arcuate arteries and afferent arterioles ($\rightarrow$ 3). The muscle cells deteriorate, and the media appears as a smooth red ring. Secondarily, amyloid is deposited in the pericapillary interstitial tissues and the tubular basement membranes. Many of the proximal convoluted tubules are dilated and contain casts which are Congo red negative ($\rightarrow$ 4). Hyalin droplet degeneration occurs frequently (compare with Fig. 225). The amyloid kidney often becomes contracted due to the glomerular involvement and the subsequent atrophy of the tubular system and the proliferation of interstitial connective tissue. This is particularly common in association with amyloidosis of the splenic pulp (lardaceous spleen, Fig. 266).

Macroscopic: The kidney is large, firm, white and waxy. The cut surface is dry and translucent; the medulla is usually reddish and the line of demarcation from the swollen cortex is preserved. The contracted amyloid kidney is small and gnarled, but usually smooth.

The nephrosis described on pages 142–145 can thus have different origins and different causes: 1) renal, as in primary injury of the glomeruli, 2) extra-renal, as in patients with abnormalities of their plasma proteins or circulatory upsets as in hypoxic nephrosis and 3) direct toxic injury of the tubular cells, for example, in chemical nephrosis.

Oxygen lack (e. g., renal infarct, shock kidney) or *acute toxic injury* (e. g., mercuric bichloride nephrosis), both lead to uptake of water by the cells (see p. 7) which manifests itself electron microscopically by edema of the ground substance (either as a diffuse decrease in density or as vacuolation), marked swelling of mitochondria (cloudy swelling) and vacuolar mitochondrial transformation. Eventually, cytolysis may develop (TOTOVIC, 1966).

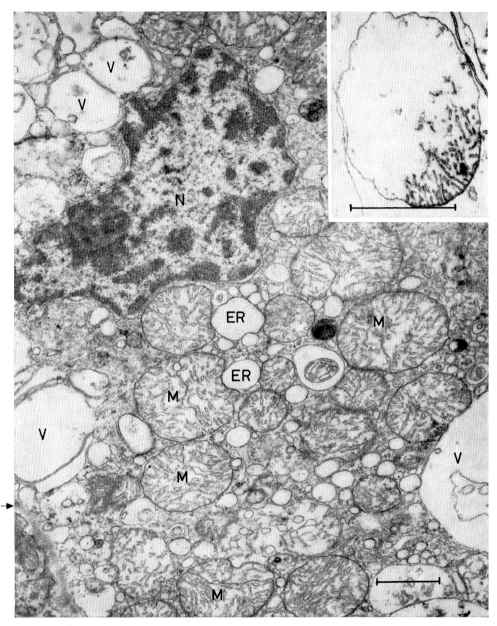

Figure 231 shows a section of a proximal tubular cell (experimental renal infarct, rat, 28 hours after ligation of the renal artery). The mitochondria (M) are swollen (matrix type). The endoplasmic reticulum (ER) is widened by vacuoles (especially marked at V = vacuolar degeneration). → = basement membrane. N = nucleus showing marginal hyperchromasia (beginning pyknosis). Inset at upper right: marked vacuolar transformation of a mitochondrion. 17,000 ×, inset 28,000 × (TOTOVIC, 1966).

Fine Structure of Tubular Degeneration

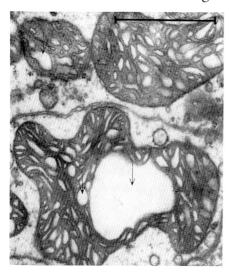

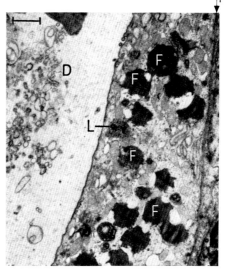

Fig. 232. *Mitochondrial swelling of cristae type* in an experimental renal infarct. The cleavage spaces of the cristae are greatly widened (→), the matrix is dense. The ground substance is loosened by edema. 27,000 × (Dr. TOTOVIC).

Fig. 233. Fatty degeneration (metamorphosis) of a collecting duct. F = osmiophilic fat droplet. L = lysosome with splintered membranes, → 1 is the basement membrane, D = cellular detritus in the lumen. 8,500 × (Dr. TOTOVIC).

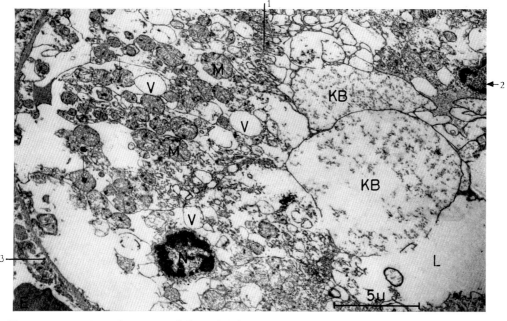

Fig. 234. Decomposition of a necrotic tubular epithelial cell (cytolysis in an experimentally produced renal infarct, 8 hours). L = lumen of a proximal tubule, KB = so-called apical vesicle, from the fusion of which marked swelling of the apical cytoplasm develops, → 1 remnants of the brush border of an adjacent cell, N and → 2 = pyknotic nuclei, V = vacuole in the ground substance, M = mitochondria with matrix aggregates (→ in the picture), → 3 = basement membrane from which the necrotic cell has already become detached, E = erythrocyte. 45,000 × (Dr. TOTOVIC).

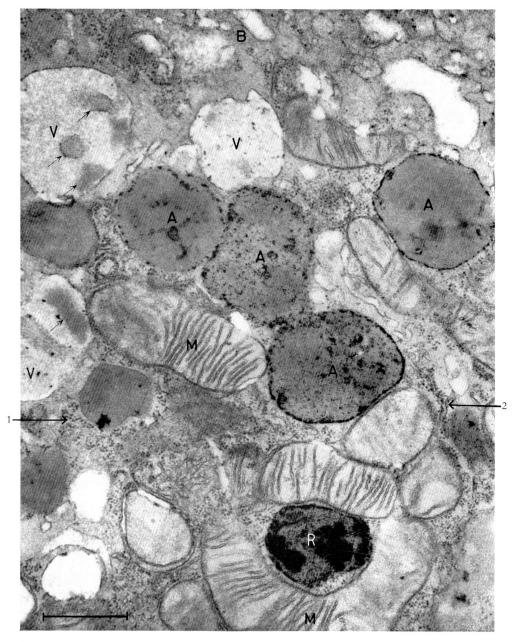

Fig. 235. Reabsorption of hemoglobin. Section from the apical region of a cell (B = under portion of the brush border) of the proximal tubule of the kidney (mouse, 1 hour after intraperitoneal injection of ox hemoglobin). All stages of the uptake and concentration of the hemoglobin can be followed in this picture from the top to the bottom. The vacuoles (V) contain in addition to granular protein, hemoglobin droplets (→ 1). In the absorption droplets (A) the hemoglobin is concentrated into bodies limited by a single membrane. The black particles are precipitates of lead phosphate (= histochemical evidence of an acid phosphate [Gomori's method, see Pearse, 1960]). These organelles can be thus identified as lysosomes. R = body with strong acid phosphatase activity and marked concentration of hemoglobin, M = mitochondria, → 1 ribosomes and polysomes, → 2 rough endoplasmic reticulum, 24,000 × Miller et al., 1964).

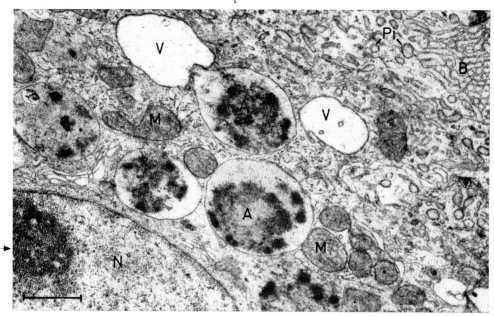

Fig. 236. Protein reabsorption droplets in the proximal tubule in protein nephrosis in man. Part of a tubular epithelial cell with a section of the brush border (B). There are pinocytotic vesicles (Pi) in the ground substance. These represent reabsorption vacuoles (V) of the protein. The protein reabsorption droplets (A) develop from these. M = mitochondria, N = nucleus, → nucleolus. 16,000 × (THOENES, 1965).

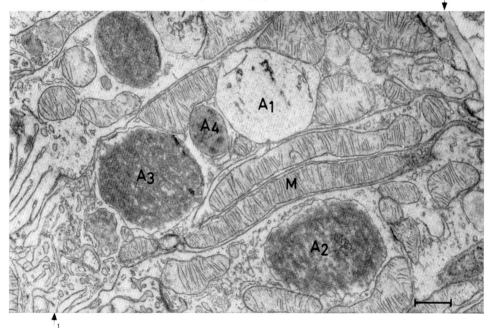

Fig. 237. Protein reabsorption droplets (protein storage cytosomes) in the proximal renal tubular epithelium in lead poisoning of the rat (5 weeks after intraperitoneal administration of a single dose of 50 mg. lead acetate). Large bodies bounded by a single membrane and with a fine granularity (A 1) as well as contents of increased electron density (A 2 – A 4), M = mitochondria, numerous pinocytotic vacuoles at the base of the brush border (→ 1), → 2 = peritubular basement membrane. 10,500 × (Dr. TOTOVIC).

149

Vascular Disorders of the Kidney

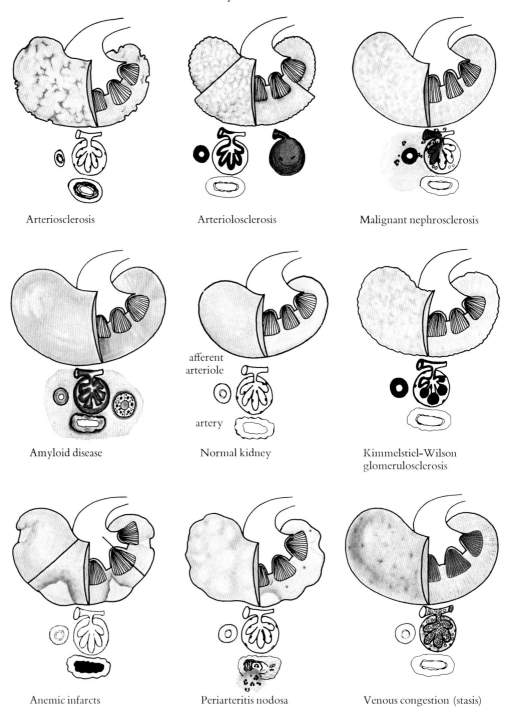

Arteriosclerosis

Arteriolosclerosis

Malignant nephrosclerosis

Amyloid disease

afferent
arteriole

artery

Normal kidney

Kimmelstiel-Wilson
glomerulosclerosis

Anemic infarcts

Periarteritis nodosa

Venous congestion (stasis)

Fig. 238. Schematic representation of the gross and microscopic changes encountered in vascular disorders of the kidney.

Vascular Renal Disorders

Vascular diseases in the kidney (Fig. 238) involve either the main arteries or the arterioles. The glomeruli almost always become involved secondarily, and ultimately the tubules.

Arteriosclerosis (Fig. 239) may uncommonly involve the main *renal arteries* at the junction with the aorta, and the resulting obstruction lead to ischemia of the kidney and renal hypertension *(Goldblatt mechanism).* Involvement of arteries of the interlobular and arcuate type is manifested by concentric fibrosis and elastosis. The severity of the glomerular lesion (hyalin degeneration) depends upon the extent of the arterial sclerosis.

Macroscopic: The surface is red and shows isolated small scars.

Arteriolosclerosis or arteriolar nephrosclerosis (see Figs. 240, 241) usually shows hyalinization of *afferent arterioles* with narrowing of the lumens (compare Fig. 32). Decreased vascular perfusion leads to hyalinized thickening of the capillary loops, terminating in complete obliteration of the glomerulus. Marked involvement leads to contraction of the kidney: *red granular atrophy (primary contracted kidney).* Arteriosclerosis and arteriolosclerosis frequently occur together (arterio-arteriolonephrosclerosis).

Macroscopic: Fine granularity of the surface with small reddish scars, resulting eventually in marked shrinkage of the entire organ, notably the cortex (primary contracted kidney, red granular atrophy). When combined with arteriosclerosis, the scars are large and red.

Malignant nephrosclerosis (see Fig. 242) is interpreted as an unusually intense variant of arteriolar nephrosclerosis, which has either been superimposed on pre-existing arteriolar nephrosclerosis or has arisen de novo in unaffected vessels. Characteristically, the *afferent arterioles and glomerular capillary loops show fibrinoid necrosis.*

Macroscopic: The kidney is slightly enlarged, with a variegated, spotted surface; in many cases, it is combined with an arteriolar nephrosclerosis.

Amyloidosis (see Figs. 230, 253) cannot rightly be considered a vascular renal disorder, but it is considered here so as to allow comparison with the gross and histologic pictures of other renal disorders.

Kimmelstiel-Wilson glomerulosclerosis (Fig. 243) represents a special sort of arteriolar nephrosclerosis. It goes hand in hand with hyalinization of the afferent and efferent arterioles, as well as with diffuse hyalin thickening of the capillary loops, thereby giving rise to the characteristic hyalin nodules in the glomerular loops. The gross appearance usually resembles arteriolar nephrosclerosis.

An **anemic infarct** (Fig. 244) most commonly results from embolic occlusion of an artery. There is a wedge-shaped, sharply demarcated, pale yellow area of necrosis that becomes depressed, contracted and white with increasing scar formation.

The acute stage of **periarteritis nodosa** (Fig. 64) in the kidney shows a yellowish gray mottled pattern. Eventually, fine, speckled, contracted scars develop (older areas of necrosis). There is fibrinoid necrosis of the arteries, with glomerulitis and scarring.

The **congested kidney** is enlarged, dusty red, particularly in the medula, and the surface veins are spider-like. The glomeruli are congested and there are protein deposits in Bowman's space. In addition, there is interstitial edema.

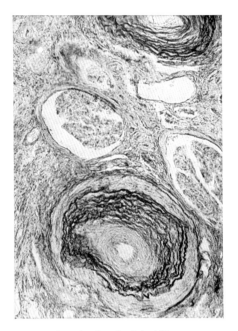

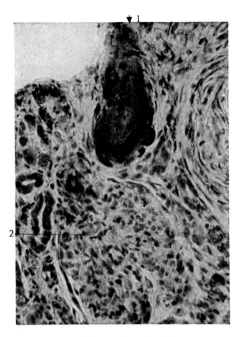

Fig. 239. Arteriosclerosis of the kidney; elastica-van Gieson stains, 70×.

Fig. 240. Arteriolar nephrosclerosis; Sudan-hematoxylin, 380×.

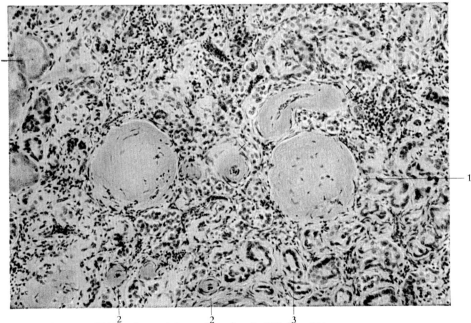

Fig. 241. Contracted kidney in arteriolar nephrosclerosis; H & E, 156×.

Arteriosclerosis of the kidney (Fig. 239). Histologically, this is actually the same process that we observed in arteriosclerosis in the heart vessels (compare with p. 60), although the lesion is not crescent-shaped, but rather has a concentric configuration. At first glance, one notices the very thick walls of the larger arteries, especially in the medulla. Medium magnification reveals hyperplastic proliferation of the elastica in the intima. This is due not only to multiplication and splitting of elastic fibers (black in the section) but also to an increase of acellular fibrous tissue (sclerosis), all of which lead to marked narrowing of the lumen. Glomeruli are partially hyalinized and the corresponding tubules have atrophied, with resulting fibrosis and lymphocytic infiltration. Local hyalinization of several glomeruli with concomitant atrophy of tubules leads to interstitial fibrosis and formation of contracted surface scars (arteriosclerotic scar). It is difficult for the beginner to differentiate arteriosclerotic scars and the associated lymphocytic infiltration from chronic pyelonephritis – but the striking arterial changes and comparatively scant lymphocytic infiltration should lead to a correct interpretation.

Arteriolosclerosis (Fig. 240, see also Fig. 32 and p. 56). In arteriolosclerosis (arteriolarsclerosis) hyalin appears between the intima and media with lumenal narrowing and medial atrophy. The changes are the same in the kidney as in the brain, cardiac muscle or spleen. Hematoxylin and eosin stains reveal red, homogeneous and anuclear arteriolar walls (see Fig. 241). The hyalinized vessels become very conspicuous when stained for fat. Inspection of the section with the scanning lens reveals several reddish dots in the cortex that can be identified, with higher magnification, as afferent arterioles ($\rightarrow$ 1), the wall of which is infiltrated by neutral fats. The media is markedly atrophic – isolated nuclei are still visible in the outermost parts of the media (see also Fig. 241, $\rightarrow$ 2). The lumen of the arteriole, barely discernible by means of a few preserved endothelial cell nuclei, is markedly narrowed. Note the deposits of fat in the glomerular connective tissue ($\rightarrow$ 2: mesangium). Tubules in the proximity of affected glomeruli have atrophied.

Contracted kidney in arteriolar nephrosclerosis (Fig. 241). If hyalinization of the afferent arterioles progresses so that a majority of the vessels are affected and if, in addition, there is concomitant sclerosis of medium-sized arteries, obliteration of large numbers of glomeruli and tubules will follow. Examination with a scanning lens discloses thinning of the cortex as well as numerous reddish discoid lesions that higher magnification shows to be glomeruli with eosinophilic concentric laminations containing a few isolated nuclei ($\rightarrow$ 1). The afferent arterioles surrounding these glomeruli have characteristic lesions in the wall ($\times$) – the intima is greatly thickened, the lining endothelial cells are barely discernible and the lumen is narrowed. The muscle fibers of the media are markedly atrophic or have disappeared. With hematoxylin and eosin stains, the appearance of the tissue resembles that found in amyloidosis. The Congo red stain, however, is negative, and van Gieson's stain brings out the red hyalinized glomeruli and arterioles (fresh hyalin is yellow, see Table 3, page 10). Figure 241 shows a longitudinally sectioned lesion in an afferent arteriole ($\times$ upper right); $\rightarrow$2 and $\times$ in the center point to arteriolar lesions cut in cross section. As a result of hyalinization of the glomeruli, there is atrophy of the dependent tubular system ($\rightarrow$3), shown by shrunken tubules with narrow lumens and atrophy of lining epithelium. Several tubules have been obliterated. There is compensatory proliferation of interstitial fibrous tissue and lymphocytic infiltration (scars). Areas of the cortex that contain intact glomeruli have undergone compensatory hypertrophy ($\rightarrow$ 4). Grossly, such areas can be seen as projecting nodules.

Clinical: Benign hypertension (essential hypertension), in which the arteriolosclerosis is considered by some authors, but not by others, to be the result rather than the cause of raised blood pressure.

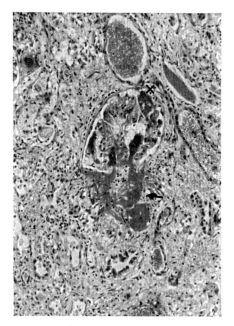

Fig. 242. Malignant nephrosclerosis:
H & E, 120×.

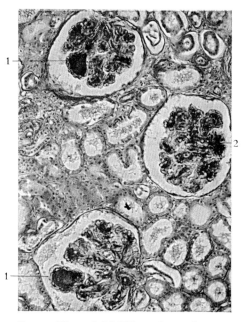

Fig. 243. Kimmelstiel–Wilson glomerulosclerosis; van Gieson, 125×.

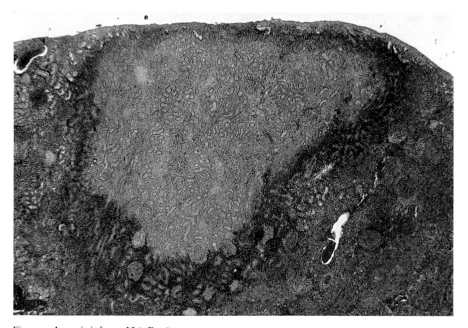

Fig. 244. Anemic infarct; H & E, 28×.

Malignant nephrosclerosis (Fig. 242) *consists of a rapidly progressive arteriolosclerosis with fibrinoid necrosis of the walls of afferent arterioles and glomerular loops.*
Histologically, the arterioles seem to undergo diffuse hyalinization, so that the walls appear homogeneous and the lumens are narrowed (→). The hyalin material stains very bright red with H & E. With van Gieson's stain, it is yellow (compare with Table 3, pages 10, 21, 23). There is nearly always an accompanying polymorphonuclear infiltration although it may be very slight. Frequently there are erythrocytes in the fibrinoid material indicative of rapid intrusion of blood into the vessel wall. The fibrinoid necrosis almost always involves adjacent glomerular loops (×), so that either single loops of the glomerulus or groups of them are affected. Should malignant nephrosclerosis be superimposed upon arterio- or arteriolonephrosclerosis, there will be a combination of sclerosis of medium-sized vessels and hyalinization of arterioles in addition to the foci of fibrinoid necrosis.

Macroscopic: Variegated, speckled kidney with indistinct gray-white foci on a reddish background. *Clinically*, when malignant hypertension develops in young people it follows a rapidly fatal course, leading to uremic or apoplectic death. Older patients (50–60) may manifest malignant hypertension as a sequel to a previously benign course, in which case the histology shows a combination of arteriolosclerosis and malignant nephrosclerosis.

Kimmelstiel-Wilson glomerulosclerosis (Fig. 243) *occurs as a complication in approximately 20% of cases of diabetes mellitus. Typically, there is hyalinization of the glomerular loops. Clinically, the patients have proteinuria, hypertension and sometimes slight renal failure.*
Histologically, there is a very characteristic lesion. Numerous glomeruli show hyalinization of single or several capillary loops, resulting in the formation of rounded ball-like structures (van Gieson red or yellowish red, → 1). The remaining glomerular loops are either free of any changes or else show the early stages of hyalinization. Some glomeruli also exhibit a diffuse thickening of the capillary wall (→ 2). The basement membranes are often frayed. In addition, the hyalinization frequently involves the afferent and *efferent arterioles*. Electronmicroscopically there is thickening of basement membranes, especially in the mesangium.

Macroscopic: Finely granular, slightly contracted kidney.

Anemic infarct (Fig. 244). *This is caused by embolic obstruction of a branch of the renal artery, resulting in a wedge-shaped area of coagulation necrosis* (see pp. 146, 147).
Examination of the section with a scanning lens reveals a pale red, wedge-shaped area, surrounded by a bluish, highly cellular zone outside of which there is a thin red rim. Observation of the central portion of the wedge-shaped area reveals the typical signs of *necrosis:* the nuclei are achromatic and the cytoplasm is homogeneous or finely granular. The nuclei in the interstitium and the glomeruli appear as shadows of their former shapes. On the whole, early infarcts will still show the faint outlines of tubules and glomeruli. Higher magnification reveals *polymorphonuclear leukocytes* in the *peripheral cellular zone* as well as all the phases of nuclear disruption: pyknosis, rhexis, lysis and finely scattered nuclear debris. Surrounding the cellular zone there is usually a *zone of reactive hyperemia:* however, this is not conspicuous in our section. Note the thin, subcapsular strip of preserved parenchyma which receives its blood supply from the capsular vessels.

Macroscopic: Yellow, dry, firm area. Older foci are contracted (reabsorption by granulation tissue), the final result being a deeply contracted, white scar. The emboli most frequently come either from a verrucous endocarditis, a mural thrombus in the heart (e. g., myocardial infarct) or from the aorta.

Inflammations of the Kidney

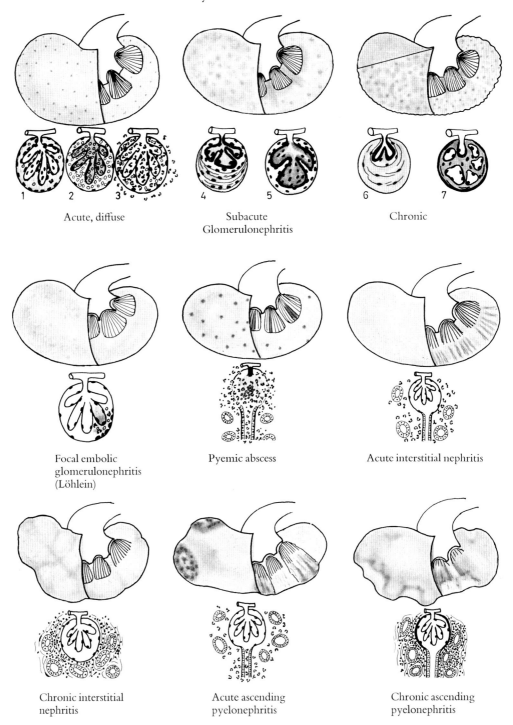

Acute, diffuse

Subacute
Glomerulonephritis

Chronic

Focal embolic
glomerulonephritis
(Löhlein)

Pyemic abscess

Acute interstitial nephritis

Chronic interstitial
nephritis

Acute ascending
pyelonephritis

Chronic ascending
pyelonephritis

Fig. 245. Diagrammatic survey of the gross and histological characteristics of inflammatory renal diseases.

Inflammations of the Kidney

In the kidney, inflammation occurs either in the **glomeruli** (focal, diffuse) or in the interstitial tissues (Fig. 245).

In the **acute stage,** three *different forms of* **diffuse glomerulonephritis** can be distinguished: 1) *membrano-proliferative* (or simply *membranous,* Fig. 252c or *proliferative,* Fig. 254); 2) *hemorrhagic-necrotizing;* and 3) *exudative glomerulonephritis* (see Fig. 246).

In **subacute** and **subchronic glomerulonephritis** there is an *extracapillary* (No. 4 in Fig. 245) as well as an *intracapillary form* (No. 5 in Fig. 245). The *extracapillary form of glomerulonephritis* (clinically, there is usually hypertension, Type I nephritis of ELLIS) is characterized by crescent-shaped proliferation of the parietal capsular epithelium (see Fig. 247), whereas the *intracapillary* variety only affects the glomerular loops, causing proliferation of the endothelial cells (see Fig. 248). Clinically, a nephrotic syndrome develops frequently (Type II nephritis of ELLIS).

The extra- and intracapillary varieties can sometimes be recognized as the starting point of the **chronic stage** of glomerulonephritis *(secondarily contracted kidneys,* see Fig. 249). The capillary loops, although hyalinized and thickened, are still discernible in chronic intracapillary glomerulonephritis (No. 7 in Fig. 245), whereas hyalinized crescents can still be distinguished in the extracapillary variety (No. 6 in Fig. 245).

Macroscopic: Acute: Large, edematous kidneys with petechiae. *Subchronic:* Either large white or variegated yellowish red, mottled kidneys. *Chronic:* Small, smooth, grayish white (intracapillary) or granular, mottled kidneys (extracapillary glomerulonephritis).

Table 6. Comparison of the morphological and clinical features of the different sorts of glomerulonephritis (modified from ROTTER, 1965).

	Clinical	Morphology
Ellis Type I	Preponderant hypertension High antistreptolysin titer (streptococcal infection) Acute onset, postinfectious 82% of cases heal	Acute exudative glomerulonephritis Progression to subacute or subchronic extra- capillary glomerulonephritis Acute proliferative glomerulonephritis (rarely pro- gression to intracapillary glomerulonephritis)
Ellis Type II	Preponderant nephrotic course Is not post-infectious Low antistreptolysin titer Insidious onset (primarily chronic) only 5% of cases heal	Acute membranous glomerulonephritis Progression to chronic membranous glomerulo- nephritis (= lipid nephrosis) Subacute or subchronic intracapillary glomerulo- nephritis Mixed type: membranous and proliferative with the appearance of intracapillary glomerulonephritis

Focal glomerulonephritis (see Fig. 250) shows patchy fibrinoid necrosis of single glomeruli or groups of glomeruli.

Macroscopic: Slightly enlarged kidney with discrete petechiae.

Pyemic abscesses (see Fig. 251) are due to infected emboli which have impacted in the glomeruli.

Macroscopic: Diffusely scattered yellow foci surrounded by a zone of hyperemia.

If the bacteria have gained access to the medullary parenchyma, there are numerous yellow, linear streaks which microscopically resemble elongated abscesses with bacterial colonies.

Acute interstitial nephritis may be either *suppurative or nonsuppurative* (see Fig. 256). The interstitial tissues are distended by exudate (e. g., in burns), or show streak-like infiltration of lymphocytes and histiocytes.

Macroscopic: Enlarged, yellowish gray kidney.

Chronic interstitial nephritis (Fig. 257) is characterized by the infiltration of lymphocytes, histiocytes and plasma cells. There is accompanying proliferation of connective tissue.

Macroscopic: Grayish red, gnarled, contracted kidneys.

Ascending pyelonephritis, acute or chronic (Fig. 255), results in damage to one or more kidney segments. The inflammation spreads upward from the tips of the pyramids. In the acute stage, there are widely scattered focal abscess formation and yellow streaks of exudate in the parenchyma. The necrotic areas are replaced by contracted grayish white scars in the chronic stage.

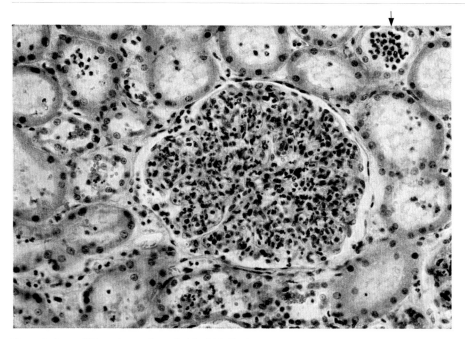

Fig. 246. Acute diffuse glomerulonephritis; H & E, 281 × .

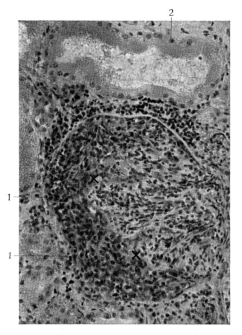

Fig. 247. Subacute extracapillary glomerulonephritis;
H & E, 169× .

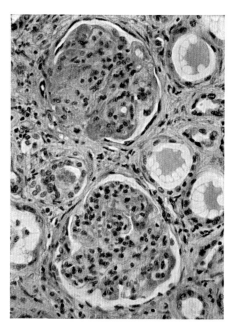

Fig. 248. Subacute, intracapillary glomerulonephritis;
H & E, 269× .

Glomerulonephritis

Glomerulonephritis is a diffuse inflammatory condition of the glomeruli that develops when the body becomes sensitized by an antigen-antibody reaction (following scarlet fever, for example). The chronic progressive inflammation seen in chronic glomerulonephritis is thought to be explained by the development of autoimmunity.

Acute diffuse glomerulonephritis. The acute stage of glomerulonephritis may show any of three or four principal forms (see Fig. 245 and Table 6).

1. **Acute exudative glomerulonephritis** (follows an infection, raised antistreptolysin titer, acute onset, good prognosis, progression to subacute extracapillary glomerulonephritis. Ellis Type I). This is an acute inflammatory reaction of the glomerular tufts with obstruction by engorgement with leukocytes and proliferated endothelial and epithelial cells.

Figure 246 shows the **acute stage of exudative glomerulonephritis.** Only the magnification provided by a scanning lens is needed to see the enlarged, highly cellular glomeruli. Bowman's space is completely filled by the glomerular tuft. The capillary loops are dilated and filled with neutrophils. In addition, the endothelial cells and, to a slighter degree, the epithelial cells are larger and more numerous. The basement membrane is swollen. Erythrocytes, protein and polymorphonuclear leukocytes are present in both the capsular spaces and the tubules (→). The interstitium is edematous and swollen and contains a few isolated leukocytes. The tubular epithelial cells are enlarged and often show cloudy swelling.

Macroscopic: The kidneys are swollen and the cut surfaces bulge beyond the edges of the tense capsule. Petechiae may be present on the surface.

2. **Acute hemorrhagic and subsequently necrotizing glomerulonephritis** is characterized by marked circulatory disturbances in the glomeruli, leading to hyperemia of the tufts, stasis, formation of fibrinous thrombi and hemorrhage into the capsular space. The lesion is probably a variant of acute exudative glomerulonephritis with a poor prognosis.

3. **Acute proliferative glomerulonephritis** (clinically similar to acute exudative glomerulonephritis; see 1. above and Table 6). Only rarely progresses to intracapillary glomerulonephritis. In addition to distinct thickening of the basement membrane (see Fig. 254), there is marked proliferation of endothelial cells and the cells of the mesangium.

4. **Acute membranous glomerulonephritis** (does not follow an infection, primarily chronic, poor prognosis, low antistreptolysin titer. Ellis Type II nephritis). The prominent changes are swelling and thickening of the basement membrane of the glomerular tufts, resulting in increased permeability for plasma proteins. The epithelial cells of the glomeruli are swollen (see Fig. 252c). In mixed membranous and proliferative forms, transitions occur to intracapillary glomerulonephritis or to lipid nephrosis.

Subacute extracapillary glomerulonephritis (Fig. 247). Although hypercellularity of the glomeruli is a conspicuous feature, the outstanding change is marked proliferation and increase in size of the parietal epithelial cells of Bowman's capsule, resulting in the formation of *crescent-shaped adhesions* composed of large, elongated cells having oval nuclei (→ 1 and × × show the extent of the crescent). The capillary loops are compressed by the rapid cellular overgrowth. The loops themselves show dense proliferation of the epithelium. The basement membranes are already thickened. The crescents show beginning collagen deposition and the glomeruli early hyalinization. Serous exudate and slight leukocytic emigration have caused swelling of the interstitium. The proximal tubules show hyalin degeneration (→ 2) and often fatty degeneration. This type of glomerulonephritis can be reproduced experimentally in rabbits (Masugi-nephritis).

Macroscopic: The kidneys are large and show red and yellow mottling.

Subacute intracapillary glomerulonephritis (Fig. 248). The most prominent changes are seen in the basement membrane. Cellular proliferation is not conspicuous. High magnification reveals marked thickening of the basement membrane, so much so that the capillary lumens can hardly be recognized. There is, in addition, proliferation of enlarged endothelial cells and increase in interstitial connective tissue.

Macroscopic: Enlarged, grayish white kidney.

159

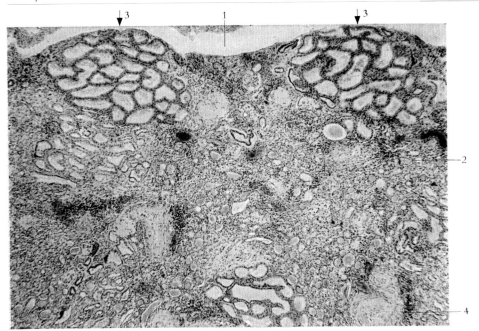

Fig. 249. Chronic glomerulonephritis; H & E, 41 ×.

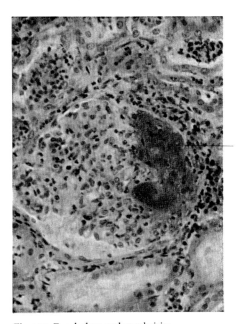

Fig. 250. Focal glomerulonephritis;
H & E, 280 ×.

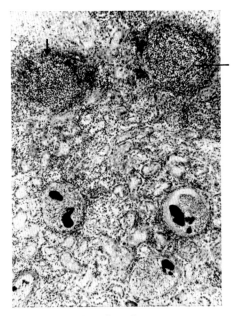

Fig. 251. Embolic kidney abscess;
H & E, 72 ×.

Chronic glomerulonephritis (Fig. 249). Survey of the preparation with a scanning lens reveals noticeable thinning of the cortex. Some areas show scarring of the surface and accumulations of inflammatory cells, while other areas show small cystic spaces and cellular paucity. Under medium magnification, most of the glomeruli are seen to have been replaced by hyalinized nodules. Frequently, the crescent-shaped lesions of extracapillary glomerulonephritis are still preserved. The attached tubules are markedly atrophic (→ 1), lined with flattened epithelium and filled with hyalin casts (→ 2). The interstitial tissue is correspondingly increased in amount and infiltrated by lymphocytes. In addition to areas of scarring (resulting in irregularity of the surface, → 1), there are also areas of compensatory hypertrophy (→ 3), with fully preserved glomeruli and dilated tubules lined with cuboidal epithelium. Aside from the completely hyalinized glomeruli, there are also some in which the inflammatory changes are recent. The vessels often shown arterio- and arteriolosclerosis (→ 4). In the end stages, it is difficult to differentiate between intra- and extracapillary glomerulonephritis. Kidneys contracted by arterio- or arteriolonephrosclerosis may also be difficult to differentiate.

Macroscopic: Small, firm kidneys with yellow or gray granular surfaces. Sometimes, the surface may be smooth, especially in cases of chronic intracapillary glomerulonephritis.

In **focal embolic glomerulonephritis** (Fig. 250), *there is inflammation of isolated loops of single glomeruli. It is seen particularly in cases of subacute bacterial endocarditis.* In the acute stages, there is fibrinoid necrosis of isolated capillary loops. They appear as homogeneous, anuclear, eosinophilic masses (→). Erythrocytes can often be seen in the fibrinoid material. This material involves the wall of the glomerular loops and also actually lies in the loops (fibrin thrombi). The unaffected loops are intact, showing, at most, slightly increased cellularity and thickening of the basement membrane. Bowman's space and the tubules contain granular casts, possibly containing erythrocytes and polymorphs. Healing of the lesions leads to focal scar formation and fusion of the loops with the parietal epithelium.

Macroscopic: The kidneys are slightly enlarged and present a flea-bitten appearance.

Embolic renal abscesses (Fig. 251). *Hematogenous spread in septicemia or pyemia leads to the formation of abscesses in the cortex and focal, streak-like suppuration in the medulla.* The scanning lens reveals scattered, highly cellular lesions in the cortex. Medium high power reveals near individual glomeruli, focal agglomerations of polymorphs invaded by wisps of connective tissue (→: abscesses). In other parts, there are clusters of bacteria in the capillary loops, and the surrounding parenchyma is infiltrated by leukocytes and invaded by connective tissue. The interstitial connective tissue also contains leukocytes. The proximal tubules contain granular casts.

The *foci of suppuration in the medulla* result from passage of bacteria through the glomeruli and their accumulation in the medulla, where they form streak-like abscesses containing central bacterial colonies (blue), frequently surrounded by an area of necrosis and a peripheral zone of leukocytes.

Macroscopic: Large yellow or gray abscesses are scattered throughout the cortex, on the surface of the kidney and as streaks along the medullary rays.

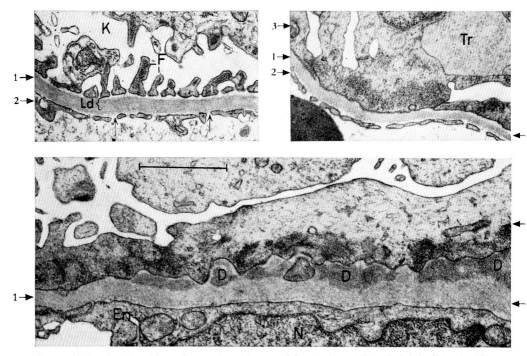

Fig. 252. a) *Normal rat glomerulus.* → basement membrane with lamina densa (Ld), endothelial cell (→ 2) with pores (→), foot processes (F) of the epithelial cells (podocytes) and capsular space (K). 22,000 × (Dr. THOENES). b) *Amino-nucleoside nephrosis* in the rat to illustrate the glomerular changes in glomerulonephrosis. Unaltered basement membrane (→ 1) and endothelial cell projection (→ 2), swollen epithelium (→ 3) with marked thickening of the foot processes, Tr. = droplets of absorbed protein in the epithelium (see also the inset in Fig. 225). 22,000 × (Dr. THOENES). c) Human *membranous glomerulonephritis* (clinically a case of pure nephrosis) with marked dense deposits (D) (see Fig. 254) on the epithelial side (→ 2 epithelial cell) of the thickened basement membrane (→ 1). Below is a section of an endothelial cell (En) with nucleus (N). The endothelial cells in this particular specimen have remained unchanged for a long time, while the epithelial cells (→ 2), because of the transformation of the foot processes, have formed broad obstructing plaques. 22,000 × (Dr. THOENES).

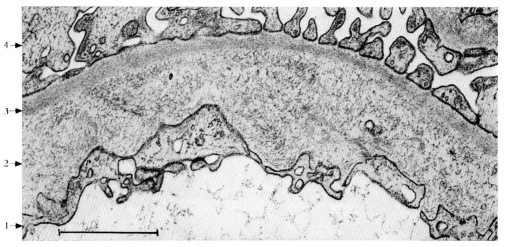

Fig. 253. Amyloidosis of a glomerular loop (golden hamster). Finely fibrillar amyloid (→2) lies between the endothelium (→1) and the basement membrane (→3). Foot processes of an epithelial cell (→4). 28,000 × (Dr. CAESAR, Dr. SCHNEIDER).

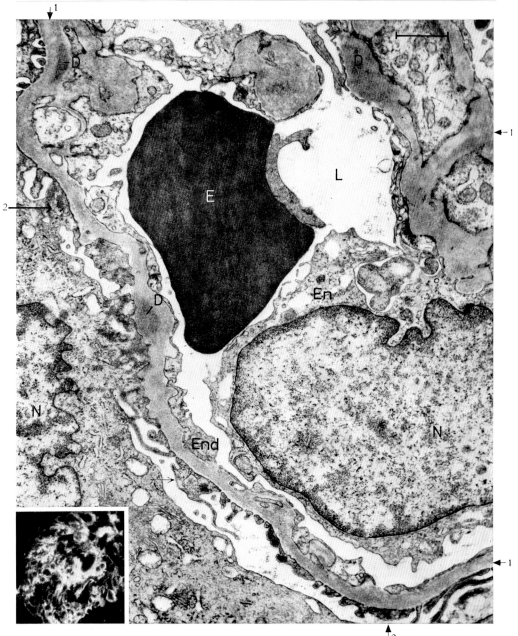

Fig. 254. *Acute proliferative postinfectious glomerulonephritis* (needle biopsy). The conspicuous histological features are thickening of the basement membrane, swelling and increased numbers of endothelial and mesangial cells. In addition, there are deposits of dense material (D) in the region of the basement membrane which contain antigen-antibody complexes. The figure shows a moderately thickened basement membrane (→ 1) and the deposits (D). An enlarged endothelial cell (En) with its nucleus (N) containing loose chromatin is seen. The processes of the endothelial cells are tightly attached without pores to the inner side of the basement membrane. To the left in the picture is an epithelial cell with its nucleus (N) and foot processes (→ 2), of which only an occasional one is thickened. An erythrocyte lies in the lumen (L) of the glomerular loop. 13,500 ×. Human gamma globulin can be demonstrated by fluorescence microscopy in the region of the basement membrane (inset at lower left of the figure), which is further evidence of the presence of an immune complex (Dr. Thoenes and Dr. Schäfer, 1965).

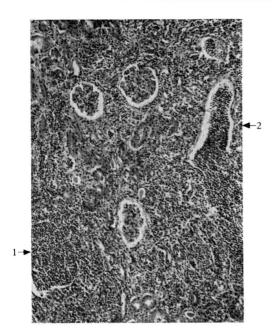

Fig. 255. Ascending pyelonephritis;
H & E, 9×.

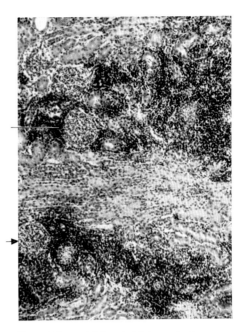

Fig. 256. Interstitial nephritis in scarlet fever;
H & E, 66×.

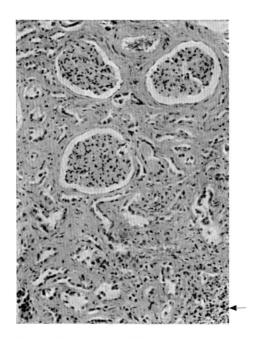

Fig. 257. Chronic interstitial nephritis;
H & E, 144×.

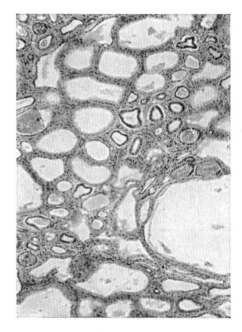

Fig. 258. Cystic kidney;
H & E, 72×.

Ascending pyelonephritis (Fig. 255). *Lower urinary tract infection (e. g., E. coli) may ascend to the kidney via the tubules or lymphatics. It usually results from obstruction, e. g., in prostatic hypertrophy or ureteric constriction and leads to suppurative inflammation of the cortex and the medulla. Pyelonephritis can also follow hematogeneous spread from a distant infection.* Very low magnification reveals streak-like areas in one or more of the medullary pyramids and increased cellularity of the adjacent cortical segments. Higher magnification shows numerous polymorphonuclear leukocytes in the collecting tubules (→ 2) and interstitial tissues. The exudate is distributed in a streaked pattern. The tubular epithelium is largely flattened and the lumen contains protein. As the disease progresses, abscesses develop in the cortex (→ 1). Healing of the acute stage may result in the complete deterioration of both glomeruli and tubules, accompanied by proliferation of interstitial connective tissue and lymphocytic infiltration. The process is always limited to a pyramid and its corresponding cortical segment, so that, in contrast to hematogenous renal abscesses, the lesions are focal.

Macroscopic: Clusters of abscesses or flat, depressed, gray scars, depending upon the age.

The disease proceeds at a lingering pace for years, with secondary renal insufficiency and hypertension developing in 40% of cases. Uremia appears in 30% of cases. Peri- and paranephric abscess can occur as complications.

Interstitial nephritis in scarlet fever (Fig. 256). Nonsuppurative inflammation with serous exudation and emigration of lymphocytes in the interstitial tissues occurs mainly *during* infectious diseases, e. g., in about 7 days after onset of scarlet fever; in contrast to glomerulonephritis which occurs 3 weeks after onset. Microscopically, the interstitial tissues are focally or diffusely infiltrated with lymphocytes and later with histiocytes and plasma cells which displace the renal tubules. The glomeruli are not affected (→). For the most part, it is a serous interstitial inflammation.

Macroscopic: Enlarged, dull, grayish white kidney.

Chronic interstitial nephritis (Fig. 257). The connective tissue surrounding the tubules is infiltrated by a chronic inflammatory exudate. There is interstitial fibrosis. The tubules are pushed apart and their lumens, which are compressed, are lined with flattened epithelium. The basement membrane of the tubules is frequently thickened. Localized collections of lymphocytes and histiocytes are seen, especially at the corticomedullary junction (→). This type of nephritis can also be observed in cases of phenacetin poisoning. The pathogenesis of these cases is usually accounted for on the basis of toxic renal damage concomitant with ascending or descending inflammation. The chronic sclerosing form is thought to have a hematogenous origin.

Macroscopic: Gnarled kidney surface.

Cystic kidney (Fig. 258). *This is most commonly a bilateral, congenital disorder, with formation of multiple cysts. Cases with small cysts have been observed in neonates.* Microscopically, the prominent feature is the presence of numerous cysts in the medulla or cortex which may be either empty or filled with homogeneous, eosinophilic material. The larger cysts have a flat, endothelium-like lining and the smaller cysts a lining of cuboidal tubular epithelium. In some cysts, glomeruli can still be made out although disrupted by pressure atrophy. A few strips of intact, but atrophic, parenchyma are still evident between the cysts.

Macroscopic: In juveniles and adults, the cysts are large and closely clustered. The parenchyma shows varying degrees of atrophy. Recent research (POTTER and coworkers, 1964) has disclosed that either isolated tubular segments may undergo cystic dilatation (small cystic kidney of the neonate, uremic death) or the ureteric buds may undergo partial obstruction at an early stage, leading to cyst formation in every part of the nephron (cystic kidney of the adult).

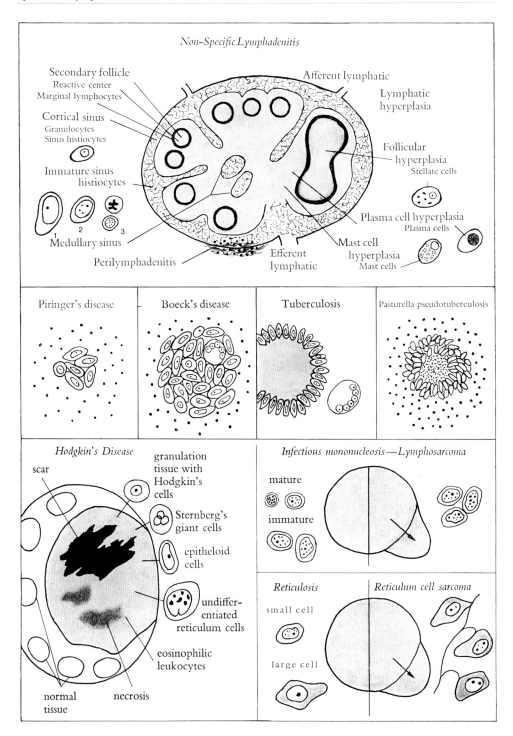

Fig. 259. Diagram of the most important diseases of lymph nodes.

Spleen and Lymph Nodes

Diseases of the spleen and lymph nodes are usually accompanied by organic structural alterations. In the **spleen,** these are manifested in changes in the integrity of the trabeculae and of the red and white pulp. Notice should be taken of the fibrous stroma, the degree of vascularity, the number and kinds of cells, as well as any pathological deposits. **Lymph nodes** (Fig. 259) should be examined first with a scanning lens so as to permit general architectural orientation. The capsule in particular should be inspected in this way. This low-power inspection should be followed by a detailed appraisal of the sinuses (numbers and kinds of cells) and the follicles (size and kinds of cells). Alterations of the normal architecture are often best demonstrated with silver stains which reveal the argyrophyl fibers. Giemsa stain is valuable for differentiating the various kinds of cells (LENNERT, 1961, 1964). **Reticulum cells** (R): *small lymphoid reticulum cells* (like lymphocytes, but having a storage function). *Medium sized reticulum cells* (= histiocytes, pale, round to oval nucleus, weakly basophilic cytoplasm). *Large reticulum cells* (finely granular chromatin, oval, often crenated, nucleus, with a distinct nucleolus). *Fixed macrophages, stellate cells,* with chromatin fragments in the cytoplasm (phagocytosis, also storage of pigment and fat). *Epithelioid cells* (wet preparations: oval to round nucleus; dry preparations: in the form of a cat's tongue. Eosinophilic cytoplasm). Function: phagocytosis, synthesis of argyrophilic fibers. **Basophilic stem cell :** (finely reticulated chromatin, large nucleolus, basophilic cytoplasm = stem cell of the pulp lymphocytes? Antibody producers?) **Lymphopoiesis :** primitive or stem cells (light, round nucleus, colorless nucleolus, scanty basophilic cytoplasm). *Lymphoblasts:* light nucleus, more basophilic cytoplasm than lymphocytes (carriers of tissue antibodies, metamorphosis to plasma cells and histiocytes?). Histiocytes probably originate from blood monocytes (LEDER, 1967). **Plasma cells :** eccentric nucleus, with spoke-like structure, basophilic cytoplasm. Derived from lymphocytes, produce humoral antibodies. **Mast cells :** metachromatic granules, heparin, histamine.

Non-specific lymphadenitis (Fig. 259): The structure of the lymph node is preserved. Polymorphonuclear leukocytes are found in the sinuses as well as histiocytes (detached sinus lining cells, see p. 173). There are also *immature sinus histiocytes*, both mature large histiocytes (1 in Fig. 259) and immature histiocytes (2 in Fig. 259). The histiocytes occur in the sinuses, together with leukocytes and lymphocytes (3 in Fig. 259). Non-specific lymphadenitis may also occur in infectious mononucleosis and Piringer's lymphadenitis. **Lymphoid hyperplasia :** enlargement of the secondary follicles with clearly demarcated reaction centers and so-called stellate cells, germinoblasts and large reticulum cells. The follicles may fuse (see Fig. 259). In *diffuse lymphatic hyperplasia,* the lymphocytes of the pulp are increased, in *plasma cell hyperplasia,* there are plasma cells in the medulla, in *mast cell hyperplasia,* mast cells in the medulla. The *tertiary follicles* are enlarged (rich in reticulum cells and basophilic stem cells). *Perilymphadenitis* (edema of the capsule, leukocytic infiltration).

Focal small epithelial cell reaction of Piringer (Fig. 271). Small groups of epithelioid cells and foci of nonspecific lymphadenitis are found in toxoplasmosis (adults), in immature cell sinus histiocytosis, in nodes draining an underlying carcinoma, and in the portal lymph nodes. In addition, it may be seen in the very early stages of Hodgkin's disease.

Boeck's sarcoid (Boeck's sarcoidosis) (Fig. 273): This is an epithelioid cell granuloma (larger cells than in Piringer's lymphadenitis), often with Langhans giant cells but lacking caseation.

Caseating tuberculosis : Caseation (necrosis) delimited by epithelioid cells, granulation tissue and Langhans giant cells (see pp. 98, 174).

Pseudotuberculosis : This includes:
1. *Pseudotuberculosis* (MASSHOFF), Pasteurella pseudotuberculosis. Mesenteric lymph nodes are predominantly involved.
2. *Tularemia* (Pasteurella tularensis). Carried by wild game (fur handlers, wild animal handlers).
3. *Cat scratch fever* (virus of the Miyagawanella group).
All three forms have the same appearance. Foci of reticulum cell proliferation develop first. Secondarily, there is central necrosis and infiltration of polymorphonuclear leukocytes. Finally, the lesion is bordered by epithelioid cells.

Hodgkin's disease (see p. 176). The chief finding is destruction of the lymph node pattern by specific granulation tissue showing characteristic cell types. In the granulation tissue, there are areas of necrosis and scarring.

Lymphadenosis – Lymphosarcoma (Figs. 280, 289), see p. 177.

Reticuloses : Definition: malignant generalized proliferation of reticulum cells (LENNERT, 1964) involving particularly spleen, bone marrow, lymph nodes and liver.

Small cell lymphoid reticulosis: existence disputed. *Medium cell reticulosis* with spill into blood: monocytic leukemia, see Fig. 292. Since monocytes arise from promyelocytes this may become a myelocytic leukemia. *Large cell reticulosis:* proliferation of large reticulum cells.

Acute infantile reticulosis (LETTERER-SIWE): Generalized proliferation of reticulum cells (all organs) with giant cells of osteoclastic type (children under 2 years). *Eosinophilic granuloma* (proliferation of reticulum cells with giant cells of osteoclastic type and eosinophilic leukocytes).

Hand-Christian-Schüller disease: like the preceding. Secondary cholesterol deposits.

Reticulum cell or reticuloendothelial sarcoma: focal, infiltrating malignant tumor of reticulum cells and fibers (Figs. 275, 276).

167

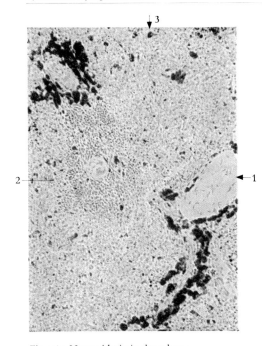

Fig. 260. Hemosiderin in the spleen;
Berlin blue reaction, 111×.

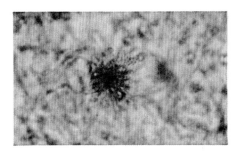

Fig. 261. Hematoidin crystals in a splenic
infarct;
H & E, 380×.

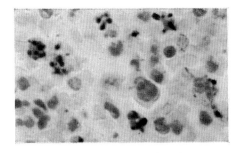

Fig. 262. Formalin pigment in the spleen;
Nuclear fast red 950×.

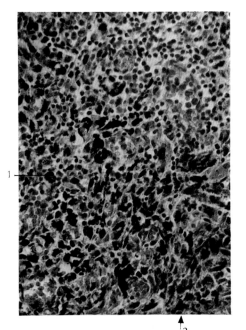

Fig. 263. Anthracosis of lymph nodes;
H & E, 304×.

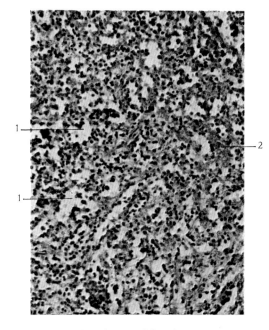

Fig. 264. Fibroadenosis of the spleen;
H & E, 187×.

Siderosis of spleen (Fig. 260). In increased erythrocytic destruction (hemolytic anemia, repeated blood transfusions) and after large parenteral iron supplements, iron pigment is stored in the reticulum cells of the spleen (see Figs. 13, 357). Histologically, low-power examination of sections stained with Berlin blue shows foci of greenish blue, layered masses in the red pulp and trabeculae (→ 1), (→ 2: follicles). High power shows that the siderin, which is stained blue by the Berlin blue reaction, lies within the cytoplasm of reticulum cells. To see this clearly, look for a part of the section in which the pigment is not so thick and where individual cells can be recognized (→ 3).

Macroscopic: The spleen is brownish red. Small hemorrhages and infarcts organized by connective tissue are present, as well as focal deposits of iron and calcium encrustations, so-called Gandy-Gamna nodules.

Hematoidin crystals in a splenic infarct (Fig. 261). These consist of crystals of bilirubin in the form of red or orange needles or rhomboid plates. When blood is broken down and not removed by cellular resorption, for example, as may occur in the center of a hematoma or splenic infarct as shown in Figure 261, iron-free pigment is formed from the hemoglobin freed from the erythrocytes (compare Fig. 14).

Formalin pigment (Fig. 262) is an artifact. The dark brown, granular, doubly refractile deposits are grouped together. They arise from the reaction of formaldehyde with unbound hemoglobin (probably protoporphyrin). The pigment gives a positive benzidine test and is soluble in weak acid.

Macroscopic: With formalin fixation, the blood appears brown or brownish black.

Anthracosis of lymph node (Fig. 263): Inhaled carbon pigment leaves the lung by way of the lymph channels and travels to the hilar lymph nodes, whence it can be carried even farther to the para-aortic lymph nodes. Rupture of markedly anthracotic lymph nodes into blood vessels in the hilus of the lung can result in spread via the blood stream and thus give rise to so-called pigment metastases in various organs.
In the hilar lymph nodes, the granular carbon pigment is first phagocytized by the sinus endothelium. With further accumulation, pigment is also found in the reticulum cells of the cortical and medullary pulp, especially around the lymphoid follicles. Higher magnification shows the carbon granules to be in individual reticulum cells and to surround and compress the nucleus (→ 1). Progressive atrophy of lymphoid tissue occurs, and finally fibrosis of the node. Figure 263 shows the atrophy of the lymphocytes → 2.

Macroscopic: Early, there is diffuse or mottled gray discoloration of the lymph nodes; later, they are homogeneous black (the cut surface is moist in contrast to silicosis).

Fibroadenosis of spleen (Fig. 264): This term is used to describe chronic congestive induration of the spleen in portal hypertension; for example, in cirrhosis of the liver. Following dilatation of the sinus from acute congestion, hyperplasia of reticulum cells and reticular fibers develops between the sinusoids and increases with the duration of the stasis. Collagenization of the reticular fibrils ensues. The sinusoids, which are largely free of erythrocytes in the illustration (→ 1), become surrounded by thick, rigid walls (→ 2). Simultaneously, the white pulp atrophies.

Macroscopic: Marked splenic enlargement. The spleen frequently weighs more than 500 Gm. The splenic capsule is thickened by fibrosis and often hyalinized. The spleen has a tough, elastic consistency. The cut surface is dark red. After hemorrhage, for example from esophageal varices, the organ is light red, firm but elastic.

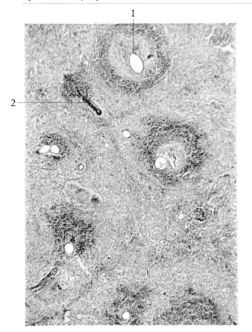

Fig. 265. Follicular amyloidosis of the spleen; Congo red stain, 25×.

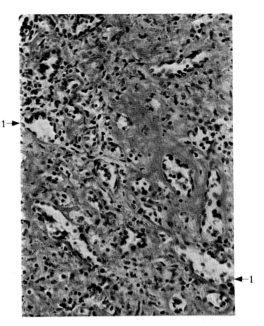

Fig. 266. Amyloidosis of the splenic pulp; Congo red stain, 263×.

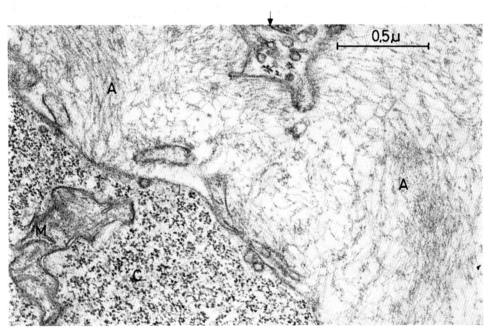

Fig. 267. Experimental amyloidosis of the mouse after giving sodium caseinate. A = fibrous amyloid outside the cytoplasm (C) of a reticulum cell of the spleen. In the cytoplasm, there are numerous aggregates of ribosomes (polysomes), an indication of high protein synthesis. M = fusion of mitochondria (giant mitochondria), → part of a neighboring cell. 49,000× (Dr. CAESAR).

Amyloidosis

Amyloid is a glassy, translucent, homogeneous substance of firm consistency which stains red with eosin and positively with Congo red (see p. 10). The composition of amyloid is 90% protein (by amino acid analysis this is γ globulin) and 1% carbohydrates (chondroitin sulfate and neuraminic acid). The binding of Congo red probably takes place with the carbohydrate component of amyloid in which a distance of 10 Å of the reactive groups of the stain is required (similar to cellulose, PUCHTLER et al., 1965). The fact that after staining with Congo red the amyloid is doubly refractile is proof of direct deposition of the stain on the amyloid fiber. Electron microscopically, amyloid shows fibers about 80 Å (50–150 Å) thick (Figs. 267, 268), which, with the usual techniques, show no internal structure (CAESAR, 1961). However, with special techniques, it has now been observed that these fibers consist of 2 fibrils, each 25 Å in diameter, forming a double helix with a space 25 Å between them. The two fibrillar strands are wound around each other, producing a transverse striation with 40 Å periodicity (BOERÉ et al., 1965). According to BENDITT and co-workers, 1966, there is a globular sub-unit 30–37 Å diameter. Amyloid is formed by mesenchymal cells (reticulum cells, endothelial cells, COHEN and co-workers, 1965) in which the high content of ribosomes speaks for marked protein synthesis (SCHNEIDER, 1964, see Fig. 267). COHEN et al. also have seen amyloid fibrils in the cytoplasm of cells and concluded that the fibrils are formed intracellularly.

Typical and atypical forms of amyloidosis are distinguished according to location. **Typical:** a) *Sago spleen type* (follicular amyloidosis, Fig. 265). Liver (pericapillary location, Fig. 187), intestinal mucous membrane,

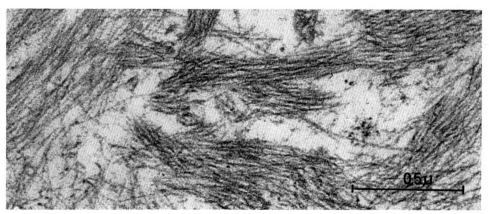

Fig. 268. Amyloid fibers without distinct internal structures, experimental amyloidosis in a mouse. 63,000× (Dr. CAESAR).

afferent arterioles of kidney, medulla of adrenal gland. b) *Lardaceous spleen type* (pulp amyloidosis, Fig. 266), liver (hepatic artery), small intestine (submucosal arteries), kidney (predominantly glomerular Figs. 230, 253), adrenal cortex (Fig. 288) (TERBRÜGGEN, 1948). **Atypical amyloidosis** (para-amyloidosis): heart, tongue, musculature, skin, brain, lungs. **Primary amyloidosis** is hereditary, for example, in familial Mediterranean fever (recessive), and occurs in typical amyloidosis or in experimental animals such as mice. **Secondary, acquired amyloidosis** is encountered in chronic infections (tuberculosis, osteomyelitis, bronchiectasis, etc.). It resembles typical amyloidosis. Experimentally, amyloidosis can be produced in mice by feeding casein (Fig. 267).

Follicular amyloidosis (Fig. 265). Low magnification of a section stained with Congo red demonstrates the red-colored follicles which are seen as red circles or little disks sometimes with a central artery (→ 1). → 2 amyloid in an artery in the pulp. The follicles contain no lymphocytes, the pulp is poor in cells.

Macroscopic: Multiple small glassy nodules = Sago spleen.

Pulp amyloidosis (Fig. 266): Low magnification shows red homogeneous tissue and focal round pale areas corresponding to the follicles. Higher magnification shows the amyloid lying between dilated sinuses lined by large endothelial cells (→ 1).

Macroscopic: Enlarged, firm spleen of wooden consistency and having homogeneous, reddish, lardaceous glassy cut surfaces.

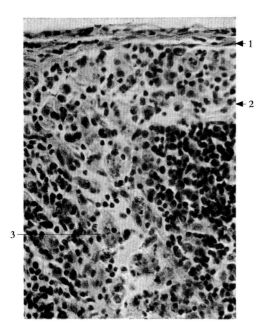

Fig. 269. Acute non-specific lymphadenitis
(sinus catarrh);
H & E, 360×.

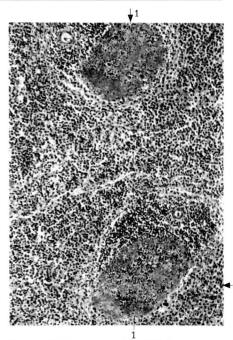

Fig. 270. Follicular necrosis in diphtheria;
H & E, 108×.

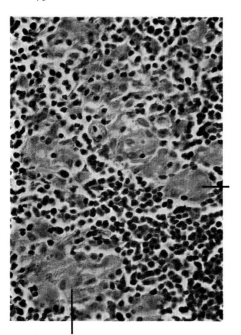

Fig. 271. Piringer's lymphadenitis (focal small
epitheloid cell reaction);
H & E, 420×.

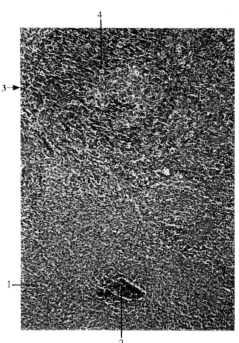

Fig. 272. Suppurative reticulocytic lymphadenitis;
H & E, 80×.

Acute non-specific lymphadenitis (sinus catarrh) (Fig. 269) is one histological form of lymphadenitis (see p. 166). The histological feature of sinus catarrh is proliferation of the reticulum cells of the sinus due to their exposure to increasing amounts of resorbable substances (protein breakdown products, as from nearby cancers, bacteria, toxins, etc.). The proliferating reticuloendothelial cells become detached in large numbers and lie in the lumen of the sinus as isolated, round or oval histiocytes with a pale eccentric nucleus: *sinus histiocytosis*. Figure 269 shows the cortical sinus of a lymph node with non-specific lymphadenitis. The sinuses are wide (→ 1 and → 2: border of the sinus) and filled with large cells with abundant cytoplasm which are detached reticulum cells containing cytoplasmic nuclear fragments (→ 3). Single lymphocytes and leukocytes are also present.

Follicular necrosis in diphtheria (Fig. 270). A particularly pronounced lymphadenitis with necrosis of the germinal centers of the secondary follicles occurs in diphtheria (direct toxic effect). Histologically, the reactive centers of the follicles are changed into necrotic eosinophilic masses (→ 1) in which nuclear debris can still be seen. The peripheral zone of lymphocytes is preserved. The remainder of the lymph node is acutely inflamed and frequently hemorrhagic (→ 2). Also seen in the mesenteric lymph nodes of small children with acute enteritis (non–diphtheritic).

Macroscopic: Enlarged lymph node with red, speckled cut surfaces.

Piringer's lymphadenitis (Fig. 271). In most cases, Piringer's lymphadenitis (PIRINGER-KUCHINKA, 1953) is due to toxoplasmosis (see p. 226), and occurs preferentially in the lymph nodes of the neck (75%). The characteristic histological changes are small focal collections of epithelioid cells, proliferation of immature histiocytes in the sinuses, hyperplasia of lymphoid follicles having large germinal centers, and perilymphadenitis. Figure 271 shows several groups of 4–8 large epithelioid cells with abundant pale eosinophilic cytoplasm (→). The nuclei of these cells are oval or shaped like a cat's tongue and possess a loose chromatin structure.
Similar foci of small epithelioid cells may be found in lymph nodes in the early stages of Hodgkin's disease, in infectious mononucleosis, and in lymph nodes draining degenerating tumors.

Macroscopic: Non-specific, swollen lymph nodes with oozing grayish red cut surfaces.

Suppurative reticulocytic lymphadenitis (MASSHOFF, Fig. 272). This type of lymphadenitis occurs in various infections: Pasteurella pseudotuberculosis infection of mesenteric and ileocecal lymph nodes which, in children, mimics the clinical picture of appendicitis (MASSHOFF, 1953): infections with Pasteurella tularensis and the agent of cat scratch fever (virus) which attack the lymph nodes regional to the infection (primary complex), especially in juveniles.
All these infections of lymph nodes show a similar histological picture. In the fully developed stages, there is extensive focal reticulum cell proliferation (→ 1) with areas of destruction of tissue (abscess → 2) surrounded by polymorphonuclear granulocytes. Next to the abscess and the cuff of reticulocytes there is a secondary follicle with a distinct reaction center (→ 3) and several so-called stellate cells (→ 4). Other changes seen in this disease – not represented in the illustration – are considerable perilymphadenitis, endophlebitis and endarteritis of neighboring blood vessels.

Macroscopic: Enlarged lymph node with grayish white foci.

173

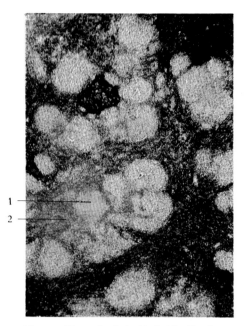

Fig. 273. Hyperplastic (epithelioid cell) tuberculous lymphadenitis;
van Gieson stain, 44×.

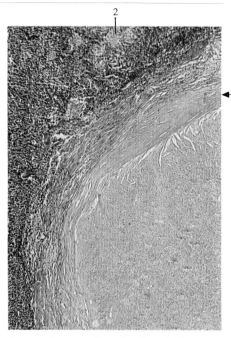

Fig. 274. Caseous tuberculous lymphadenitis;
H & E, 20×.

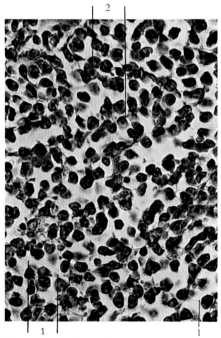

Fig. 275. Reticulum cell sarcoma;
H & E, 440×.

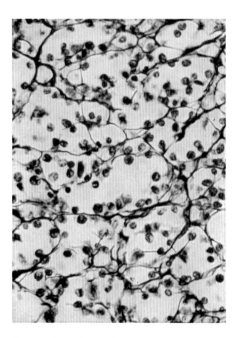

Fig. 276. Reticulum cell sarcoma;
Bielschowsky's silver stain, 480×.

Tuberculous lymphadenitis (Figs. 273, 274). There are two morphological types of tuberculous lymphadenitis: *hyperplastic*, or *epithelioid cell* tuberculosis, and *caseous* tuberculosis. In the former, the disease frequently runs an unusual course and is known as *Boeck's sarcoid*.

In **hyperplastic tuberculous lymphadenitis** (Fig. 273), the microscopic section shows numerous, closely packed tubercles containing chiefly epithelioid cells. The rounded, frequently confluent lesions are conspicuous under low-power magnification. Slightly higher magnification reveals typical epithelioid cells (see Fig. 141, p. 98) and solitary Langhans type giant cells. There can be secondary central necrosis (→ 1) but this is unusual. In older lesions, a good deal of hyalin connective tissue may appear (→ 2) and finally lead to scar formation.

Macroscopic: A slightly enlarged lymph node with translucent gray nodules on the cut surface.

In **caseating tuberculosis of lymph nodes** (Fig. 274), necrosis completely dominates the histological picture, and the specific granulation tissue is visible only as a narrow border or, as in this illustration, is for the most part replaced by a fibrous capsule (→ 1). With the unaided eye, large homogeneous eosinophilic masses (caseation) are seen to have replaced the lymphoid tissue. Higher magnification shows extensive finely granular areas of necrosis without remnants of the original tissues. Peripheral to the focus of caseation there are non-caseating granulomas of epithelioid cells (→ 2).

Macroscopic: Compartmented cut surface with focal or map-like, dry, yellow areas.

Reticulum cell sarcoma (Figs. 275, 276) (Synonyms: reticuloendothelial sarcoma, reticulosarcoma, reticuloendothelioma). Reticulum cell sarcoma is a malignant tumor consisting of an overgrowth of reticulum cells. It occurs in lymph nodes or bone marrow (Ewing's sarcoma). Reticulum cell sarcoma of the lymph nodes is probably the most frequent tumor of the lymphatic tissues; 60–70% begin in the cervical lymph nodes or tonsils.

Histologically, the node shows general enlargement due to proliferation of medium-to-large cells, and loss of the characteristic lymph node pattern. Ewing's sarcoma is composed of small cells. In parts, the tumor consists of densely packed bands of tissue with now and then tubule-like fissures reminiscent of epithelial structures. In other parts, there are cords of reticulum cells which frequently show differentiation into capillary-like spaces. The tumor cells are variously shaped: partly rounded, partly shaped like many pointed stars. In differentiating this tumor from lymphosarcoma, it is helpful to keep in mind the rule of thumb that with Giemsa's stain the cells of reticulum cell sarcoma have pale nuclei and strongly basophilic cytoplasm. The cells of lymphosarcoma have darker nuclei and paler cytoplasm (LENNERT, 1963). Mitoses are numerous. The nuclei in reticulum cell sarcoma that are not dividing are oval or round. They are pale and vesicular and most contain a distinct nucleolus, occasionally even two or three.

Figure 275 shows a section of a reticulum cell sarcoma, in which the tumor cells are strung on delicate fibrils. The resulting cleavage spaces are bridged over by the pointed cytoplasm (→ 1). In many places, the vesicular nature of the nucleus and the nucleoli is distinct even in H & E preparations (→ 2).

The peculiarity of reticulum cells, that is, to form reticulum fibers, is present in highly differentiated reticulum cell sarcomas. The identification of such reticular fibrils is important for confirmation of the diagnosis, since they occur frequently in this tumor. Figure 276 shows the reticular fibers stained with silver according to the method of *Bielschowsky*. Mostly, the reticular fibers run tangentially in a row, as do the silvered nuclei, thus producing a picture resembling catkins lined up on a willow branch.

Macroscopic: Marked enlargement of the involved lymph nodes which have a white or grayish white, oozing cut surface resembling fish flesh. Because of the infiltrating type of growth, the nodes are adherent to surrounding structures. Tumor masses may also develop in other organs.

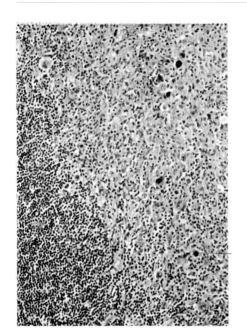

Fig. 277. Hodgkin's disease;
H & E, 160×.

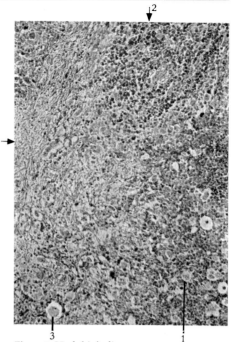

Fig. 278. Hodgkin's disease;
Giemsa stain, 64×.

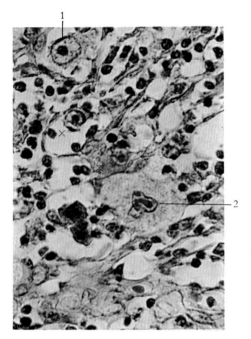

Fig. 279. Hodgkin's disease;
Giemsa stain, 400×.

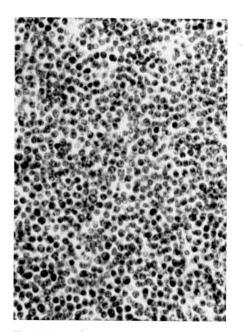

Fig. 280. Lymphosarcoma;
H & E, 438×.

Hodgkin's disease (Figs. 277, 278 and 279), *Hodgkin's disease (lymphogranulomatosis)* is a common disease of lymph nodes. It is thought by many to be neoplastic. It consists of proliferating invasive tissue that resembles granulation tissue (Fig. 277) and has specific characteristics.

The histological picture is not uniform in the different stages of the disease. In the earliest stages, there is predominantly an increase in lymphocytes (diffuse lymphatic hyperplasia, as, for example, in the lower left of Fig. 277) and increase in reticulum cells (reticulocytosis). In addition, there are small foci of epithelial-like cells similar to those seen in Piringer's disease (Fig. 271).

The characteristic cell type for the disease, the Hodgkin cell, arises from reticulum cells ($\times$ and $\rightarrow$ 1 in Fig. 279, see also Fig. 388). Hodgkin cells have a striking pale vesicular nucleus with a distinct nuclear membrane. The nuclei lie in the middle of the cytoplasm, which is basophilic, stains with Giemsa and has indistinct margins. The cytoplasm is not particularly abundant. The nucleus contains a rather large nucleolus (Figs. 278 $\rightarrow$ 1, 279 $\rightarrow$ 1 and $\times$). From such Hodgkin cells, the multinucleated Sternberg giant cells are formed. Their nuclei, which are also vesiculated, partially overlay each other and the cytoplasm is abundant (Fig. 277 $\rightarrow$, Fig. 278 $\rightarrow$ 3, Fig. 279 $\rightarrow$ 2). In fully developed stages of the disease, the reticulum cell proliferation with Hodgkin cells and Sternberg giant cells dominates the histological picture (upper right of Fig. 277). Dense infiltration of eosinophilic granulocytes (Fig. 278 $\rightarrow$ 2) and lymphocytes (Fig. 279) also occurs. Focal, circumscribed necrosis develops in the areas of reticular proliferation. The end stages of the disease are characterized by collagenous fibrous tissue scarring which may involve most of the node (Fig. 278 $\rightarrow$ 4).

Aside from this typical form of Hodgkin's disease, which has an average duration of about 2 years (several months to over 10 years from the recognition of the disease until death in individual cases), there is a form with a more benign course called **Hodgkin's paragranuloma.** In this form, the life span may be as long as 40 years. Histologically, the lymph node shows a predominantly lymphocytic infiltration with accompanying typical Hodgkin cells and small foci of epithelioid cells. A more malignant variant of Hodgkin's disease is **Hodgkin's sarcoma.** This consists of neoplastic proliferation of atypical reticulum cells. The diagnosis is usually made with the knowledge that there was preceding Hodgkin's disease.

Macroscopic: Cervical lymph nodes are most often affected, less frequently mediastinal and abdominal lymph nodes, spleen (porphyry spleen), liver, bone marrow; occasional involvement of lung, kidney, heart, intestinal tract, skin, meninges, etc. The affected lymph nodes are enlarged and adherent. *Cut surface:* the medulla is grayish white due to the proliferating granulomatous tissue and contains yellow foci or map-like areas of necrosis. With cicatrization, the gray color increases and the consistency becomes dense and fibrous.

Lymphadenosis – Lymphosarcoma. Two sorts of lymphadenosis can be recognized:
a) *mature well differentiated lymphadenosis:* with an aleukemic, subleukemic or leukemia blood picture (chronic lymphatic leukemia, Fig. 289). Course: months to years. *Histology:* lymphoblasts and lymphocytes (some cases may become less differentiated with time and show a variety of both mature and immature cells). b) *immature or undifferentiated lymphadenosis* (leukosarcoma) with moderately marked leukemic blood picture (lymphoblastic leukemia, Fig. 291). Course: 6–12 months. *Histology:* monotonous proliferation of large lymphoblasts (one cell type).

Macroscopic: In both sorts the lymph nodes, bone marrow, spleen and liver (periportal areas) are diffusely infiltrated.

Lymphosarcoma (see also Fig. 384): No leukemia. *Histology:* Uniform proliferation of immature lymphoblasts forming tumor nodules in the involved lymph nodes. Cytologically resembles b) above.

Macroscopic: nodular growths. Lymph nodes become fused. Sarcomatous nodules in liver, spleen, bone marrow. Combinations of a) and b) occur in lymphosarcoma (malignant lymphadenosis).
Fig. 280 is from a patient with a **mature form of lymphadenosis** (lymphatic leukemia) showing diffuse infiltration of a lymph node. There are cells with large nuclei having a porous appearance (lymphoblasts) as well as cells with small nuclei and dense chromatin (lymphocytes). The capsule may be infiltrated.

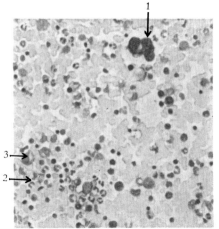

Fig.281. Bone marrow smear (normal);
Giemsa stain, 480×.

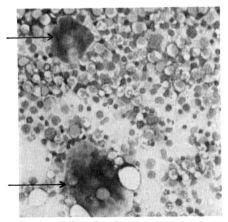

Fig.282. Polycythemia vera;
Giemsa stain, 480×.

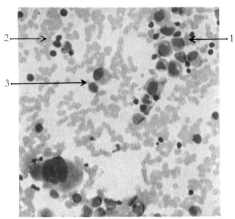

Fig.283. Agranulocytosis;
Giemsa stain, 480×.

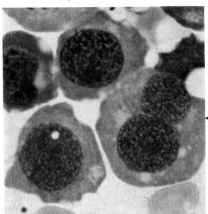

Fig.284. Pernicious anemia;
Giemsa stain, 1,200×.

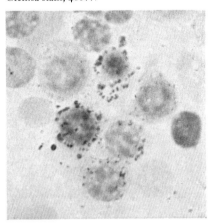

Fig.285. Sideroblastic or siderochrestic anemia;
Berlin-blue reaction, 1,200×.

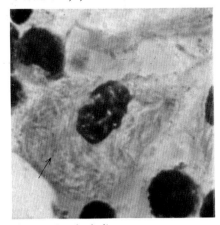

Fig.286. Gaucher's disease;
Giemsa stain, 1,200×.

Bone Marrow and Blood

The bone marrow reacts as an organ or well-defined system under both physiological and many pathological circumstances. Upon this knowledge rests the significance of diagnostic bone marrow biopsy. In the evaluation of a bone marrow aspiration, the same procedure is used as for the evaluation of a histological slide. Low power is used for orientation with respect to cell content and distribution. Medium power gives a general survey of the relation of the different kinds of mature cells and allows identification of unusual cells or groups of cells. Cytological details are observed and recorded under the highest magnification (oil immersion). It should be noted that quantitative assessment of cells in a smear is possible only within limits, since the number of cells depends, among other things, upon the way the puncture is done and the technique of smearing. The qualitative findings have more validity. For reasons of space, only those disease entities will be considered in which the morphological findings have diagnostic significance or provide information of clinical value. Giemsa stain shows cellular details best (Figs. 281–292).

Normal bone marrow smear (Fig. 281). The megakaryocytes are the largest cells seen in bone marrow smears and can be recognized even at low magnification ($\rightarrow$ 1). The cells of the erythropoietic series have round, deeply stained nuclei. Cells of the granulopoietic series are seen in all stages of maturity ($\rightarrow$ 2 leukocyte with a segmented nucleus, $\rightarrow$ 3: myelocyte). This illustration is shown for the purpose of comparing and evaluating the cellular contents.

Polycythemia vera (Fig. 282). *In this disease, there is an increase of all three blood-forming systems: erythropoietic, granulopoietic and the megakaryocytes.* The megakaryocytes are ordinarily distinctly larger than in normal marrow smears ($\rightarrow$). Observe that, by comparison with Figure 281, the cells are densely compacted. Myelopoiesis = cells with large pale nuclei; erythrocytopoiesis = cells with round dark nuclei.

Agranulocytosis (Fig. 283). *In agranulocytosis, only granulopoiesis is depleted. Frequently, it is produced by medication (Pyramidon. Allergy to drugs)* Panmyelopthisis: *The marrow is empty and all blood-forming cells have disappeared.* In Figure 283, only the very early stages of granulopoiesis can be seen (promyelocytes and myelocytes $\rightarrow$ 1). Mature forms are lacking. There are also interspersed round nucleated elements some of which are lymphocytes $\rightarrow$ 2 and some undifferentiated blasts ($\rightarrow$ 3: vesicular nuclei, scanty cytoplasm). The lack of mature leukocytes lessens the resistance of the host, and necrotic inflammation of the mucous membranes develops (mucous membranes of the mouth and large intestine).

Pernicious anemia (Fig. 284). *This results from defective absorption of vitamin B_{12} caused by lack of intrinsic factor (atrophic gastritis, autoantibodies).* The typical megaloblasts (pathological erythroblasts $\rightarrow$: binuclear forms) have a large round nucleus with loose chromatin, which corresponds in a general way to proerythroblasts in the normal stage of development. The cytoplasm, however, appears more mature (contains hemoglobin). The granulopoietic series of cells show analogous alterations of the nucleus (giant metamyelocytes and band nuclei). The megakaryocytes are distinguished by oversegmentation of the nuclei. Similar changes are found with lack of folic acid, in certain forms of erythemia and in erythroleukemia.

Refractory sideroblastic or siderochrestic anemia (Fig. 285). *In this condition, there is a disturbance of porphyrin synthesis with defective uptake of iron. It is seen in lead poisoning, among other conditions.* With the Berlin-blue reaction, the iron is visible in the form of large granules in the cytoplasm of the erythroblasts (sideroblasts, see Fig. 13 for siderin).

Gaucher disease (Fig. 286). This is a genetically dependent lipid storage disease (enzyme defect). All cells of the RES (predominantly in the spleen and bone marrow) store kerasin. Microscopically, the cytoplasm shows a striated fibrillary pattern reflecting the storage of lipid in the membranes of the endoplasmic reticulum ($\rightarrow$, see also Table 4).

179

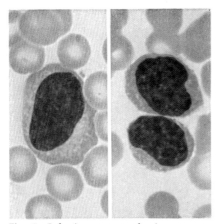

Fig. 287. Infectious mononucleosis;
Giemsa stain, 1,200×.

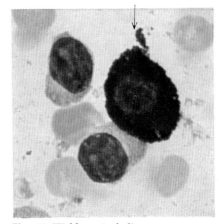

Fig. 288. Waldenström's disease;
Giemsa stain, 1,200×.

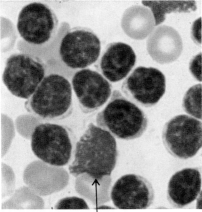

Fig. 289. Chronic lymphatic leukemia;
Giemsa stain, 1,200×.

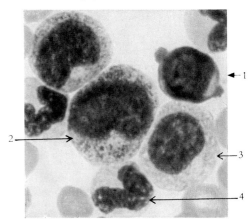

Fig. 290. Chronic myelogenous leukemia;
Giemsa stain, 1,200×.

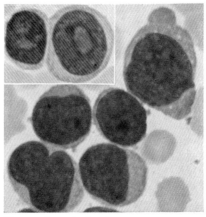

Fig. 291. Acute leukemia;
Giemsa stain, 1,200×.

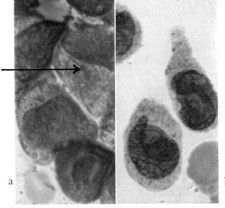

Fig. 292. a) Promyelocytic leukemia,
b) Monocytic leukemia; Giemsa stain, 1,200×.

Infektious mononucleosis (Fig. 287). *This is probably a viral disease Oral. Angina is frequently present.* The peripheral blood contains up to 90% lymphoid cells which come from the lymphatic tissues. They are distinguished from normal lymphocytes by more marked cytoplasmic basophilia and large often indented nuclei. All variations from normal lymphocytes to monocytoid cells are found (this is characteristic).

Waldenström's disease (Fig. 288). *This disease belongs in the group of the paraproteinoses (see also plasma cell myeloma). Chemical analysis of the proteins of the blood serum reveals macroglobulin of the γM-globulin type.* The bone marrow (also lymph nodes) contains cells which, morphologically, are between lymphocytes and plasma cells. The nucleus is similar to that of lymphocytes and has a distinct nucleolus; the cytoplasm is markedly basophilic like that of a plasma cell. Frequently, the tissue mast cells are increased ($\rightarrow$).

Chronic lymphatic leukemia (Fig. 289, see also Figs. 209, 250). *The chronic mature cell type of lymphatic leukemia has a relatively good prognosis.* Elderly men are chiefly affected (over 60 years). The peripheral blood shows small lymphocytes with scanty cytoplasm, which may appear smudged ($\rightarrow$: smudged cells).

Clinical: Enlargement of lymph nodes and spleen.

Chronic myelogenous leukemia (Fig. 290, also Fig. 208). *Clinically, middle-aged persons are affected predominantly. Splenic enlargement is present but lymph adenopathy is often lacking.* The peripheral blood picture is characterized by an outpouring of cells of all stages of granulopoiesis, including increased numbers of basophilic and eosinophilic granulocytes ($\rightarrow$ 1: myeloblast $\rightarrow$ 2: promyelocyte $\rightarrow$ 3: myelocyte $\rightarrow$ 4: band cell). In the differential diagnosis, osteomyelosclerosis or a leukemoid reaction must be considered. In chronic myelogenous leukemia, the cytoplasmic alkaline phosphatase is reduced or absent in the neutrophils but increased in leukemoid reactions. Is osteoporosis, biopsy of the bone marrow shows fibrosis and thickening of the spongiosa (fibrosis alone = myelofibrosis).

Acute leukemia (Fig. 291). *Leukemia with immature cells (so-called blast cell leukemia) is found in all age groups. It accounts for more than 98% of all childhood leukemias.* The cytological differentiation of the various cell types is difficult. Most frequently, there are pleomorphic, undifferentiated blasts (so-called paramyeloblasts, Fig. 291). In childhood, lymphoblastic leukemia predominates. The small picture inserted in the upper part of Figure 291 shows two lymphoblasts in a case of acute leukemia (lymphoblastic leukemia).

Promyelocytic leukemia (Fig. 292). Clinically, there is a prominent hemorrhagic diathesis. Blood smears show distinct azurophilic (reddish) granulation of the cytoplasm of the abnormal cells and occasionally the pathological equivalent of these granules, crystal-like bodies (Fig. 292a). This is a leukemia with immature cells and is frequently aleukemic.

Monocytic leukemia is difficult to separate from other forms of leukemia with the ordinary stains. Figure 292b shows atypical monocytes with indented nuclei, fine granular chromatin, and irregular grayish blue cytoplasm. Clinically, the oral mucous membranes are infiltrated frequently. Monocytic leukemia is distinguished histochemically from other leukemias by the presence of nonspecific cytoplasmic esterase (LÖFFLER, 1963).

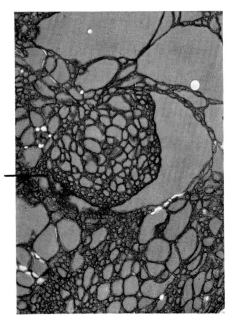

Fig. 293. Nodular colloid goiter;
H & E, 38×.

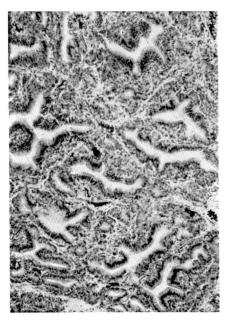

Fig. 294. Simple goiter;
H & E, 99×.

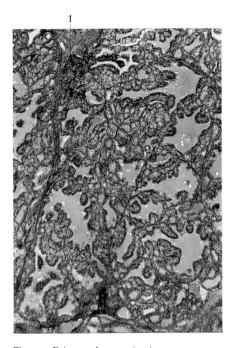

Fig. 295. Primary thyrotoxicosis;
H & E, 38×.

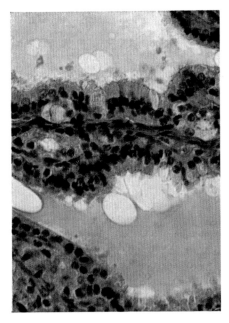

Fig. 296. Primary thyrotoxicosis;
H & E, 396×.

Endocrine Glands – Reproductive Organs

Consideration of disturbances of the endocrine glands and reproductive organs will be limited to illustrations of a few typical cases, since a thorough description would exceed the scope of this book. Moreover, the pathological manifestations of clinical endocrine gland disease are quite uniform. Hyperfunction is ordinarily associated with hyperplasia, the proliferation and enlargement of the cells and nuclei ultimately bringing about an adenomatous appearance. Hypofunction, on the other hand, is associated with atrophy of the organ, hypoplasia of cellular elements and interstitial fibrosis. In addition to these disorders, the usual specific and nonspecific inflammations and circulatory disturbances also occur.

Nodular colloid goiter (Fig. 293). *Nodular thyroid hyperplasia and thyroid adenomas appear to be endemic in certain regions (e. g., the Great Lakes region, Switzerland) and are usually regarded as compensatory hyperplasia due to iodine insufficiency* (amino acid deficiency?, inhibition of thyroxin synthesis?). The illustration (Fig. 293) shows a section of a macrofollicular nodular colloid goiter. A survey of the microscopic section with the scanning lens shows that the nodules are composed of many different-sized follicles and are surrounded by a dense fibrous capsule. The follicles are filled with colloid and lined with flat cuboidal epithelium. Higher magnification reveals cushion-like excrescences of epithelium, which may be so pronounced that new follicles arise within the excrescence (→). Degenerative changes (e. g., central necrosis, cysts, hemorrhages, scars, calcifications) arise as a result of vascular insufficiency and compression of the proliferating colloid nodules against the connective tissue capsule in which lies the nutrient vasculature (oxygen deficiency).

Macroscopic: Enlarged, nodular thyroid. The cut surface shows glistening nodules and focal yellow lesions (degenerative changes).

Simple goiter (Fig. 294). *This occurs particularly in young people up to the age of puberty in endemic areas.* Most commonly, it progresses to colloid goiter. As the name indicates, there is glandular proliferation without colloid storage. Microscopically, the thyroid lobules are enlarged and contain ramified glands with tall columnar epithelium or solid masses of cells, separated by connective tissue septa. Colloid is lacking.

Primary thyrotoxicosis or exophthalmic goiter (Figs. 295, 296). *In this condition, hyperfunction of the gland produces increased amounts of thyroid hormone (thyrotoxicosis). The etiology is not very clear (increased TSH production by the hypophysis? Disturbance of the thyroid gland itself?).* With the scanning lens, the histological section (Fig. 295) reveals large and small, highly branched follicles of various shapes with little or no colloid. The irregular configuration of the follicles is due to the cushion-like overgrowth of the epithelium (pseudopapillary proliferation) which, in places, shows fibrous stalks (papillary proliferation). The colloid, particularly near the surface of the epithelial cells, contains numerous vacuoles. Isolated foci of lymphocytes are quite characteristic (→ in Fig. 295).

High magnification (Fig. 296) shows tall columnar epithelium with pale cytoplasm and basally placed nuclei. In some places, the epithelium is stratified (→ in the picture). The so-called resorption vacuoles stand out clearly in this picture. These are artifacts of fixation, indicating that the colloid has a thin consistency.

Macroscopic: The thyroid is enlarged, with yellowish gray, liver-like cut surfaces devoid of colloid.

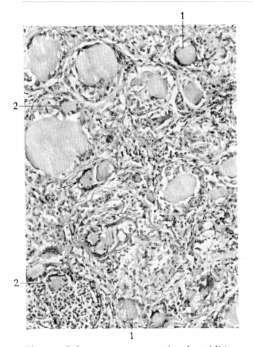

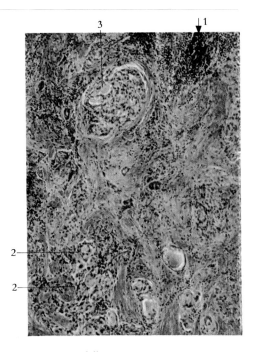

Fig. 297. Subacute, nonsuppurative thyroiditis (de Quervain); H & E, 160×.

Fig. 298. Riedel's struma; van Gieson, 102×.

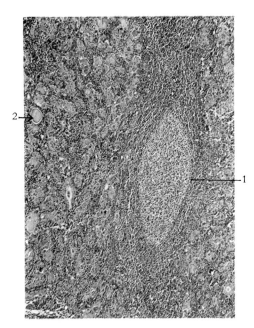

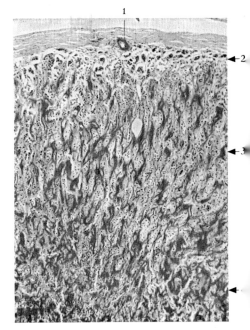

Fig. 299. Hashimoto's struma (struma lympho-matosa); H & E, 60×.

Fig. 300. Amyloidosis of the adrenal gland; Congo red, 120×.

Thyroiditis

The nonspecific inflammations of the thyroid, although rare, do present an impressive and characteristic histological picture. In addition to *acute or subacute suppurative and nonsuppurative inflammations* (*thyroiditis* of De Quervain, 1936), there are two types of *chronic thyroiditis* – chronic hypertrophic thyroiditis or *Riedel's struma* (Riedel, 1896) and *struma lymphomatosa* (Hashimoto's disease or lymphadenoid goiter, 1912).

Subacute nonsuppurative thyroiditis (De Quervain) (Fig. 297). Histologically, there are follicles of different sizes lined by cuboidal to columnar epithelium, which, in part, has a cushion-like appearance. Scattered about are smaller follicles without colloid. The relatively viscous colloid and colloid masses (→ 1) have been resorbed by giant cells partly derived from epithelium and partly from mesenchyma (→ 2). Small numbers of lymphocytes, plasma cells and occasional polymorphonuclear leukocytes can be seen between the follicles.

Chronic hypertrophic thyroiditis or Riedel's struma (Fig. 298). This form of chronic thyroiditis is accompanied by thyroid enlargement. The organ is firm and the cut surface reveals dense, white sclerotic scar tissue. The predominant features, microscopically, are hyalinized streaks of scar tissue and focal lymphocytic infiltration (→ 1). The follicles, except for some small remnants, are destroyed. A few isolated groups of intact follicles (→ 2) may undergo regenerative proliferation, thus giving rise to small adenomata (→ 3). An important diagnostic feature is the extension of the chronic sclerosing inflammation into the soft tissues of the neck, in particular, the muscles.

Struma lymphomatosa (Hashimoto) (Fig. 299). This is a chronic, progressive inflammation characterized by lymphocytic infiltration and atrophy of thyroid follicles. Figure 299 shows diffuse interstitial lymphocytic infiltration (often there are plasma cells), with formation of a typical lymphoid follicle having a reaction center (→ 1). The thyroid follicles are small and some contain inspissated colloid (→ 2).

Clinical: Hypothyroidism, sometimes myxedema.

Macroscopic: Slightly swollen, firm, brownish cut surface flecked with white.

Pathogenesis: 65% of the cases of chronic thyroiditis show autoantibodies against thyroid tissue when tested immunologically (autoimmunity). It can be shown in animal experiments that injection of thyroid extract causes a thyroiditis that histologically resembles very closely struma lymphomatosa (Witebsky, 1962). A similar mechanism has been suggested for many other diseases: allergic encephalitis, lupus erythematosus, immune hemolytic anemia, agranulocytosis, thrombopenia, chronic glomerulonephritis, cirrhosis of the liver?, myasthenia gravis, ulcerative colitis.

Amyloidosis of the adrenal gland (Fig. 300). *Amyloid deposition in the adrenal cortex occurs regularly in cases of general amyloidosis (kidney, spleen, liver). Clinical adrenal cortical insufficiency can develop in severe cases.* The section shows a small artery (→ 1) in the capsule, in the wall of which a homogeneous, red-stained deposit can be seen. In the cortex, the amyloid is deposited around capillaries. The zona glomerulosa is unaffected (→ 2). Broad bands of amyloid in the zona fasciculata (→ 3) and reticularis (→ 4) have caused pressure atrophy of the cortical cells.

Macroscopic: The adrenals are enlarged and appear glassy.

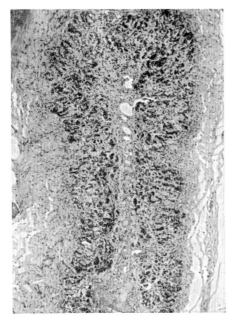

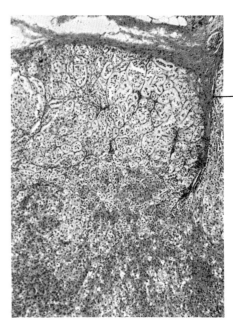

Fig. 301. Atrophy of the adrenal cortex;
H & E, 66×.

Fig. 302. Hyperplasia of the adrenal cortex in
Cushing's disease;
H & E, 64×.

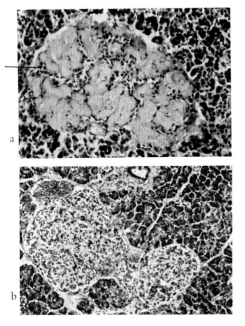

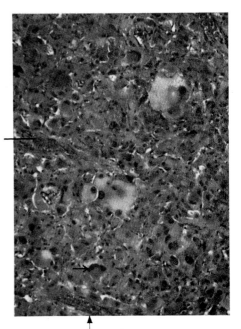

Fig. 303 a. Hyalinization of an islet of Langerhans (diabetes mellitus); H & E, 170×.
Fig. 303 b. Islet hyperplasia (newborn of a
diabetic mother); H & E, 127×.

Fig. 304. Pheochromocytoma;
H & E, 130×.

Atrophy of adrenal cortex (Fig. 301). Adrenal insufficiency may result from primary disease of the adrenal cortex (tuberculosis, cytotoxic contraction, hemorrhage, etc.), so-called *primary adrenal insufficiency*. Clinically, the picture is that of *Addison's disease*. On the other hand, adrenal insufficiency may be *secondary to insufficient hypophyseal stimulation* (ACTH deficiency) as in postpartum pituitary necrosis or scarring (SHEEHAN, 1955), or after infections or trauma.

Figure 301 is from a patient with *Sheehan's syndrome and secondary cortical atrophy*. The cortex is much reduced and the various zones are completely disorganized. The cortex consists solely of clumps and groups of cells, the arrangement of which is faintly reminiscent of the zona glomerulosa. There is also proliferation of interstitial fibrous tissue.

Macroscopically, the adrenal gland is paper-thin. *Clinically*, there is panhypopituitarism, so-called Simmond's disease.

Adrenal cortical hyperplasia in Cushing's disease (Fig. 302): In Cushing's syndrome, there is overproduction of adrenocortical hormone (glucocorticoid), with metabolic transformation from protein manufacture to production of glucose and fat. In 60% of cases, the adrenal cortex shows hyperplasia which is dependent upon increased ACTH production by a basophilic or chromophobic pituitary adenoma. Usually, no pituitary tumor can be found, however (primary hyperplasia of unknown cause). True adrenal cortical adenomas (or carcinoma in children) may also cause the syndrome.

Figure 302 shows great widening of the adrenal cortex (compare this with Fig. 301, which is at the same magnification), which is so great that only a portion of the cortex can be shown. The zona fasciculata extends to the connective tissue capsule →, in the upper part of which there are fat-laden cells (the fat has been dissolved in preparation of the section), arranged in ball fashion, →: radiating septum of connective tissue (beginning adenoma formation, nodular hyperplasia).

Macroscopic: Enlarged adrenals, showing a wide yellow cortex and nodular hyperplasia or adenomas.

Clinical: Obesity of the trunk, full-moon visage, thick neck, striae, hypertonus, osteoporosis, diabetes.

Islet hyalinization in diabetes mellitus (Fig. 303 a). Hyalinization of the capillaries of the islets of Langerhans may be found, particularly in diabetes in elderly persons (not in young persons!). Whether this is the cause or the consequence of the diabetes is disputed. The hyalin material is deposited in the wall of the capillaries, obstructs the lumen and secondarily causes atrophy of the islet cells (→).

Islet hyperplasia (newborn of a diabetic mother) (Fig. 303 b). This is considered an adaptation hyperplasia of the islets of Langerhans of the fetus to the hyperglycemia of the diabetic mother. The richly cellular giant islets can be easily seen under low magnification. Higher magnification shows, in addition, greatly enlarged nuclei and often multinucleated giant cells (β-cell hyperplasia).

Pheochromocytoma (Figs. 304, 305). This is usually a benign tumor (malignant examples are rare) of the adrenal medulla (most unilateral, 40–50 years). Most have endocrine activity (periodic outpouring of adrenalin and noradrenalin. *Clinical:* Increase in blood pressure, hyperglycemia).

The histological picture shows epithelial tumor tissue arranged in strands or cellular balls, often situated perivascularly (→: vessel). The cells are large, round or polygonal and pleomorphic and frequently have eccentrically situated nuclei. Giant cells are seen frequently (→). Expanding hemorrhage is common. The brown color produced by the chromate reaction (dichromate salts) demonstrates adrenalin (fine granules) and noradrenalin producing cells (large granules) (Fig. 305). Noradrenalin can be identified with potassium iodide (KRACHT et al., 1958; WEBER, 1949; SHERWIN et al., 1965). Commonly there is hemorrhage and resulting deposition of hemosiderin (Fig. 305).

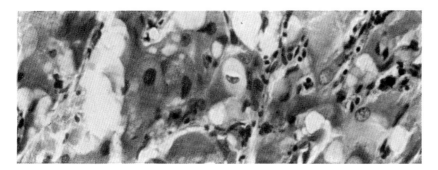

Fig. 305. Pheochromocytoma after chromation; H & E, 375×.

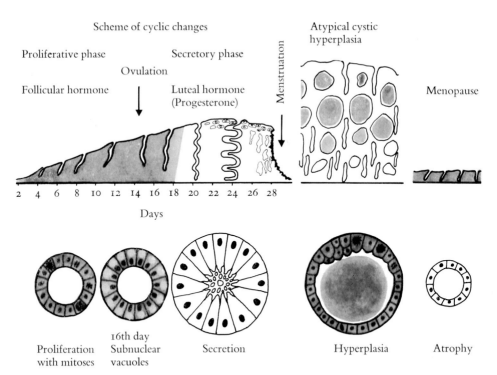

Scheme of cyclic changes

Atypical cystic hyperplasia

Proliferative phase

Secretory phase

Ovulation

Follicular hormone

Luteal hormone (Progesterone)

Menstruation

Menopause

2   4   6   8   10   12   14   16   18   20   22   24   26   28

Days

Proliferation with mitoses

16th day Subnuclear vacuoles

Secretion

Hyperplasia

Atrophy

Fig. 306. Schematic representation of the histological changes occurring in the endometrium during the menstrual cycle and in various endocrine disorders.

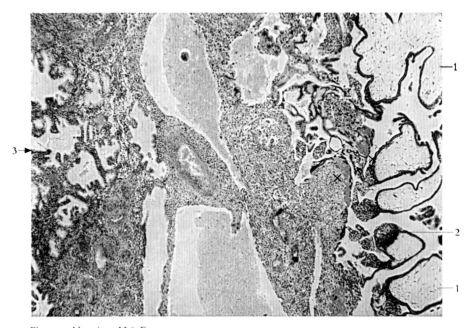

Fig. 307. Abortion; H & E, 50×.

Endometerium

Figure 306 is a schematic representation of the changes occurring in the endometrium during the normal menstrual cycle as well as during endocrine disorders.

In the normal cycle, *estrogens* (estradiol, follicular hormone) elicit progressive growth of the uterine mucosa (endometrium), including *glandular proliferation* (4th–14th day). The glands are deep and become slightly tortuous toward the end of the proliferative phase. After ovulation (14th day), the *secretory phase* begins with the secretion of the corpus luteal hormones, and *subnuclear vacuoles* (glycogen) appear in the glandular epithelium as the first sign of the progesterone effect. With increasing secretion, the nuclei take a more basal position in the cell, while bud-like *secretory granules* collect at the apex of the cell. Droplets can be demonstrated in the glandular lumina. On the whole, the cytoplasm is clear (compare with the dark epithelial cells of the proliferative phase). The glands are now markedly tortuous, and the stromal cells larger. In the uppermost layers of the mucosa (compacta) there appear large stromal cells that resemble the decidual cells seen in pregnancy *(pseudodecidual transformation)*. *Regressive changes* make their appearance at the 24th–26th day. The glandular nuclei become pyknotic. The stroma becomes loosened until, during *menstruation*, the hemorrhagic mucosa is sloughed off. Regeneration begins again from the glandular remnants in the basalis.

When endocrine dysfunction occurs, as, for example, in *overproduction of estrogens* (persistent follicle, granulosa or theca cell tumor of the ovary), the endometrium becomes hyperplastic, and numerous, rather characteristic, dilated and cystic glands develop which are lined with stratified, cuboidal epithelium *(atypical cystic hyperplasia)*. *Hypofunction* of the ovary leads to *atrophy of the mucosa* similar to that seen physiologically after the menopause.

Abortion (Figs. 307, 308). Histologic examination of shed material from an abortion (expulsion of the fetus within the first 28 weeks of pregnancy) provides an opportunity to study the placental tissues and the uterine mucosa of pregnancy. The remnants of the placenta consist of chorionic villi (→ 1 in Fig. 307) composed of a loose core of mucoid tissue and connective tissue fibers covered by the Langhans cell layer and the syncytial cell layer (without sharp cell boundaries), which is interspersed with islands of giant-cell-like proliferation (→ 2). Later, the syncytial layers undergo fibrinoid transformation (×, homogeneous, eosinophilic material), as does the decidua (secondary so-called white infarcts of the placenta).

Decidual transformation of the endometrium (Fig. 308) consists of marked enlargement of the stroma cells which acquire large, round nuclei and a large amount of cytoplasm. The mucosal glands (→ 3 in Fig. 307) are very tortuous. The epithelium appears as tall, pale, non-secretory cells. A lack of chorionic villi should suggest the possibility of ectopic pregnancy.

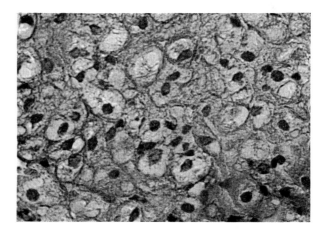

Fig. 308. Decidua; H & E, 512 ×.

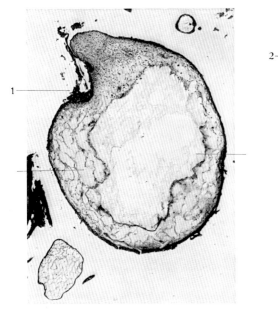

Fig. 309. Hydatidiform mole;
H & E, 31×.

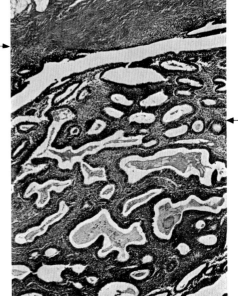

Fig. 310. Endometriosis of the abdominal wall;
H & E, 48×.

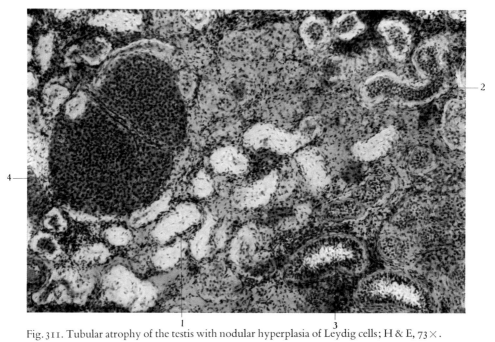

Fig. 311. Tubular atrophy of the testis with nodular hyperplasia of Leydig cells; H & E, 73×.

Hydatidiform mole (Fig. 309). *Hydatidiform mole is a translucent, mucoid, cystic swelling of the chorionic villi of unknown etiology. It is conjectured that the changes are due to a "missed abortion" of a poorly viable ovum. As a result of incomplete or absent development of fetal vasculature, coupled with unimpeded activity of the trophoblasts, swelling of the villi and changes in the chorionic epithelium occur after about 8 weeks. The contents of the cysts correspond to normal chorionic fluid. (These statements are based on findings of early abortions and of placentas with regional circulatory abnormalities.)* Microscopically, there is marked swelling of the chorionic villi and the stroma is loose and myxomatous (→). At the same time, there is proliferation of chorionic epithelium (→ 1: Langhans and syncytial cell layers). Invasion of the uterine wall *(chorioadenoma destruens)*, as well as malignant change *(chorion carcinoma, Fig. 429, p. 252)*, can result, depending upon the degree of proliferation and differentiation. Less frequently, deposits of hydrophic vesicular villi are found in the adnexa or lungs as well as other organs.

Macroscopic: Large, vesicular, grape-like structures. Following curettage, it is important clinically to follow the urinary chorionic gonadotropin in order to detect possible recurrent proliferation or malignant transformation as early as possible.

Endometriosis of the abdominal wall (Fig. 310). *Endometriosis is the growth of endometrial tissue outside the uterine cavity.* Histologically, there are typical endometrial glands and a small cell stroma (→ 1). Notice the difference from adenocarcinoma (proliferation of glands without typical stromal cells). The glands in endometriosis show focal cystic dilatation and contain coagulated protein. The mucosa shows cyclical activity *(clinically, pain occurs at four weekly intervals but in the middle of the period)*. Frequently, hemosiderin is found in the stroma and points to previous bleeding. The nodule illustrated here occurred in the anterior abdominal wall. There is a capsule of fat and connective tissue (→ 2).

Sites: In the wall of the uterus, where the condition is called adenomyosis uteri, the walls of the fallopian tubes, the external genitalia, laparotomy scars, the navel or in the inguinal region.

Macroscopic: Brown or bluish black nodules.

Tubular atrophy of the testis with focal nodular hyperplasia of Leydig cells (Fig. 311). *A great number of conditions (mumps and other inflammations, heart disease, irradiation, pressure, hypoxia, etc.) can lead to scarring or complete atrophy of the testes.*
The germinal epithelium is very sensitive and is destroyed first. Figure 311 shows complete sclerosis of the tubules (→ 1) and marked fibrosis of the tunica propria. A few nuclei are seen in the nearly totally obliterated lumens. In some regions, the process has not progressed so far. Sertoli cells have been spared (→ 2). In a few tubules, spermatogenesis is almost normal (→ 3). A conspicuous feature of testicular atrophy from any cause is localized, almost adenomatous, *proliferation of Leydig interstitial cells* (→ 4). The cause of the testicular atrophy is not clear in most cases.
Testicular atrophy can be caused by endocrine disturbances or have a genetic basis, as in sclerosing tubular degeneration (Klinefelter syndrome: tall men with eunuchoid growth characteristics, gynecomastia and sterility. Most have 3 sex chromosomes – XXY). Hormonal factors are also involved in testicular atrophy accompanying cirrhosis of the liver or the use of hormone therapy for carcinoma of the prostate.

Macroscopic: Small, firm testes with brown cut surfaces. The testicular tubules do not separate as easily as normally.

191

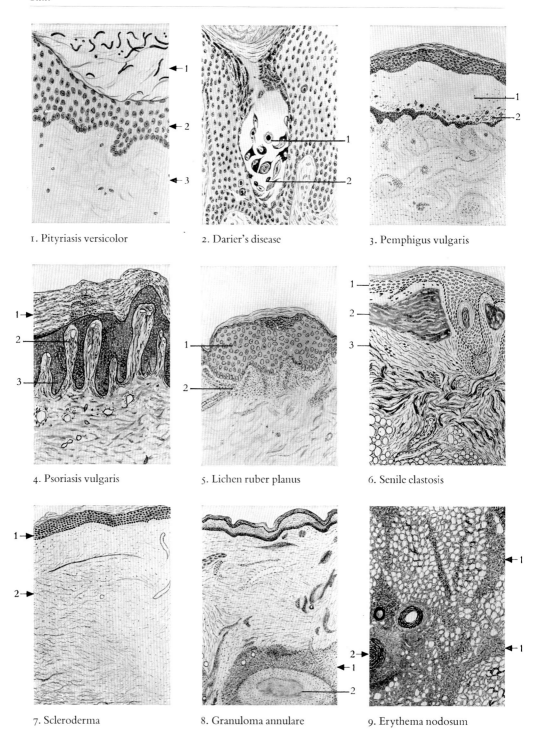

1. Pityriasis versicolor 2. Darier's disease 3. Pemphigus vulgaris

4. Psoriasis vulgaris 5. Lichen ruber planus 6. Senile elastosis

7. Scleroderma 8. Granuloma annulare 9. Erythema nodosum

Fig. 312. Diagram of examples of the different sorts of skin alterations.

Skin

The histopathology of the skin constitutes a difficult and complicated area of knowledge and those who are especially interested should consult the special books written on the subject, such as LEVER.

Figure 312 (1–9) depicts in diagrammatic form some of the many diseases of the skin. They are shown from the standpoint of their localization in the various layers of the skin: a) disturbances of cornification, b) of the epidermis, c) of the epidermis and corium, d) of the corium and e) of the subcutis.

a) Cornified layer: Pityriasis versicolor (Fig. 312/1). This is a fungal disease manifested by reddish brown spots. The causative agent (Microsporum furfur) is found in the stratum corneum ($\rightarrow$ 1) in the form of hyphae and spores. The epidermis ($\rightarrow$ 2) and corium ($\rightarrow$ 3) are not involved. **Darier's disease** (Fig. 312/2). This is a hereditary skin disease manifested by brownish red kerato-follicular papules, most of which occur in groups. Histologically, there is follicular and para-follicular hyperkeratosis and dyskeratosis with "corps ronds" ($\rightarrow$ 1) and "grains" (kernels $\rightarrow$ 2). Lacunar, mostly sub-basal, spaces or vesicles also develop. **b) Epidermis: Pemphigus vulgaris** (Fig. 312/3). Vesicles developed on otherwise unaltered or occasionally faintly reddened skin (mucous membranes may also be affected). Microscopically, there are intraepidermal ($\rightarrow$ 1) and sub-basal acantholysis (= lysis of the epidermal cement substance) and vesicles containing degenerated epithelial cells ($\rightarrow$ 2). **c) Epidermis and corium: Psoriasis vulgaris** (Fig. 312/4). A familial, progressive disease which presents as sharply delimited erythematous, maculopapillary eruptions overlaid with pale silver scales. The microscopic picture shows parakeratosis (= nucleated scales, $\rightarrow$ 1), acanthosis (= prolongation of the epidermal columns $\rightarrow$ 3) and papillomatosis ($\rightarrow$ extension of the papillary bodies, including the connective tissue and blood vessels of the corium, nearly to the horny layer, $\rightarrow$ 2). Dilated vessels, perivascular edema and infiltration of lymphocytes, histiocytes and leukocytes are seen in the stratum papillare and stratum reticulare. The microabscesses, which are not always found, contain compacted neutrophilic leukocytes in the epidermis. **Lichen ruber planus** (Fig. 312/5). This is a dermatosis accompanied by marked itching, irregularly marginated livid red papules and a waxy sheen (variants: verrucous lichen ruber, follicular and pemphigoid lichen ruber). The principal histological feature is a so-called mixed papule consisting of thickened, hyperkeratotic epidermis ($\rightarrow$ 1) and a band-like infiltrate composed predominantly of lymphocytes. It occurs in the basal cell layer, which shows vacuolar degeneration and has a moth-eaten appearance. **d) Corium: Senile elastosis** (Fig. 312/6). This develops in exposed areas of the skin (strong solar radiation) in seamen and farmers and in elderly men. It is a dermatosis marked by atrophy, yellowish pigmentation and wrinkling (cutis rhomboidalis), especially in the region of the forehead, zygomatic arch, bridge of the nose and neck. Histologically, the picture is that of senile elastosis with flattened epidermis ($\rightarrow$ 1) and degeneration of the elastic fibers (thickened, fragmented) which, along with the collagen fibers, stain intensely with elastica dyes ($\rightarrow$ 2). $\rightarrow$ 3 = atrophy of the collagenous fibers of the connective tissue. **Scleroderma** (Fig. 312/7). Clinically, the disease occurs in circumscribed and diffuse forms, both of which are characterized by decreased elasticity and hardening (pachydermia) of the skin. The diffuse form is progressive and involves internal organs (e. g., lung, esophagus, gastrointestinal tract). Microscopically, both forms of the disease show similar changes. Apart from the erythema and edema at the onset, the full-blown picture is recognized by the narrow epidermis ($\rightarrow$ 1) and the greatly widened corium ($\rightarrow$ 2). Broad, interlacing collagen fibers, destruction of pre-existing elastic fibers, newly formed delicate collagen and elastic fibers, vascular dilatation and contraction as well as a slight inflammatory infiltrate, especially around vessels, are the essential features. **Granuloma annulare** (Fig. 312/8). In this condition, the skin shows pea-sized areas of discoloration; occasionally it is white or yellowish, in the center of which sits a slightly depressed papule forming a complete or incomplete ring shape (the lesions occur usually on the extremities, particularly of children). Microscopically the corium shows round or oval nodules of granulation tissue ($\rightarrow$ 1), lymphocytes, histiocytes, fibroblasts, occasional giant cells and central necrosis ($\rightarrow$ 2). The cells of the granulation tissue are often arranged radially from the center of the nodules. **e) Subcutis: Erythema nodosum** (Fig. 312/9). The lesions appear on the extensor surfaces of the lower legs. They are raised, discoid, reddish, infiltrated lesions covered with smooth skin and sensitive to pressure. The essential histological findings are localized in the subcutaneous fat tissue and neighboring corium. Nodular and streak-like infiltrates ($\rightarrow$ 1, along the septa of the fat tissue) of lymphocytes, histiocytes, leukocytes and occasional eosinophils without necrosis, make up the tissue changes. Small radially arranged collections of regimented histiocytes and fibroblasts may also be seen. Here and there, blood vessels are involved in the inflammatory process. Endophlebitis may develop ($\rightarrow$ 2).

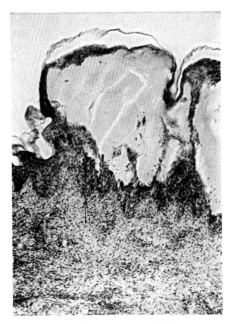

Fig. 313. Vesicular eruption in chickenpox (varicella); H & E, 60×.

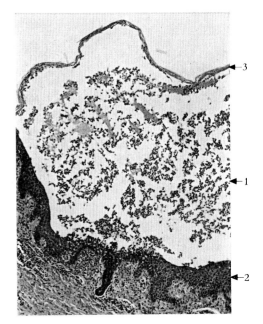

Fig. 314. Subcorial pustule; H & E, 80×.

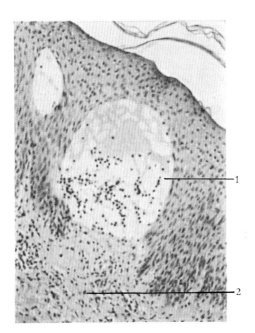

Fig. 315. Dermatitis herpetiformis; H & E, 125×.

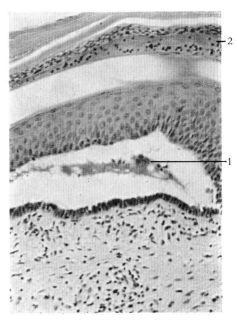

Fig. 316. Pemphigus erythematosus (seborrheic pemphigus); H & E, 125×.

Vesicular eruption in chickenpox (Fig. 313). *This is a virus disease characterized by a generalized vesicular and pustular exanthem.* Histologically, there is intraepidermal vesicle formation just as in smallpox, herpes zoster and herpes simplex. Figure 313 shows such a vesicle containing homogeneous protein material. The uppermost epidermal layer forms the outer margin, and a thin basal layer (→) delimits the vesicle from the dermis. The dermis is slightly infiltrated with lymphocytes. The intraepidermal vesicle is formed from the deterioration of epidermal cells. Intranuclear inclusion bodies are present (viral inclusion bodies?). Similar vesicles, but without inclusion bodies, are seen in the skin in burns and freezing. Vesicular inflammation is often complicated by suppuration, in which case the lesion is termed a pustule.

Macroscopic: Vesicles with clear, serous contents or pustules and a hemorrhagic rash.

Subcorial pustule (Fig. 314). This disease, which attacks women more frequently than men, is a relapsing, progressive dermatitis (Sneddon-Wilkinson's disease) and involves the skin of the trunk, shoulders, groin and proximal portions of the extremities. Histologically, there are vesicular or bullous spaces filled with neutrophils and eosinophils (→ 1). The epidermis (→ 2), which is partly loosened, forms the base, and the horny layer (→ 3) the roof of the pustule. The upper corium that is adjacent to the base of the pustule shows a perivascular chronic inflammatory infiltrate.

Macroscopic: Grouped, yellowish white pustules of pepper corn or pea size showing erosion and crusting.

Dermatitis herpetiformis (Fig. 315). *This is a dermatitis of allergic origin (Duhring-Brocq's disease) which causes an irritating pruritus. The disease involves particularly the trunk, buttocks and scalp.* In contrast to pemphigus vulgaris and seborrheic pemphigus (which show intraepidermal vesicles, see p. 193 and Fig. 316), the microscopic picture of dermatitis herpetiformis consists of subepidermal vesicles or bleb formations (→ 1). In the vesiculo-bullous eruptions, many eosinophilic leukocytes are found. The dermal connective tissue forming the floor of the vesicles shows a marked inflammatory reaction (→ 2). Edema, dilated blood vessels, eosinophilic leukocytes and lymphocytes are present.

Macroscopic: The clinical picture is pleomorphic. Erythema, urticaria, vesicles and bullae occur. Often, the eruption is herpetiform. A symmetrical distribution is often apparent.

Pemphigus erythematosus or seborrheic pemphigus (Fig. 316). This is a clinically important variant of pemphigus vulgaris (Fig. 312/3) described by SENEAR and USHER. It localizes on the scalp, the face and in the sweaty folds of the anterior and posterior skin of the trunk.
Histologically, just as in pemphigus vulgaris, there is formation of intraepidermal vesicles resulting from acantholysis with so-called Tzanck cells (→ 1) in the vesicular spaces. In contrast to pemphigus vulgaris, however, the intraepidermal changes are often discrete and the vesicles are shallower, often consisting merely of clefts. Also, the follicles (the ostia of the follicles are dilated) and the epithelium of the sebaceous glands are involved. There may be a superimposed parakeratotic change in the stratum corneum (→ 2). The corium is scantily infiltrated with lymphocytes and histiocytes in the early stage, but in older lesions there is a marked infiltrate of these cells.

Macroscopic: There is often a secondary impetigenous, seborrheic eczema, or the disease may localize in the face as an erythema (for this reason, it is called pemphigus erythematosus or erythematodes). The disease picture consists of loose vesicles, scales, crusts and erythema.

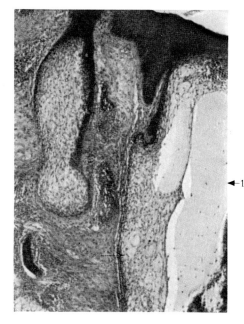

Fig. 317. Psoriasis vulgaris; histochemical reaction for non-specific esterase; 75×.

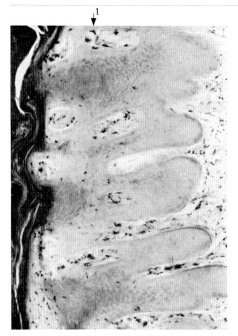

Fig. 318. Follicular mucinosis; H & E, 50×.

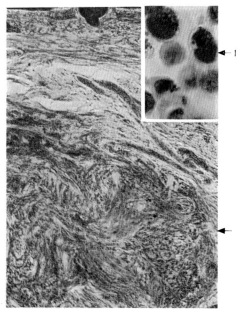

Fig. 319a. Xanthoma tuberosum (xanthofibroma); Sudan-hematoxylin stain, 50×. Inset: H & E, 480×.

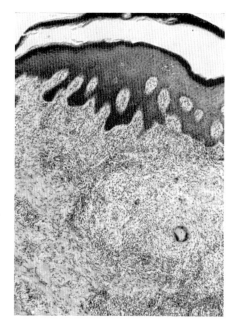

Fig. 320. Tuberculosis (lupus vulgaris); H & E, 60×.

Psoriasis vulgaris (Fig. 317, also Fig. 312/4). A characteristic feature of the histological picture of psoriasis is the non-specific esterase reaction. Numerous esterase-positive cells are present in the papillary and subpapillary strata. The parakeratotic horny layer is strongly positive (normally it is positive only in the so-called intermediate zone). There are numerous histiocytic elements, so-called lipophages (→ 1), which are already present during the ripening of the psoriatic papule. The clinical features and the general histological findings are shown on pages 192, 193.

Follicular mucinosis (Fig. 318). *This is a disease of hair follicles and sweat glands. One form is of unknown etiology and is manifested by flat or raised brownish red nodules (on hairy regions of the skin it is known as alopecia mucinosa of Pinkus). Another form occurs as a part of mycosis fungoides and reticulosis of the skin.*

Figure 318 shows the hydropic-vacuolar degeneration of the follicular epithelium and sebaceous glands which leads to disintegration of the attachments of the cells (→ within the picture) and cyst formation (→ 1: a cystically dilated hair follicle filled with mucin). The affected cells and the cysts stain red with mucicarmine and contain positive alcian blue material (acid mucopolysaccharides).

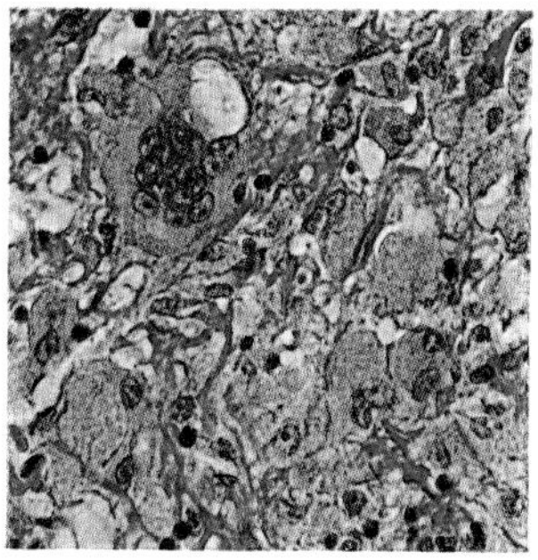

Xanthoma tuberosum or Xanthofibroma (Fig. 319a). These patients show a reddish yellow, nodular eruption (sites of predilection: elbows, patella, hands, Achilles tendon, buttocks) accompanied by either hypercholesterolemia (clear blood serum) or hyperlipemia (milky serum). New nodules show a preponderance of histiocytes with variegated, markedly foamy cytoplasm (foam or xanthoma cells → 1). Frequently, there are Touton-type giant cells (see Fig. 319b). The giant cells have centrally located nuclei and frequently the cytoplasm is vacuolated. Typical foamy cells occur in the lesions. Older lesions show, in addition, fibroblasts and fibrocytes showing fiber formation. With the Sudan stain, reddish or orange deposits of fat are seen

Fig. 319b. Touton type giant cells and foam cells; Azan stain, 500×.

both intracellularly and extracellularly (→). Histochemical analyses of the fatty material as well as investigations with the polarizing microscope, even without knowledge of the blood biochemical findings, permits provisional division of xanthomas into those with hypercholesterolemia (excess cholesterin is demonstrable in the tissues) and those with hyperlipemia (excess neutral fats).

Tuberculosis of skin (lupus vulgaris) (Fig. 320). Of the different forms of cutaneous tuberculosis and tuberculoid lesions, *tuberculous lupus vulgaris* will be discussed here. Histologically, it is restricted mainly to the upper layer of the dermis. The lesions are not unusual, resembling ordinary epithelioid cell granulomas (compare with tuberculous lymphadenitis, Fig. 273). Figure 320 shows a small epithelioid cell granuloma with one Langhans giant cell containing almost circularly arranged nuclei. There is slight lymphocytic infiltration at the periphery of the granuloma, with extension far into the adjoining tissues. Collagen fibers have also proliferated. The epidermis shows hyperkeratosis and acanthosis (longer rete pegs). Precancerous lesions and even basal cell carcinoma may develop, especially following therapeutic x-radiation *(lupoid carcinoma)*.

Macroscopic: Red or brownish red nodules appearing mostly on the face. Ulceration of the epidermis and secondary infection may develop.

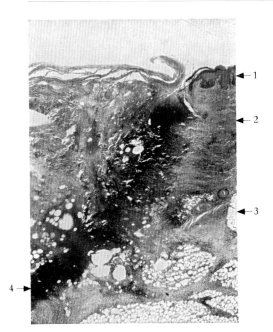

Fig. 321. Decubitus;
H & E, 15×.

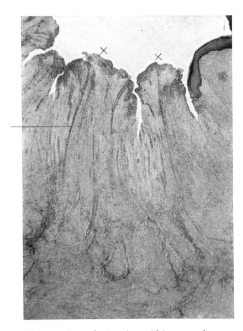

Fig. 322. Granulation tissue (skin wound),
healing by second intention;
H & E, 15×.

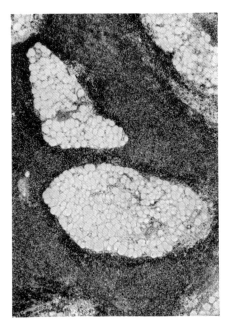

Fig. 323. Acute phlegmonous inflammation of
subcutaneous fat tissue (cellulitis);
H & E, 42×.

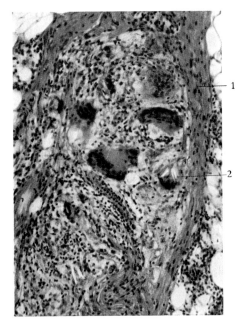

Fig. 324. Foreign body granuloma;
H & E, 150×.

Decubitus (Fig. 321). *This is an example of cutaneous necrosis due to local tissue death resulting from prolonged pressure. This type of necrosis occurs most frequently over the ischium in bedridden patients and is due to compression of blood vessels and eventual ulceration.* The histological picture reveals preserved epidermis (top right in Fig. 321 → 1), corium (→ 2) and subcutaneous tissues (→ 3). A blue-staining zone of leukocytes and cellular debris cuts transversely through the section (→ 4). This blends into another necrotic, anuclear zone on the left hand side of the picture, in which fat tissue is still faintly recognizable and local hemorrhage has occurred. Secondarily, granulation tissue can infiltrate and replace the necrotic tissue, producing an ulcer.

Granulation tissue (skin wound) (Fig. 322). Immature, new connective tissue accompanied by proliferating capillaries (angioblasts), fibroblasts and histiocytes as well as by infiltration of varying numbers of lymphocytes and plasma cells act to resorb and replace injured and necrotic tissues of the host. Resorption is a prominent feature of chronic inflammation and the granulation tissue contains large numbers of inflammatory cells (compare Fig. 471). Replacement of tissue, however, is achieved principally by proliferation of new capillary loops and fibroblasts (e. g., in a cutaneous defect or gastric ulcer). The section shows healing of a cutaneous injury, in which the granulation tissue has already grown to the level of the epidermis. It also shows individual granulations (×) composed of budding granulation tissue in which there are long, parallel nutrient vessels reaching to the surface (→). The surface is covered by a flat layer of fibrin.

Macroscopic: Raspberry-like granulations covering the surface (proud flesh).

Acute phlegmonous inflammation (cellulitis) of subcutaneous fat tissue (Fig. 323). Diffuse leukocytic inflammation of the skin has developed mainly in the loose subcutaneous fat tissue, in which it can easily spread. Histologically, there is a diffuse, dense, streak-like infiltration of polymorphonuclear leukocytes (see Fig. 173a and b). Streptococci are the usual causative agent.

Macroscopic: Gelatinous appearing, grayish white tissue. Phlegmons in the floor of the mouth are particularly liable to extend to the mediastinum. Erysipelas is usually caused by β-hemolytic streptococci.

Foreign body granuloma (Figs. 324, 325). *The inability of tissues to resorb foreign bodies stimulates the development of granulation tissue, the increased resorbing capacity of which is indicated by the appearance of giant cells. Foreign bodies frequently encountered include suture material, talcum powder, crystalline particles, injected oily solutions. Endogenous substances, such as the horny lamellae from an epidermoid cyst, cholesterol crystals or amyloid may also elicit a foreign body giant cell reaction. The giant cells engulf the foreign bodies and attempt to digest them (see p. 16).* Histologically, the section shows scar tissue (→ 1) in the periphery and proliferating capillaries, fibroblasts and lymphocytes in the central zone. Giant cells are present and contain spindle-shaped cytoplasmic crystals (→ 2) which are very clearly displayed under the polarizing microscope (Fig. 325). The nuclei in the giant cells are closely packed on the side opposite to the ingested material.

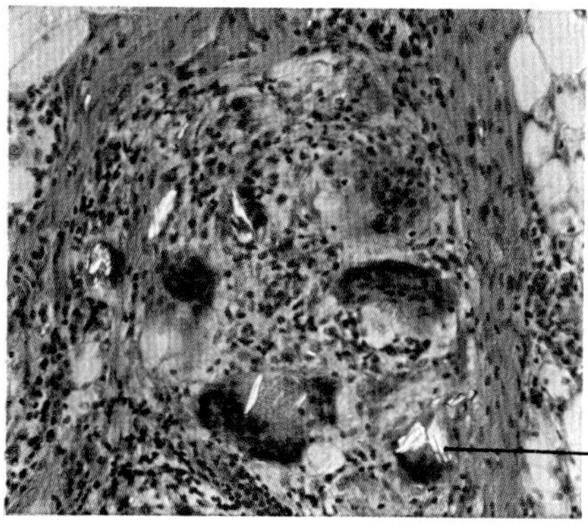

Fig. 325. Foreign body granuloma viewed with polarized light; H & E, 150×.

199

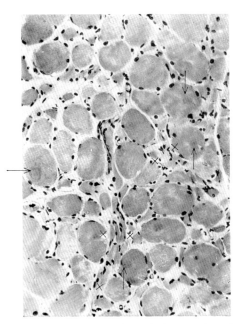

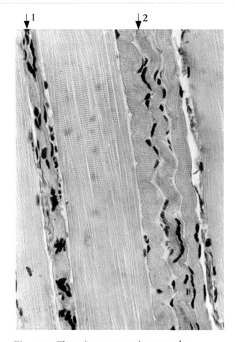

Fig. 326. Recent atrophy with degeneration of muscle fibers occurring in acute polyneuritis; H & E, 170×.

Fig. 327. Chronic neurogenic muscular atrophy in polyneuritis; H & E, 320×.

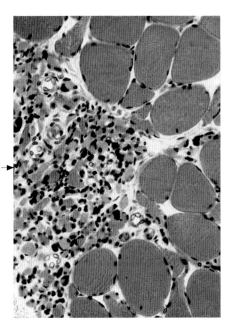

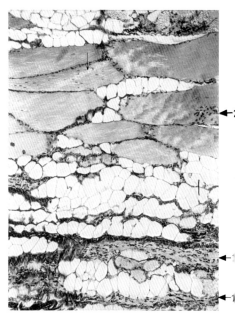

Fig. 328. Progressive spinal muscular atrophy (in early infancy); H & E, 233×.

Fig. 329. Progressive spinal muscular atrophy (pseudomyogenic form); van Gieson, 60×.

Muscles

Skeletal muscles can be affected in *generalized disease states* or they can be *affected independently*. In both cases, the result is either *degeneration of the muscle fibers* themselves or secondary involvement of the muscle from extension of primary disease of the *interstitial tissues*. In primary degenerative muscle disease, acute degenerative changes occur and lead to necrosis. They must, of course, be differentiated from chronic atrophies of muscle fibers.

Muscular atrophies are the result of neurogenic or of myogenic disease. The basis of *neurogenic atrophies* is peripheral denervation, due either to a primary lesion in the anterior horn cells *(spinal muscular atrophy)* or to a lesion along the course of the *peripheral motor nerves*.

The early stages of **neurogenic muscular atrophy** are well seen in cases of polyneuritis. Figure 326 **(recent muscular atrophy in acute polyneuritis)** illustrates the atrophy of individual muscle fibers in cross-section (between the crosses). The fibers are smaller and the nuclei lie closer together. Although the other muscle fibers seem unchanged in size, they already show early degeneration, as evidenced by the loss of their regular fibrillary cytoplasmic structure (compare this with Fig. 328) and the very characteristic localized clumps of contractile material, the so-called target fibers ($\rightarrow$).

If neurogenic atrophy develops slowly, the histological picture will consist of groups of markedly atrophic muscle fibers intermixed with essentially intact fibers. The former represent areas innervated by affected motor axons or their branches **(chronic neurogenic muscular atrophy in polyneuritis).** Figure 327 is a longitudinal section showing typical groups of atrophic muscle fibers. It can be seen that the fibers about $\rightarrow$ 1 are more severely atrophied than those about $\rightarrow$ 2. The atrophy in this case affects only small groups, corresponding to the so-called subunits of a motor unit.

Motor unit = anterior horn cell with its corresponding peripheral motor axon, its collaterals, the motor end plates and the muscle fibers. Depending upon the type of muscle involved, a motor unit is composed of 800–1,700 or more muscle fibers.

Spinal muscular atrophy, as a result of destruction of anterior horn cells, always involves entire motor units and not just subunits, leading to atrophy of all the muscle fibers supplied by a particular unit. Figure 328 **(the infantile form of progressive spinal muscular atrophy)** shows more widespread involvement of larger groups of muscle fibers ($\rightarrow$). The cross-sectional view reveals the very thin fibers and closely placed nuclei so that they seem to have multiplied (frustrated regeneration). The other muscle fibers are unaffected and have retained the integrity of their intracytoplasmic structure.

Spinal progressive muscular atrophy of adults (pseudomyogenic type) (Fig. 329). This lesion progresses very slowly so that adaptation and regeneration are prominent. The section shows a longitudinal section of a muscle bundle ($\rightarrow$ 1) surrounded by tongues of connective tissue and proliferated lipomatous tissue. The groups of intact muscle fibers undergo compensatory hypertrophy as a result of increased demand. There are increased numbers of nuclei, as well as centrally located multinuclear muscle cells ($\rightarrow$ and $\rightarrow$ 2). This fibroadipose transformation and replacement of muscle is a non-specific manifestation of chronic, progressive wasting of muscles. Similar changes to these are also seen in chronic muscular atrophy having an inflammatory or degenerative basis (Fig. 330).

I am indebted to Prof. Erbslöh (Director of the Neurology Clinic, University of Giessen) for Figures 326–332 and for his suggestions.

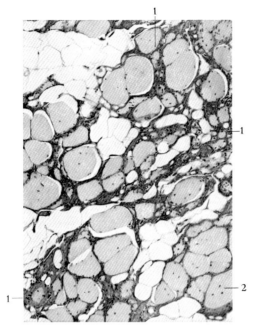

Fig. 330. Progressive muscular dystrophy (Erb);
van Gieson, 80×.

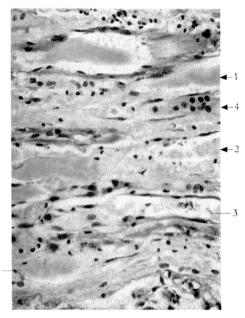

Fig. 331. Early muscular necrosis in acute
polymyositis;
H & E, 200×.

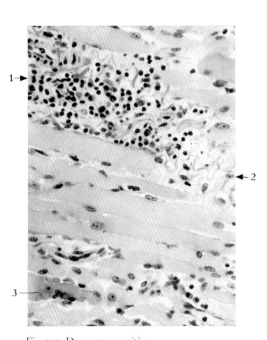

Fig. 332. Dermatomyositis;
H & E, 250×.

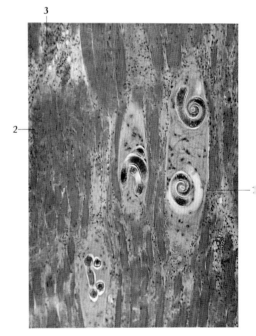

Fig. 333. Trichinosis;
H & E, 78×.

Progressive muscular dystrophy (Erb) (Fig. 330). In contrast to spinal progressive muscular atrophy, *the primary disturbance in progressive muscular dystrophy (myogenic atrophy) resides in the muscle cells themselves* (congenital metabolic disorder of unknown origin). Thus, the atrophic manifestations do not correspond to a motor unit distribution. Instead, they represent disseminated atrophy of individual fibers without regular distribution.

The section shows atrophic fibers (→ 1) adjoining numerous normal as well as hypertrophic fibers. Many have central nuclei (→ 2). In addition, the muscle fibers are surrounded by connective tissue and the degenerated and atrophic fibers have been replaced by fat tissues *(fibro-adipose replacement)*. The scar ring can produce secondarily a lobular arrangement of muscle bundles, giving a cirrhosis-like appearance.

Dystrophic muscles frequently show early stages of muscle fiber degeneration, such as occur in systemic diseases, e. g., the progressive degeneration of the abdominal musculature in typhoid. Figure 331 **(early muscular necrosis in acute polymyositis)** shows several types of degeneration that may lead to necrosis. The first change is often progressive waxy degeneration (→ 1) leading to dissolution of the fibrous proteins and cross-striations. Gradually, as the nuclei degenerate, lumpy aggregates become evident and as the sarcoplasm comes apart and vanishes, only empty sarcolemmal sheaths are left behind (→ 3) (compare Fig. 48, p. 38). Focal groups of muscle nuclei can be seen indicating a regenerative activity (→ 4).

Acute muscular degeneration of such severity often results in development of the so-called *crush-syndrome* in the kidney (see Fig. 288, p. 142). Not only does it occur with necrotizing myositis but also with *intoxications* (e. g., CO poisoning) or in severe muscle trauma.

Dermatomyositis (Fig. 332) is a *necrotizing panmyositis with dermatitis* which in the acute stages prominently displays the degenerative and necrotizing changes described above. In addition, the tissues are densely infiltrated with lymphocytes and plasma cells. In the subacute and chronic stages of this intermittently progressive disease, there is mainly interstitial infiltration (→ 1), scarring (→ 2) and tissue replacement. Additionally, there may be marked regeneration of the muscle fibers themselves (→ 3).

The clinical course of *necrotizing polymyositis* consists of extensive paralysis of the peripheral muscles, which, because of its resemblance to the muscular paralysis of trichinosis, is at times referred to as pseudotrichinosis.

Trichinosis of muscle (Fig. 333). *The embryos of Trichinella spiralis pass through the lacteals of the intestine into the blood stream, and so reach striated muscle, where they develop into spiral-shaped larvae.* Histologically, the cross-cut or tangentially cut, spiral-shaped trichinellae are surrounded by a hyalin capsule (→ 1) and can be easily seen even at low power. Adjoining muscle fibers show considerable alteration, e. g., granular and waxy degeneration (→ 2). The interstitial tissue contains aggregations of eosinophils and chronic inflammatory cells.

Macroscopic: Small white nodules.

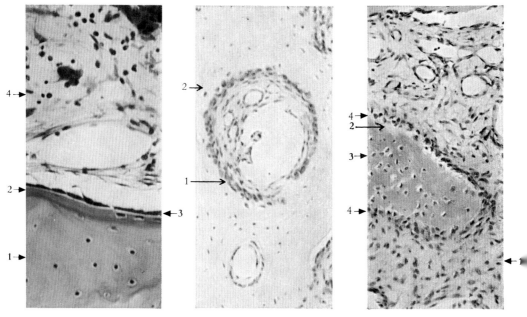

Fig. 334. Endosteal bone
formation;
H & E, 350×.

Fig. 335. Bone formation from
Haversian system;
H & E, 140×.

Fig. 336. Fibrous bone
formation;
H & E, 280×.

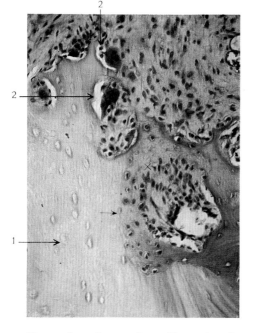

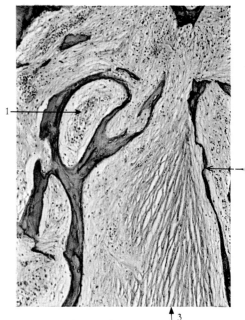

Fig. 337. Smooth resorption and formation of
lacunae in bone;
H & E, 250×.

Fig. 338. Perforating bone resorption;
van Gieson stain, 80×.

Bones and Joints

Microscopic study of bone sections necessitates knowledge of the *type of bony tissue* being examined (whether compact bone with Haversian systems or spongy bone without Haversian systems). The *quantitative relation between cancelous part and marrow space* must be evaluated (e. g., in the rarefaction due to osteoporosis) as well as the *types of cells appearing in the marrow spaces* (active hematopoietic, fatty or fibrous marrow, inflammatory infiltrates, etc.). It is important to see if the osteocytes in the *trabeculae* are stained (in bone necrosis the nuclei do not stain. Care must be exercised, however, for severe decalcification causes negative nuclear staining). The number of osteoblasts, the width of the osteoid margins, the degree of calcification of newly formed bone and the number of osteoclasts serve as an *indication of bone formation or resorption*.

In order to simplify the study of the various bone diseases, they will be considered only from the point of view of general pathology. Thus, the reaction of bony tissue to the stimulus of disease will be considered in terms either of *bone formation* or of *bone resorption*.

New bone is formed from connective tissue cells which, because of chemical or physical stimuli, differentiate to form osteoblasts. During this process of differentiation, the nuclei and nucleoli enlarge, the rough endoplasmic reticulum increases and the increased RNA causes increased basophilia. The *osteoblasts* fulfill three basic functions: 1. formation of mucopolysaccharide (MPS)-protein complexes, 2. synthesis of collagen fibers, 3. participation in mineralization. The acid and neutral mucopolysaccharides act as ion exchangers, which are destroyed by enzymatic action after mineralization.

With the light microscope, the following sites of bone formation can be differentiated: 1. *Periosteal bone formation* (proceeding from osteoblasts in the periosteum). This occurs in pathological situations, e. g., ossifying periostitis, chronic osteomyelitis, formation of a fracture callus. 2. *Endosteal bone formation* (proceeding from endosteal osteoblasts). This also is seen in pathological situations, e. g., formation of a fracture callus, chronic osteomyelitis (see Fig. 334). This type of bone formation often leads to gradual substitution of bone (see Fig. 337). Thus, there may be simultaneous bone resorption by cells with a single nucleus as well as formation of new bone. This occurs, for example, in osteitis deformans of Paget (simultaneous action of osteoclasts and osteoblasts). 3. New bone formation from the *Haversian systems* (see Fig. 335). In this case, the formation of new bone is accomplished by cells derived by differentiation from perivascular connective tissue cells. 4. Finally, *osteocytes* from the interlamellar osseous tissue can form bone (mostly when there is bone substitution and, therefore, accompanying bone resorption). In these various ways new bone is built like a shell around existing lamellar bone. However, new bone may also form without contact with bone previously formed in connective tissue, mostly in the bone marrow, (fibrous bone formation: no Haversian canals). Such fibrous bone can later convert to lamellar bone with Haversian canals.

Figure 334 shows **endosteal new bone formation.** Below, there is mineralization of bone ($\rightarrow$ 1) which is lying on a narrow zone of newly formed osteoid ($\rightarrow$ 2). Osteoid contains collagen fibers, MPS-protein complexes, but not hydroxyapatite, although there are large amounts of calcium (attached by ion binding to the acid MPS). Osteoid is formed by osteoblasts which can be seen as a single layer of cells with one nucleus ($\rightarrow$ 3). Above this is the loose connective tissue of the marrow cavity ($\rightarrow$ 4), most of which is richly vascularized. Figure 335 shows **new bone formation in the region of a Haversian canal.** Osteoblasts are forming an edge of bone in the periphery of the perivascular connective tissue ($\rightarrow$ 1). The boundary between new and old bone is marked by a cement line ($\rightarrow$ 2). **Fibrous bone** (Fig. 336). In the midst of the richly cellular collagenous connective tissue ($\rightarrow$ 1), fibroblasts differentiate to osteoblasts which become mineralized (nonmineralized intercellular substance: $\rightarrow$ 2; mineralized intercellular substance: $\rightarrow$ 3). The resulting bone trabeculae are again surrounded by osteoblasts ($\rightarrow$ 4). By special staining, it is possible to show that the collagen fibers in the surrounding connective tissue are continuous with those in the bone trabeculae.

Bone resorption results from the action of mononucleated or multinucleated connective tissue cells (osteoclasts). These cells are concerned with demineralization, enzymatic resorption of collagen (collagenase) and splitting of the MPS-protein complex (lysosomal enzymes). The most important morphological forms are: 1. *smooth resorption* (often in company with slow substitution), this is the commonest form of bone resorption by cells with a single nucleus. 2. *lacunar resorption* by multinucleated osteoclasts. These arise by fusion of cells with a single nucleus and can convert back to uninuclear cells. During the process of bone resorption, the osteoclasts develop numerous microvilli (electron microscopy) on the outer cell

Continued on page 207.

Healing of Fractures

Fracture hematoma	Temporary, provisional connective tissue callus	Temporary, provisional bony callus	Final definitive callus
1–2 days	2–8 days	1–4 weeks	4–6 weeks

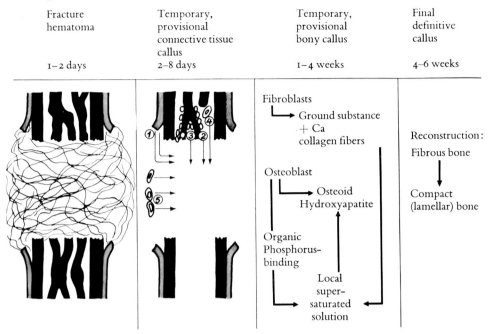

Fibroblasts
→ Ground substance
 + Ca
  collagen fibers

Osteoblast
→ Osteoid
  Hydroxyapatite

Organic
Phosphorus-
binding
→ Local super-saturated solution

Reconstruction:

Fibrous bone
↓
Compact
(lamellar) bone

Fig. 339. Diagram of the stages in the healing of fractures.

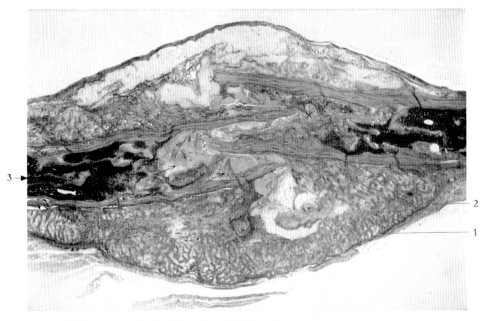

Fig. 340. Rib fracture with definitive callus; H & E, 7×.

membrane (this is morphological evidence of the increased work of resorption). Occurrence: particularly noticeable in brown tumors. 3. *Perforating resorption ("tunneling")*, which results from the action of cells of the Haversian system with one nucleus. This leads to excavations or lacunae in the bone trabeculae. Occurrence: e.g., in osteomyelitis and brown tumors.

Figure 337 shows **slow substitution** with smooth resorption and lacunar formation. In the lower left part of the picture there is necrotic bone (→ 1: empty spaces left by bone cells). At →, the old bone has been resorbed in layer fashion. In all probability, the resorption has been accomplished by the same uninucleated cells that are forming new bone at X. Bone resorption by osteoclasts (→ 2) leads to formation of lacunae (Howslip's lacunae) in resorbed bone.

Perforating resorption (Fig. 338) "tunnels" the bone trabeculae. Connective tissue cells with a single nucleus from the Haversian canals resorb the bone (→ 1). This process of resorption leaves only narrow strips of spongy trabecular (→ 2), until, finally, these also are resorbed and only poorly cellular connective tissue remains behind (→ 3).

The *regulation of bone resorption and bone formation* is accomplished under both normal and pathological circumstances by physical forces (chiefly effective locally) and chemical agents (generalized effect). For example, the operation of the piezoelectric effect, in which electric currents are formed that apparently change the cell performance (the exact mechanism of translation of electric current into the chemical "language" of the cell is still unknown). The action of parathyroid hormone is an example of a chemical agent which, along with other influences (kidney), has an effect on the cells of the skeletal system (this has been demonstrated in organ cultures) and in all probability stimulates bone resorption.

Bone Fracture

A fracture is a complete or partial break in the continuity of a bone. It sets in motion a series of regular tissue reactions, which lead to restoration of continuity. The results of these tissue reactions are depicted schematically in Figure 339. First, a **hematoma** forms between the two ends. As early as the second day, capillary loops and fibroblasts (granulation tissue) begin to grow into the hematoma. Starting points for formation of new tissue are (refer to the number in the second column of Fig. 339): 1. the periosteum, 2. the endosteum, i. e., osteoblasts, 3. the Haversian canals, 4. blood vessels in the marrow cavity, 5. blood vessels in the subcutaneous tissues and muscle. This leads to subsequent formation of a **provisional callus of connective tissue.** At the end of the first week, however, this already shows signs of being converted to a **provisional bony callus.** First, the immature connective tissue cells put down ground substance and collagen fibers. The fibroblasts develop into osteoblasts and produce osteoid, which is the organic matrix of bone. As a result of certain chemical reactions, calcium and phosphate form a supersaturated solution from which the mineralizing substance (secondary calcium phosphate hydroxyapatite) precipitates. This process constitutes the genesis of so-called *fibrous bone*, which by repeated remodeling by the action of osteoblasts and osteoclasts will give rise to *compact bone*. Only the latter can, in turn, form the **definitive callus.** Fracture healing may be regarded as the prototype of all healing processes in bony tissue.

Figure 340 (scanning lens view) shows a **rib fracture** with definitive callus formation. The fractured ends (×) are not well aligned, possibly because of the shearing forces of the respiratory or other movements. Such shearing forces produce cartilage formation (→) in the provisional callus. The healing process in the ribs is thus atypical, since the formation of the cartilaginous callus continues to progress. The fractured ends are surrounded not only by cartilaginous tissue but also by immature connective tissue and newly formed bone (→ 1) covered by periosteum (→ 2). Typical hematopoietic marrow can be seen at a distance from the fracture (→ 3).

The following *complications* of fracture or its delayed healing may occur: 1. *Fat embolism* (especially after fractures of long bones). 2. *Infection* of the reparative hematoma (osteomyelitis, especially after compound fractures). 3. Insufficient callus formation or interposition of soft tissues *(pseudarthrosis)*. 4. *Hyperactive callus formation* (exuberant callus causing pressure on soft tissues, nerves, etc.). 5. Formation of a *cartilaginous callus* (due to the development of shearing forces, leading to delayed healing of the fracture).

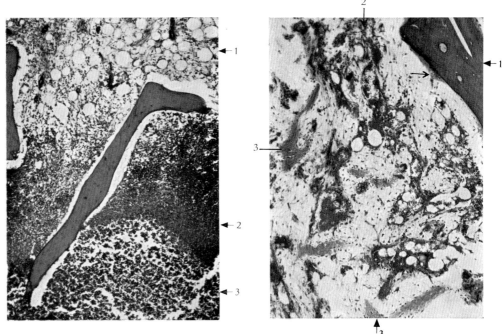

Fig. 341. Abscess of the bone marrow in acute osteomyelitis; H & E, 60×.

Fig. 342. Fibrous bone formation in chronic osteomyelitis; H & E, 95×.

Disorders in development of growing bones

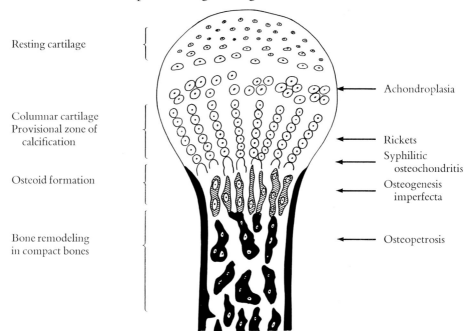

Resting cartilage

Columnar cartilage
Provisional zone of
    calcification

Osteoid formation

Bone remodeling
in compact bones

Achondroplasia

Rickets

Syphilitic
    osteochondritis

Osteogenesis
    imperfecta

Osteopetrosis

Fig. 343. Schematic representation of endochondral ossification and disorders of growing bone.

Inflammations of Bones

As in other organs, inflammations of bones can be either *non-specific* (acute osteomyelitis, chronic osteo-myelitis) or *specific* (e. g., tuberculosis, actinomycosis, syphilis). Whereas non-specific inflammations seem to have a predilection for *metaphysis or diaphysis*, specific inflammations (especially *tuberculosis*) prefer-entially affect the *epiphysis*. The regional bony structures are destroyed in the course of inflammation (loss of osteocytes, resorption by osteoclasts and blood vessels). The pieces of dead bone are partly seques-tered. In addition, new tissue grows (from the periosteum) around the dead bone (*sequestrum* of osteomyel-itis). As is to be expected, all types of inflammatory cells are found in the bone itself.

A *non-specific osteomyelitis* has been chosen as an example of a bone inflammation. Such an osteomyelitis can arise at a site of injury (e. g., in fractures or in otitis media) or it can be hema-togenous (e. g., in septicemia). Figure 341 shows a **marrow abscess** in an acute osteomyelitis of hematogenous origin. In the upper part of the picture there is fat marrow that has been infil-trated with granulocytes (→ 1). At → 2 is seen the necrotic wall containing granulocytes and fibrin. In the lower portion of the picture (→ 3) there is destruction of tissue and numerous polymorphonuclear leukocytes (abscess). Because of the necrosis, the bone trabeculae have lost their supporting matrix and are themselves necrotic. Bacterial toxins also contribute to the destruction of the osteocytes. A sequestrum of bone is formed (a piece of dead bone). In more advanced stages of osteomyelitis (chronic osteomyelitis, Fig. 342), there are dead bone trabeculae (→ 1) which can be seen in the picture to be overlaid with newly formed bone (→), thus form-ing a case for the dead bone. The marrow space shows fibrosis (loose collagenous tissue) and a perivascular inflammatory infiltrate of lymphocytes and plasma cells (→ 2). Beneath this, there is fibrous bone formation (→ 3).

Disorders in Development of Bones

Osteodystrophies are in some ways comparable to metabolic disturbances in other organs. One way to consider them is in terms of *growing* and *grown or adult bones*. Figure 343 is a **schematic representation of endochondral ossification and the possible causes of its disturbed development.** At the left are represented the various zones which normally make up the zone of ossification: Quiescent or resting cartilage, cartilage columns and the provisional zone of calcification, osteoid formation, bone remodeling into compact lamellar bone.

Disturbances can occur at any step of this complex process. *Defective or absent growth of columnar cartilage* gives rise to a disease entity known as *chondrodystrophy* (Fig. 344, p. 210). In *rickets*, the process of *calcifica-tion in the zone of provisional calcification may be deficient* (see Figs. 345, 346, p. 210). Deficient *osteoid formation* leads to *osteogenesis imperfecta* (compare with Fig. 347, p. 210). In compact bones, the disorder may be in the zone of remodeling as in *osteopetrosis*.

In most cases of disordered development, the changes are not restricted to endochondral ossification alone but also involve other aspects of bone formation (hatched areas in Table 7).

Table 7. Diagram of the different disturbances in ossification in the osteodystrophies

I. *Compensatory Bone Formation*	Chondro-dystrophy	Rickets	Syphilitic Osteo-chondritis	Osteogenesis Imperfecta	Osteo-petrosis
1. Enchondral O.					
a) epiphyseal O.	▥	▥	▥	▥	▥
b) metaphyseal O.	▥	▥	▥	▥	▥
2. Perichondral O.		▥		▥	▥
II. *Periosteal bone formation*		▥		▥	▥

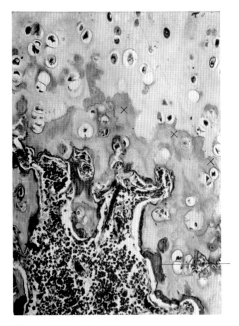

Fig. 344. Achondroplasia;
H & E, 110×.

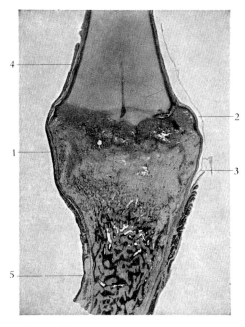

Fig. 345. Rickets;
H & E, 5×.

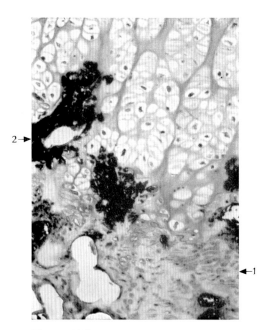

Fig. 346. Rickets;
Azan stain, 110×.

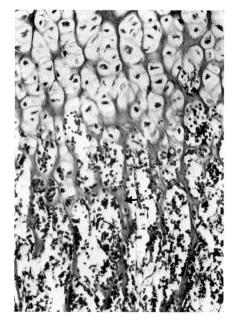

Fig. 347. Osteogenesis imperfecta;
H & E, 110×.

Achondroplasia (Fig. 344). *In achondroplasia (also called chondrodystrophy), endochondral ossification is disturbed in spite of well-developed perichondral and periosteal ossification* (see Fig. 343 and Table 7). *Short, thick bones are the result (achondroplastic dwarfs, circus clowns and the dachshund).* The disturbance can be traced morphologically, as shown in Figure 344, to deficiency or even absence of formation of the columns of cartilage. The usual characteristic columnar organization is replaced by solitary, somewhat vesicular cartilage cells. Calcification of the cartilagenous ground substance (dark gray, map-like regions, ×) is seen to be irregular. Thin shafts of osteoid are deposited (→) on the bulky projections of the zone of provisional calcification. In the lower portion of the section there are marrow spaces. Since the basic disturbance in achondroplasia occurs mainly within the zones of vesicular and columnar cartilage formation, flat bones are largely spared. This leads to a certain disproportion between the developing bones of the cranial vault (flat bone formation) and the retarded growth of the bones at the base of the skull (long bone formation).

Rickets (Figs. 345, 346). *This disease is the result of a hypovitaminosis (vitamin D deficiency), which leads to faulty mineralization of newly formed bone. For this reason, the lesions would be expected in the zone of provisional calcification and in regions where osteoid is normally mineralized.* Figure 345, from a rib, shows the altered osteochondral margin in rickets. The osteochondral margin is widened, irregular and distended (*ricketic rosary* → 1). The upper portion of the widened margin is composed of an exaggerated layer of columnar cartilage cells (→ 2). The lower portion is made up of combined chondroid and osteoid tissue (→ 3), in which remnants of cartilaginous ground substance blend irregularly with non-mineralized, newly formed bone (osteoid). (Normal cartilage, → 4, normal spongy or cancellous bone, → 5).

Under **higher magnification** (Fig. 346), the chondro-osteoid (→ 1) substance can be seen in the lower portion of the section. This newly formed osteoid does not become mineralized. The opening up of primitive marrow spaces by tuft-like vascular proliferation (→ 2), which is characteristic of rickets, can be clearly seen. Above this, there is the zone of columnar cartilage whose ground substance (also called the zone of provisional calcification) has not become mineralized. Rickets affects not only endochondral ossification but also perichondral ossification and mesenchymal bone formation (see Table 7, p. 209). In the skull, this results in deficient bone formation and insufficient mineralization of new-formed bone, giving rise to thin areas in the occipital and parietal bones, which are called *craniotabes*. Craniotabes is an important, easily detected diagnostic sign of rickets.

Osteogenesis imperfecta (Fig. 347). *If a disturbance of ossification involves the next deeper "level" (compare Fig. 343) osteogenesis imperfecta results. This disease is thus a disorder of bone formation in which there is insufficient osteoid formation and abnormal fragility of bone.* Figure 347 illustrates these relationships clearly. The orderly, well-developed columnar cartilage can be seen in the upper portion of the section. The lower portion of the picture, on the other hand, discloses the shredded remnants of cartilaginous ground substance (→). Osteoid formation is not present. Primitive marrow spaces can be seen between shafts of ground substance. All stages of bone formation are disturbed.

Many newborn children with osteogenesis imperfecta are born dead, while others die soon after birth. It is only in a very few cases, when the disease is not too pronounced, that these children survive any length of time. The prominent feature, then, is bone fragility. In some individuals, more than 100 fractures have been noted.

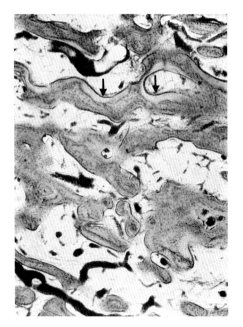

Fig. 348. Osteomalacia;
H & E, 28×.

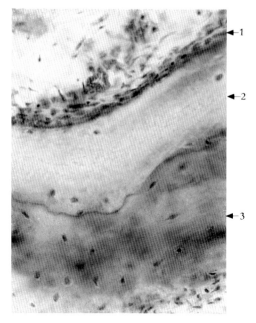

Fig. 349. Osteomalacia;
H & E, 280×.

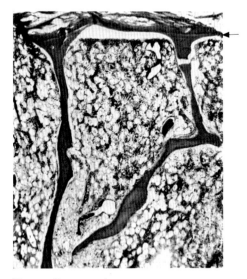

Fig. 350. Osteoporosis;
H & E, 28×.

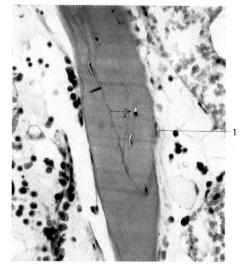

Fig. 351. Osteoporosis;
H & E, 280×.

Osteodystrophies of Adult Skeleton

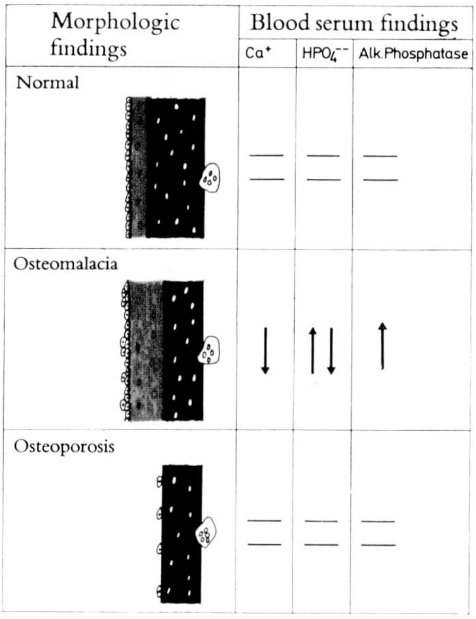

Morphologic findings	Blood serum findings		
	Ca⁺	HPO₄⁻⁻	Alk.Phosphatase
Normal	— —	— —	— —
Osteomalacia	↓	↑↓	↑
Osteoporosis	— —	— —	— —

Fig. 352. See text.

The bony changes seen in the adult skeleton are most frequently *osteoporosis*, and less frequently-*osteomalacia*. Figure 352 explains these two conditions schematically.

In *osteomalacia*, or adult rickets (Figs. 348, 349), *numerous osteoblasts are evident in the bony trabeculae, and sufficient bony substance is formed, but it does not become mineralized* (light gray zone in Figs. 348, 349). There are broad osteoid bands. In this respect, osteomalacia is the counterpart in the adult skeleton of rickets in the growing one. The serum calcium is lowered. The phosphate level varies, depending on kidney function (it is raised in case of renal damage). The alkaline phosphatase is noticeably raised.

Microscopically (Figs. 348, 349), the widening of the cancellous trabeculae can be seen even under low magnification (Fig. 348). Conspicuous light gray margins are present at the edges of the cancellous trabeculae (→). This is non-mineralized osteoid. It shows up even clearer under **higher magnification** (Fig. 349). A wide layer of osteoblasts (→ 1) surrounds the edges of the cancellous trabeculae. Next is a broad band of non-mineralized osteoid substance (→ 2) and then, set off by a line, mineralized bone (→ 3). *Osteomalacia then represents a defect of mineralization with preserved or frequently increased osteoblastic activity.* Loss of calcium salts from previously calcified bones very probably plays no role in osteomalacia.

The opposite of osteomalacia is **osteoporosis** (Figs. 350, 351). In this disease, *mineralization is mostly intact, but osteoblastic function is reduced* (see Fig. 352). Insufficient amounts of bone substance are formed to replace normal resorption. The serum values, the best indication of the mineralization process, are normal. *Microscopic* examination reveals, even with low magnification (Fig. 350), rarefaction of spongy bone with widening of the marrow spaces (→: thinned cortex). The marrow spaces may be filled with either brown or red marrow. **Higher magnification** (Fig. 351) reveals mineralized bony trabeculae and preserved osteocytes (→) but absence of osteoid bands and only scattered osteoblasts (→ 1), which lie at the edges of the trabeculae. These morphologic appearances explain why bones in *osteomalacia are soft and pliable*, whereas in the case of *osteoporosis they are brittle and fragile.*

Osteomalacia and osteoporosis are disorders of bone formation. Increased bone resorption can also accompany the osteodystrophies (see p.205). The most frequent types of *bone resorption* are:

   a) lacunar resorption (by multinucleated osteoclasts),
   b) smooth resorption (by a margin of mononucleated cells),
   c) perforating resorption (by capillary buds).

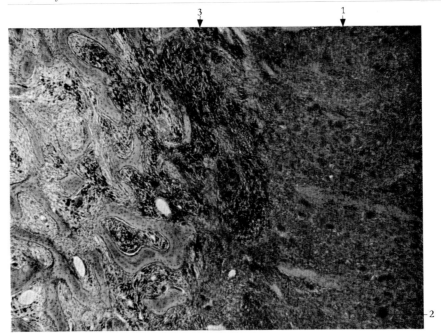

Fig. 353. Osteitis fibrosa cystica (so-called brown tumor); H & E, 40×.

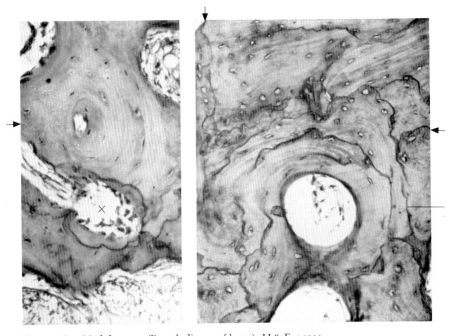

Fig. 354. Osteitis deformans (Paget's disease of bone); H & E, 152×.

Osteitis fibrosa cystica (so-called brown tumor) (Fig. 353). *Osteitis fibrosa cystica* (perhaps better named fibrous osteodystrophy) is a nodular bone disease, either localized or generalized, that leads to the destruction of the affected portion of bone. *The generalized type occurs with hyperparathyroidism (if caused by a parathyroid adenoma = von Recklinghausen's disease of bone)*[1]. Histological examination reveals proliferation of immature connective tissue, arising from the endosteum, the adventitia of medullary blood vessels and the Haversian canals. As is shown in Figure 353, there is richly cellular granulation tissue (→ 1), which on the right-hand side consists of reticulum cells, histiocytes and fibroblasts. Fine reticular fibers can be found between the cells. The numerous, bizarre-shaped, multinucleated giant cells (→ 2) are rather characteristic and probably represent frustrated capillary buds (angioblastic giant cells). It is by means of this granulation tissue that portions of bone are destroyed and reabsorbed. Hence, cysts may be seen in the bone radiologically. Frequently, hemorrhages occur in the immature connective tissue and, as a result, many histiocytes can be seen in the cytoplasm of which there are large amounts of hemosiderin (→ 3). On the left-hand side of the section there is normal cancellous bone showing medullary fibrosis.

Macroscopic: Brown nodules or cysts. The distal femur and proximal tibia are affected preferentially. Occasionally, a true sarcoma may arise from osteitis fibrosa. Localized "brown tumors" may also be seen following trauma. A similar histological picture is seen in epulis.

Osteitis deformans (Paget's disease of bone) (Fig. 354). Another example of the group of osteodystrophic diseases is *osteitis* or, better, *osteodystrophy deformans* (PAGET). Osteitis deformans *begins* as a *serous inflammation* in the marrow cavity of the affected bone. The *second phase* in the disease process is characterized by *osteomalacia*, i. e., the new-formed bone fails to calcify and the previously mineralized bone becomes demineralized *(cement lines)*. It is this "softening of the bone" that is responsible for the various bone deformations associated with osteitis deformans. *In the third phase, remodeling of the bone takes place.* Local bony structures are partially or wholly absorbed. New bone is formed simultaneously and is usually overproduced. It is deposited in crescents along preserved trabeculae, and along broken Haversian canals. This remodeling is comparable to the reconstruction of the liver seen in cirrhosis.

The *left portion* of Figure 354 contains an Haversian system (→) the lower margin of which already shows both bone destruction by osteoclasts and new bone formation by osteoblasts (×). This continuous destruction and concomitant irregular re-formation gives rise to *the characteristic mosaic appearance* of Paget bones *(picture on the right)*. The pronounced *cement lines* (→) also result from the process of remodeling. The normal lamellar bone structure is thus completely altered by this repeated remodeling. In such bones, there are also numerous arteriovenous anastomoses and, hence, these patients frequently have increased cardiac output.

Macroscopic: Patients afflicted by the generalized type have thickened, deformed bones (e. g., saber legs). The localized type occurs mainly in the skull (leontiasis ossea). In about 8% of the cases of osteitis deformans an osteosarcoma develops.

Also belonging to the group of osteodystrophies is *fibrous dysplasia*, which afflicts younger individuals. The bones are grossly expanded and deformed. The marrow cavity, instead of containing fatty or hematopoietic marrow, is filled with fibrous tissues in which fibrous bone formation takes place. X-rays reveal an opaque, glassy appearance of the bone.

---

1 Original description by ENGEL (1864).

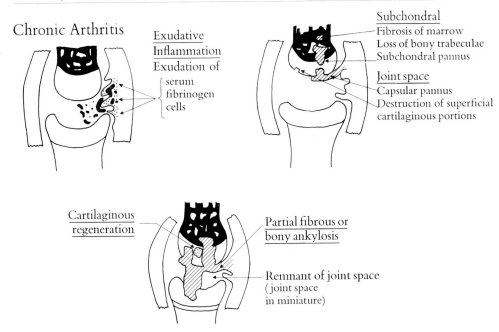

Chronic Arthritis

Exudative
Inflammation
Exudation of
{ serum
  fibrinogen
  cells

Subchondral
Fibrosis of marrow
Loss of bony trabeculae
Subchondral pannus

Joint space
Capsular pannus
Destruction of superficial
cartilaginous portions

Cartilaginous
regeneration

Partial fibrous or
bony ankylosis

Remnant of joint space
(joint space
in miniature)

Fig. 355. Diagram of the joint changes in chronic arthritis.

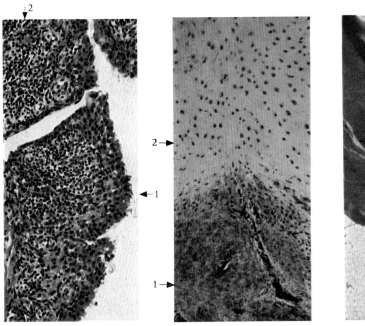

Fig. 356a. Chronic arthritis
(inflammation of the joint
capsule);
H & E, 200×.

Fig. 356b. Chronic arthritis
(destruction of cartilage by
granulation tissue);
H & E, 300×.

Fig. 357. Chronic arthritis
(fibrous ankylosis in a finger
joint);
H & E, 100×.

Inflammatory Diseases of Joints

The inflammatory joint diseases may be subdivided into:

1. *Suppurative inflammations of joints;*
2. *Rheumatic inflammations of joints*
    a) joint inflammation in rheumatic fever,
    b) chronic arthritis (arthritis deformans, osteoarthritis),
    c) ankylosing spondylitis;
3. *Rheumatoid arthritis.* (The clinical picture resembles that of rheumatic fever with its involvement of joints. The causes, however, are different; e.g., infectious diseases, tuberculosis, etc.)

In *active (febrile) rheumatic fever*, true Aschoff nodules may occur in the loose connective tissues of the joint capsule (compare with heart, Figs. 63–67, pp. 46, 47). *The large joints* seem to be preferentially affected, particularly in *young individuals.* In most instances, antistreptolysin and antistaphylolysin titers are often markedly elevated. The joint lesions ultimately regress completely. *Chronic arthritis* (see Figs. 355–357) has the morphological appearance of a non-specific chronic inflammation (in most instances, there are no Aschoff nodules in the joint capsule). *The small joints* (fingers, toes) are preferentially affected. *Older individuals* are afflicted more frequently than young persons. Very frequently results of the latex-fixation and Waaler-Rose tests are positive. Ankylosis of joints occurs as a result of the severe destructive changes.

Ankylosing spondylitis (Bechterew's disease) begins with scanty inflammatory infiltration of lymphocytes into the capsule and ligaments of the *small vertebral joints.* The prominent feature of this disease is the excessive bone formation which leads to ankylosis of the vertebral column.

Chronic arthritis (rheumatoid arthritis) can serve as an example of inflammatory joint disease. Compare the schematic drawings in Fig. 355 with the corresponding photomicrographs in Figs. 356a, b and 357.

Chronic arthritis (inflammation of joint capsule), Fig. 356a. The disease begins with inflammation of the joint capsule, as has been shown recently by study of biopsies of the capsule. There is exudation in the joint space of blood plasma and emigration of cells (granulocytes with cytoplasmic inclusion bodies containing rheumatoid factor, synovial cells, lymphocytes, plasma cells). The synovial cells covering the joint capsule are focally destroyed and the foci covered with fibrin. In other places the synovial cells proliferate ($\rightarrow$ 1). The synovial connective tissue is densely infiltrated with plasma cells and lymphocytes ($\rightarrow$ 2), which often form small lymph follicles. Occasional foci of fibrinoid may be seen.

Chronic arthritis (destruction of cartilage by granulation tissue), Fig. 356b. The stage of exudation may lead to a stage of proliferative inflammation. Richly vascularized connective tissue called a panus ($\rightarrow$ 1) from the synovium or the subarticular bone marrow may grow into the joint cartilage ($\rightarrow$ 2) and destroy it on both the joint and bone surfaces.

Chronic arthritis (fibrous ankylosis), Fig. 357. The final phase of fibrous ankylosis develops when granulation tissue proliferating from both joint surfaces meets. The subarticular portions of the bone are still intact ($\rightarrow$ 1). Only small portions of the joint cartilage are still visible and they show secondary degenerative changes. Solitary slit-like spaces remain from the former joint space ($\rightarrow$ within the picture. The articulations of the bones are fused by connective tissue ($\rightarrow$ 2).

Macroscopic: White, fibrous cartilagenous deposits (panus), ulceration of cartilage and ankylosis.
Note: 1. Subcutaneous periarticular rheumatoid nodules have diagnostic significance (excision, histopathological examination). 2. The following complications may occur: a) amyloidosis (in about 20%), b) panarteritis nodosa (in about 25%, muscle or liver biopsy may be indicated as a diagnostic measure).

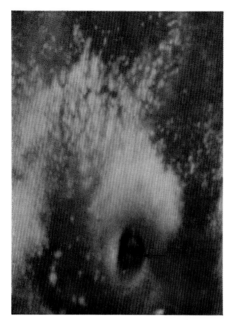

Fig. 358. Granular proteinaceous degeneration of joint cartilage; eosin stain, photographed under fluorescent light, 625×.

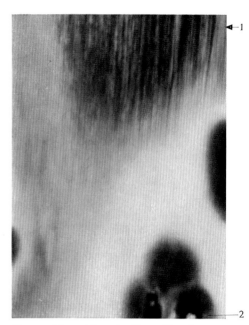

Fig. 359. Unmasking of collagen fibers in joint cartilage;
toluidine blue stain, 625×.

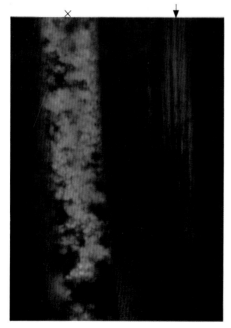

Fig. 360. Cyst formation and fibrillation of joint cartilage;
toluidine blue stain,
625×.

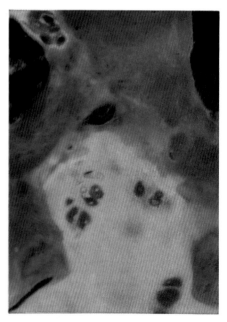

Fig. 361. Bone formation in a joint cartilage in arthritis deformans;
acridin orange stain, fluorescent light,
400×.

Degenerative Joint Disease (Osteoarthritis)

In contrast to inflammatory joint diseases, the degenerative joint disorders (e. g., *arthritis deformans, spondylosis deformans*) always begin in the joint cartilage itself. The first detectable change is mucoid or **granular proteinaceous degeneration of the joint cartilage.** Figure 358 shows a section through such a joint cartilage. In the lower part of the picture there is a preserved cartilage cell (→) surrounded by numerous yellow granules having a fan-shaped arrangement. These consist of protein or mucopolysaccharides, as can be demonstrated by histochemical techniques. These changes are interpreted as a process of disintegration in which the breakage index of the ground substance is altered, and the normally invisible collagen fibers of the hyalin joint cartilage become visible (→ 1 in Fig. 359).

Unmasking of collagen fibers in the joint cartilage (Fig. 359). This section shows that the cartilage cells (→ 2) in the vicinity of the unmasked fibers (→ 1) are still intact. Once these cells are destroyed, the lesion is described as **fibrillation** of the cartilage (Fig. 360), such as is frequently seen in rib cartilage. The portions of cartilage affected in this manner frequently develop **cysts** and in such regions cells are no longer demonstrable. Only denuded fibers (→) and elongated, cystic spaces (×) remain. Bone may arise in these cysts as a result of proliferative budding of granulation tissue. Figure 361 is stained with acridin orange and photographed under fluorescent light to show cancellous bone (green) within bright yellow cartilaginous ground substance (cartilage cells are stained red).

In summary, it is the destruction of cartilaginous tissue which is responsible for the loss of the shearing strength of the hyalin cartilage, and the increasing transfer of pressure is to the bone (Fig. 362), since it can no longer be transformed into thrust. The effect of this pressure is to stimulate **new bone formation.** This leads to overgrowth of subchondral cancellous bone (compare Fig. 362), ossification in the joint cartilage itself, and marginal bony outgrowths which finally give the afflicted joint its characteristic structure (so-called lipping of the joint).

Macroscopic: The cartilage is ulcerated and there is marginal enlargement and beading (e. g., spondylosis deformans).

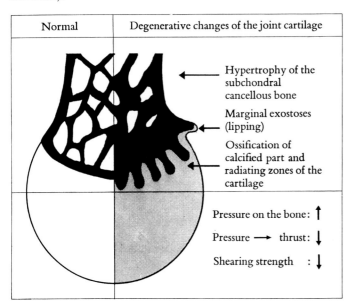

Normal	Degenerative changes of the joint cartilage

Hypertrophy of the subchondral cancellous bone

Marginal exostoses (lipping)

Ossification of calcified part and radiating zones of the cartilage

Pressure on the bone: ↑

Pressure → thrust: ↓

Shearing strength : ↓

Fig. 362. Diagram of the development of the bony changes resulting from degenerative injury of the joint cartilage.

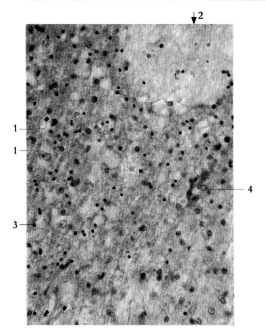

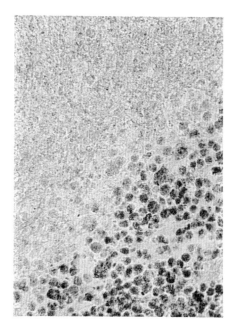

Fig. 363. Focal area of recent encephalomalacia or softening of the brain; pallid area (honeycomb area); H & E, 248×.

Fig. 364. Center of an area of encephalomalacia with granular, fat-containing phagocytic cells (Gitter cells or compound granular corpuscles); Sudan stain, 250×.

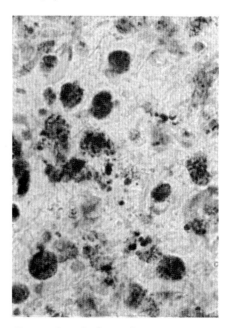

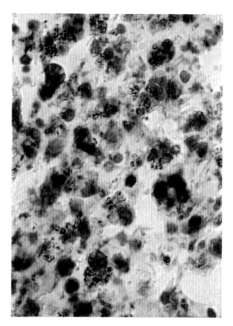

Fig. 365. Granular fatty cells; scarlet red-hematoxylin, 512×.

Fig. 366. Iron-containing phagocytic cells (pigmented granular cells) in encephalomalacia; Berlin blue reaction, 800×.

Brain and Spinal Cord

Histological examination of the brain and spinal cord should start with an investigation of the conditi on of the meninges (cellularity, vascular changes, unusual deposits). The substance of the brain and spinal cord is composed of *neurons with their cytoplasmic processes* (dendrites and axis cylinders or axons surrounded by a myelin sheath – special stains must be used to demonstrate them), *neuroglia* (*astrocytes* with relatively large round nuclei and cytoplasm which is seen well only with special stains, *oligodendroglia* with small round nuclei, and *microglia* with small fusiform nuclei) and *blood vessels*. Both the intact and injured portions of the tissue must be examined (e. g., areas of softening, foci of demyelinization). Perivascular or tissue infiltrates should be noted and the types of cells that compose them.

Encephalomalacia

This is due to **necrosis** of the brain substance followed by *liquefaction* and *secondary cavitation* (cyst formation) resulting either from occlusion of a nutrient artery (arteriosclerosis, thrombosis, embolization) of from generalized hypoxia. The process has several stages. 1. The stage of *cortical pallor* with ischemic changes in the neurons (shrinkage of both the cell body and nucleus with loss of Nissl substance). There may also be interstitial edema with fiber and nuclear degeneration (so-called honeycomb appearance) and, finally, complete *necrosis* with loss of nuclei (see Fig. 368). 2. The stage of *softening with granular fatty cells*, also called gitter cells or compound granular corpuscles (stage of resorption). 3. The stage of *cyst formation and glial scarring* (end stage).

Figure 363, which shows **focus of recent brain softening,** will serve as an example of the *first stage* (cortical pallor). There is conspicuous edema between fibers and focally around cells (→ 1), and degeneration of the myelin sheaths, resulting in their complete dissolution (→ 2). The oligodendrocytes have a shrunken appearance (→ 3). The nuclei of the macroglia stain weakly (beginning of karyolysis, → 4). In the upper portion of the picture (→ 2) there is a pale red focus in which the process is further advanced. Nuclei are almost totally lacking, the myelin sheaths dissolved.

Macroscopic: The brain tissue is of slightly soft consistency, and the gray substance is pallid.

The *second stage* (stage of *focal softening*) is characterized by resorption of the destroyed myelin substance (lipids). Figure 364 shows the center of an area of **brain softening.** Even with the unaided eye, fat stains show a red lesion that stains with Sudan, as well as a loosening of the tissues, which is discernible in the bluish red brain substance. Examination of the lesion with medium high power reveals numerous round cells, the cytoplasm of which is filled with red sudanophilic granules. High power clearly shows (Figs. 365, 367) these **granular fatty cells** with their eccentrically located nuclei (they are either phagocytic microglial cells or histiocytes derived from the sheaths of blood vessels). In paraffin sections, the fat droplets are dissolved and the cytoplasm has a vacuolated appearance. In many cases, bleeding into the tissues has occurred, in addition to the softening (*hemorrhagic softening*, frequently seen with emboli). The extravasated erythrocytes and hemoglobin are also taken up by phagocytes and stored as hemosiderin. Such phagocytic cells are called **pigmented granular cells** (Figs. 366, 369), since the cytoplasm contains brown hemosiderin granules (iron-reaction positive). In addition, granular fatty cells as well as extracellular deposits of brown pigment can be seen (*hematoidin* = iron-free hemoglobin, see also Fig. 261, p. 168 and Fig. 14).

Macroscopic: There is softening and liquefaction of brain tissue. In cases of hemorrhagic softening, there are punctate hemorrhages which show a brown discoloration when the lesion is a little older. In unstained fresh microscopic preparations, numerous granular fatty cells may be seen (granular cytoplasm with glassy granules).

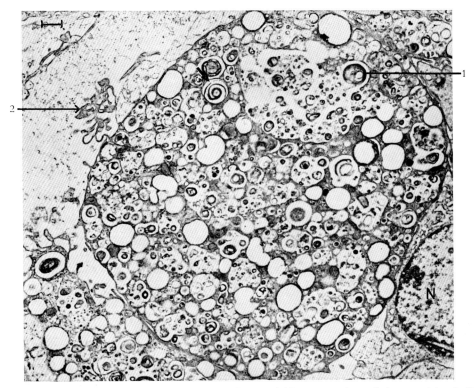

Fig. 367. Compound granular cells from the margin of an area of old experimental coagulation necrosis (cerebral infarct, 5–10 days old). The nucleus is not remarkable. The cytoplasm is filled with phagolysosomes which contain concentrically layered lipoprotein (myelin figures: → 1 and the arrow within the picture). In addition, there are vacuoles containing homogeneous osmiophilic material (fat). Bizarre processes protrude from the surface of the cell. The cytoplasm of a neighboring cell is at the lower left. N = nucleus of an adjacent cell. 5,000 × (ESCOLA and HAGER, 1964)

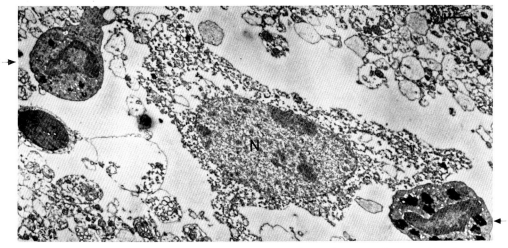

Fig. 368. Necrotic nerve cell from the cerebral cortex. The outline of the cell body is still recognizable. The nucleus (N) appears coarser and denser than normal (pyknosis). The cytoplasmic organelles, for the most part, are no longer recognizable. In their place are disorderly clumps of fragmented material. Two leukocytes (→ 1, → 2) are feeding on the necrotic cell (neuronophagia: compare Fig. 378). 6,000 × (Dr. HAGER).

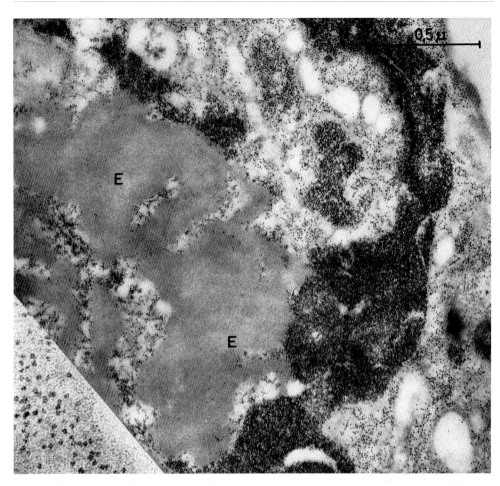

Fig. 369. Disintegration of an erythrocyte within a macrophage in an area of traumatic necrosis of the cerebral cortex. Around the disintegrating remains of the erythrocyte stroma (E) may be seen masses of tightly packed ferritin granules, which, on further resolution (lower left), can be recognized as typical ferritin building blocks (compare Fig. 13). 60,000×. Inset: 80,000×.

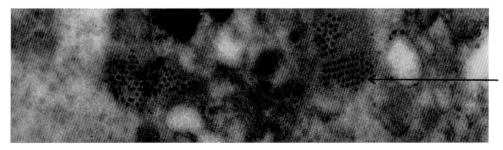

Fig. 370. Section through the cytoplasm of a polymorphonuclear leukocyte in the cerebral cortex of a mouse infected with polioencephalitis virus (parapoliomyelitis virus, Columbia-SK-group). Aggregations of virus particles of uniform size (→) are present in the cytoplasm. They have a sort of crystal lattice arrangement and are embedded in a granular matrix. 70,000× (Dr. HAGER).

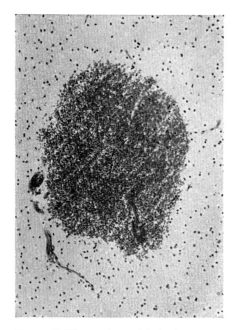

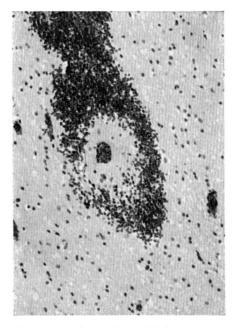

Fig. 371. Ball hemorrhage of the brain;
H & E, 120×.

Fig. 372. Ring hemorrhage of the brain;
H & E, 175×.

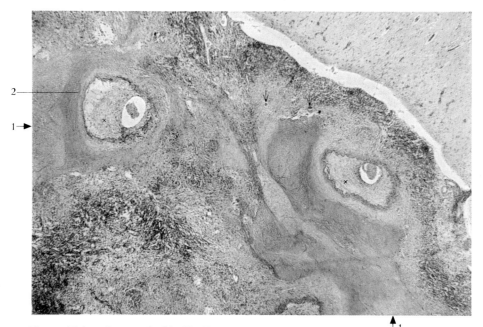

Fig. 373. Tuberculous meningitis; H & E, 33×.

Ball and ring hemorrhages of the brain (Figs. 371, 372). *These hemorrhages are due to circulatory disturbances accompanied by necrosis of the vessel wall.* Ball hemorrhages are spherical lesions composed of compactly arranged extravasated erythrocytes, in the center of which can be seen a venule with a necrotic wall (→ in Fig. 371). In **ring hemorrhages,** the center of the lesion is occupied by a vessel that is completely plugged with erythrocytes. This is surrounded by a ring of necrotic brain tissue (in this case, homogeneous myelin sheaths and an occasional cell with an intact nucleus). The outer zone consists of a ring of erythrocytes.

Macroscopic: Punctate hemorrhages, which cannot be wiped away, are present on the cut surfaces of the brain. They are common in hypertension, air embolism, heat stroke, and hemorrhagic encephalitis.

Tuberculous meningitis (Fig. 373). *Tuberculous inflammation of the meninges is hematogenous in origin, affects the base of the brain and occurs chiefly in children.* In the acute exudative stage there is a rich fibrinous and protein-rich exudate containing polymorphonuclear leukocytes that is especially prominent around blood vessels. Caseation sets in rapidly in the vicinity of the vessels. Figure 373 shows the perivascular necrosis and network of fibrin (→) and the dense cellular infiltration (mainly lymphocytes) of the neighboring tissues. In some areas, the necrosis is already delineated by epithelioid cells. Solitary Langhans giant cells (→ within the picture) are also seen *(subacute proliferative stage).* Of great importance is the fact that the caseation also affects arteries, causing partial or complete necrosis of the vessel walls (→ 2). In addition, if the caseation involves the adventitia, an arteritis develops, which, by a process of inward extension, causes marked endarteritis obliterans (×) with intimal proliferation and marked reduction of the lumen. For this reason, secondary foci of encephalomalacia may be seen in the healing stages of tuberculous meningitis.

Macroscopic: Acute: Gray, gelatinous exudate covers the base of the brain. *Subacute-subchronic:* Small yellow or grayish, white, translucent nodules. In the *end stage,* there is connective tissue proliferation with grayish white thickening of the meninges.

Suppurative meningitis (Fig. 374). *This inflammation of the leptomeninges arises either from bloodborne infection, from direct spread from suppurative infection of adjacent tissues or from penetrating wounds.* Microscopic examination with low power reveals a dense cellular exudate in the leptomeninges. Higher magnification shows that the exudate consists of densely packed polymorphonuclear leukocytes intermingled with fibrin strands (see Fig. 173 b). Frequently, the inflammation extends into the cortex (→) along blood vessels (meningoencephalitis).

Macroscopic: There is a plaque-like layer of yellowish or greenish exudate, mostly over the convexity of the brain.

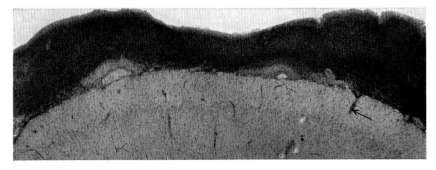

Fig. 374. Suppurative meningitis; H & E, 24 ×.

225

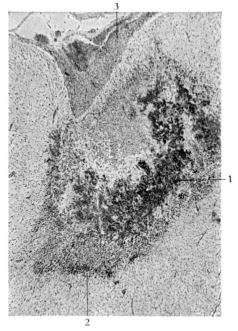

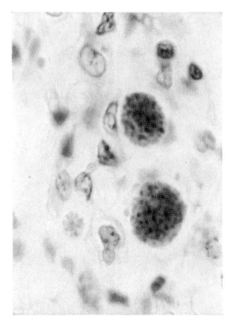

Fig. 375. Encephalitis caused by toxoplasmosis; H & E, 10×.

Fig. 376. Pseudocysts of toxoplasmosis in the brain; thionine stain, 1,400×.

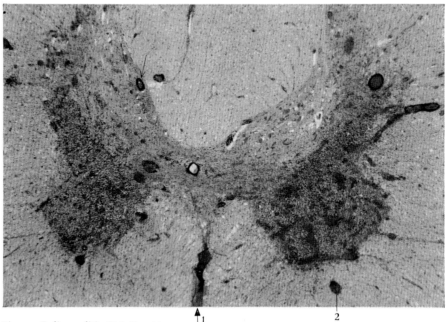

Fig. 377. Poliomyelitis; H & E, 51×.

Encephalitis in toxoplasmosis (Fig. 375). *This is a granulomatous, necrotizing and calcifying encephalitis caused by Toxoplasma gondii (a protozoon) and occurring chiefly in neonates.* Examination of the specimen with a scanning lens discloses conspicuous cellular nodules and blue-stained calcified foci in the cortex and white matter. Sometimes there are larger necrotic lesions. Closer inspection shows that the cellular nodules are granulomas consisting of lymphocytes, plasma cells, histiocytes and glial cells. Figure 375 shows such a cortical lesion with a calcified central zone of necrosis (stained blue, → 1) surrounded by a cellular infiltrate (→ 2), consisting largely of lymphocytes and histiocytes. The arachnoid (→ 3) is also infiltrated by lymphocytes.

With oil immersion, **pseudocysts** can often be seen in the granulomas (Fig. 376) consisting of intracellular colonies of the causative organisms. The infected cells are round and the cytoplasm is filled with bow-shaped toxoplasma containing small, oval inner bodies. There are histiocytes in the surrounding tissues.

Macroscopic: Brown or yellow nodular lesions are seen on the cut surface of the brain.

Poliomyelitis (Figs. 370, 377, 378). *This viral infection affects the motor neurons of the anterior horn of the spinal cord, causing cell destruction and resorption.* Examination of the section with the scanning lens shows dense cellular infiltration of the anterior horns. At the bottom of Figure 377 is the anterior median fissure in which may be seen the lymphocytic infiltration of the leptomeninges (→ 1). The central canal is clearly visible. Dilated vessels (→) in the white matter are also surrounded by mantles of round cells (→ 2). The posterior horns are uninvolved.

Under **higher magnification** (Fig. 378), leukocytes and proliferated glial cells are seen to have replaced the phagocytosed necrotic cells (*neuronophagia*, Fig. 368). In places, the shadowy outlines of nerve cells may be seen in the middle of the exudate (→ 1: phagocytosed neuron, → 2: shrunken neuron).

Macroscopic: The anterior horns are deformed.

Typhus fever encephalitis (Fig. 379). *This results from systemic infection with Rickettsia prowazeki and is characterized by a nodular form of panencephalitis.* The section shows the olive of the medulla oblongata with two cellular nodules of proliferating microglial cells. These glial cell nodules are situated perivascularly (reaction to rickettsial toxin?). The neurons are unchanged. The nodules are not specific for typhus fever and may occur in other sorts of encephalitis.

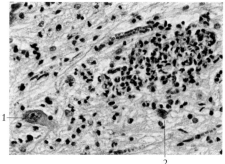

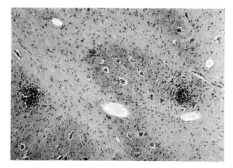

Fig. 378. Poliomyelitis;
H & E, 227×.

Fig. 379. Typhus fever encephalitis;
H & E, 60×.

227

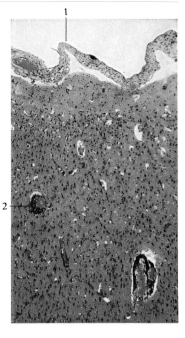

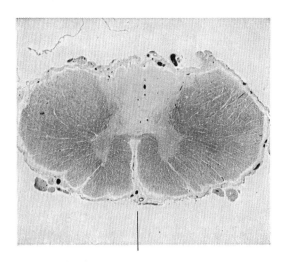

Fig. 380. Tabes dorsalis;
Heidenhain's myelin sheath stain, 10×.

Fig. 381. General paresis;
H & E, 60×.

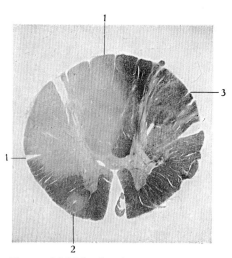

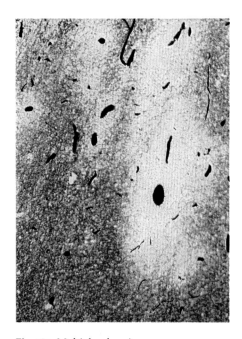

Fig. 382. Multiple sclerosis.
Sudan stain, 5×.

Fig. 383. Multiple sclerosis;
Myelin stain, 60×.

Tabes dorsalis (Fig. 380). *In the tertiary stage of syphilis, a chronic, slowly progressive meningitis may develop, with injury of the dorsal roots of the spinal cord and secondary degeneration of posterior columns.* The histological appearance in sections stained for myelin is very typical. With the histological section oriented according to the deeply indented anterior longitudinal fissure (→), the lack of myelin stain in the region of the posterior columns and dorsal roots is immediately apparent. The gray matter (neurons and unmyelinated fibers of the anterior gray horns) is of almost identical hue. Under higher magnification, individual preserved myelin sheaths or sheaths with clumped degenerated myelin may still be recognized. In the florid stages, sections stained for fat show tissue disintegration and granular fatty cells. The meninges are fibrotic and thickened and infiltrated by lymphocytes.

Macroscopic: The meninges are opaque, especially in the thoracic region, and the spinal cord is shrunken and the posterior columns are discolored gray.

General paresis, also called general paralysis of the insane or dementia paralytica (Fig. 381). This is a *chronic syphilitic encephalitis with frontal lobe atrophy and deposits of iron in the brain tissue.* In contrast to *luetic meningoencephalitis,* in which there is a predilection for the base of the brain with secondary progression of the inflammation along vascular channels to the cortex, *paresis* affects primarily the *frontal lobes* (insular cortex and temporal lobes) and encephalitis is more marked than is meningitis. The leptomeninges (→ 1) are thickened by fibrosis and sparsely infiltrated by lymphocytes and plasma cells. The most conspicuous feature is in the cortex, where the adventitia of the small vessels is infiltrated by lymphocytes and plasma cells (→ 2) which, even under low-power magnification, may be seen as bluish cuffs. In addition, there is a diffuse increase of microglial cells which contain cytoplasmic hemosiderin, as do the macrophages derived from the perivascular tissues.

Macroscopic: Atrophy of the convolutions of the frontal lobe with opaque, thickened meninges.

Multiple sclerosis (Figs. 382, 383). *A chronic, progressive, focally disseminated, demyelinating disease of the brain and spinal cord of unknown etiology.* Myelin stain or Sudan stain (Fig. 382) demonstrates the demyelinated lesions clearly. A cross section of the spinal cord shows a well-demarcated, pale round lesion located mostly in the vicinity of the dorsal roots (between → 1 in Fig. 382). However, there are isolated smaller lesions (→ 2) that are not restricted to anatomically distinct fiber tracts (compare this to the picture of tabes dorsalis, Fig. 380). The spreading of the demyelinating process has been compared to an ink stain on a blotter. An early stage may also be seen in Figure 382, in which there is resorption of the myelin substance by granular fatty cells (→ 3). Even under low power, the light red stain of the neutral fats stored in macrophages is conspicuous, and under higher power these prove to be typical granular fatty cells (Fig. 367).

The **myelin stain** (Fig. 383) shows that the demyelinating process proceeds from the vessels, but nevertheless does not correspond to the area of distribution of the vessel.

Axons are preserved. A glial scar forms secondarily, consisting of a network of glial fiber and slightly increased numbers of glial cells (sclerosis). The myelin stain colors the erythrocytes in the vessels a deep blue.

Macroscopic: Old lesions appear gray, more recent lesions are salmon colored.

Tumors

Tumors may be defined as abnormal growths with autonomous characteristics. Tumors differ from such regular growth processes as regeneration and hyperplasia by not conforming to the ordinary individual growth pattern of the host organism.

A *classification* of tumors for diagnostic purposes should take into consideration the fate of the host and the essential biological behavior of the tumors (whether *benign* or *malignant*). However, this cannot be fully accomplished by morphological methods alone. To do this, we must make use of knowledge learned in retrospect as to whether a tumor behaves in a benign or a malignant fashion. For this reason, knowledge of the site of the tumor and the age and sex of the patient are of considerable importance in diagnosing a tumor. Equally important is the positional relation of the tumor to the normal tissues. A first principle of taking a biopsy, therefore, is to include surrounding normal tissue in the specimen.

The *incongruity that exists between the morphological structure and the biological behavior* becomes very apparent when we examine the morphological criteria for distinguishing benign and malignant tumors, as is made clear by the following table (Table 8).

Table 8. Some differences between benign and malignant tumors

	Benign Tumors	**Malignant Tumors**
Growth	Slow, expansile, compressing normal tissues	rapid, invasive
Structure	Homologous, typical of the tissue of origin, mature	heterologous, atypical, immature
Metastasis	—	+
Recurrence	+	+

Some tumors *deviate from these rules.* Thus, there are tumors of infiltrative growth, like carcinoid and basal cell carcinoma, that do not ordinarily metastasize. However, a change in the malignancy of certain tumors such as carcinoids leading to metastasis does occur *(malignant carcinoid).* On the other hand, well-matured, homologous tumors occur, such as the adenomas of salivary glands, that have a morphologically benign appearance, but nevertheless invade the veins in the area and metastasize *(metastasizing salivary gland adenoma).* (Lit.: P. DENOIX, 1967.)

In order correctly to diagnose a tumor, that is, to determine whether it is *benign or malignant,* as well as to put it into its proper place in the classification – either *epithelial or mesenchymal – the necessary first step* is to consider its *histological pattern.* For this purpose, *always* use the *low-power lenses* of the microscope.

Epithelial tumors show an *organoid structure* so that *parenchyma and stroma* are clearly distinguishable from each other. In contrast, *tumors of connective and supporting tissues* usually consist of one sort of tissue (variously differentiated mesenchyma) and are said to have a *histioid structure.*

The second step in making a diagnosis is to consider the *relationship between the tumor and the neighboring tissues.* Is it sharply circumscribed (encapsulated) or invasive? For this purpose, it may be necessary to use medium magnification.

The third step in diagnosis is to determine whether the tumor is composed of epithelial or mesenchymal tissue. As a basis for judgment, it is helpful to remember that tumors are "caricatures" of normal tissues; e. g., in a cornified squamous cell carcinoma, the various epithelial layers are present but are a distorted imitation of the normal.

In the fourth and last step in making a diagnosis, high magnification is used in order to study the structure of the cells. The following points should be considered (Table 9).

Table 9. Review of some cytological features of tumors

	Benign Tumors [1]	Malignant Tumors	
Nuclei			
Size	uniform	various sizes; large and small nuclei	Pleo-morphism
Shape	round, oval, spindle	irregular	
Chromatin	finely granular, evenly divided	coarsely lumpy, un-evenly divided, increased	Hyper-chromasia
Chromosome number	euploid	abnormal as a rule	
Chromosome shape	uniform	(non-euploid); enlarged or shrunken; e.g., V-form chromo-somes	
DNA content	normal-euploid	deviating, non-euploid, great scattering	
Number of mitoses	few	increased, atypical mitoses	
Nucleolus	regular, small	enlarged, deeply stained	
Nucleus/cytoplasm ratio	normal	altered (nucleus relatively larger)	
Cytoplasm			
RNA	normal	increased, strongly basophilic	
Mitochondria	normal	decreased, greatly altered	
Ergastoplasm	orderly arrangement	disorderly arrangement	
Specific functions	mostly preserved	usually lacking	

All tumors, so far as is known, have similar characteristics whether measured by morphological, biochemical or histochemical methods. Among these the following may be noted: most have an increased growth rate with increase in RNA, DNA and chromosomal deviations, and show disturbances of the enzyme patterns, glycolysis, cytoplasmic organization (see p. 232), and an immunological defect (loss of tissue-specific antigens, etc.). Tumors are known to follow the application of such potent carcinogenic agents as aromatic hydrocarbons, azo dyes and other chemical agents, as well as radiant energy and viruses (see p. 232).

The action of a **carcinogen** may be explained by any of the following possibilities:

a) transformation of normal cells into cancer cells.

b) selection of pre-existing clones of tumor cells. In this case, the carcinogen becomes toxic for normal cells but not for cancer cells ("clonal selection" theory).

c) activation of a latent virus.

The direction of recent work is to the question of whether the carcinogen acts primarily on the cytoplasm **(protein deletion theory)** or on the nucleus **(mutation theory)** – see the reviews by V. R. POTTER, 1964 and BERNHARD *et al.* 1963.

It is probable that a simultaneous attack on both the cytoplasm and nucleus is necessary. In the nucleus, carcinogens cause a change in the genetic material, which leads to failure to synthesize protein (AMBROSE and ROE, 1966). In the cytoplasm, binding of a carcinogen to proteins alters the control mechanisms that normally regulate DNA, RNA and protein synthesis and the mitotic rate. Examples of such a failure of regulation in the early stages of the development of a cancer (e.g., in experimental hepatoma) are: 1. **on the enzyme level :** failure of feedback arrest of thymidinkinase in the DNA synthesis pathway. 2. on the **transcription level** (DNA → messenger-RNA): alteration of transcription by excess methylation of DNA and transfer-RNA. 3. on the **translation level** (polysomes, messenger-RNA, protein): alteration of the life cycle of messenger-RNA for definite enzymes.

---

1 Chiefly the same cytological features as in normal tissues.

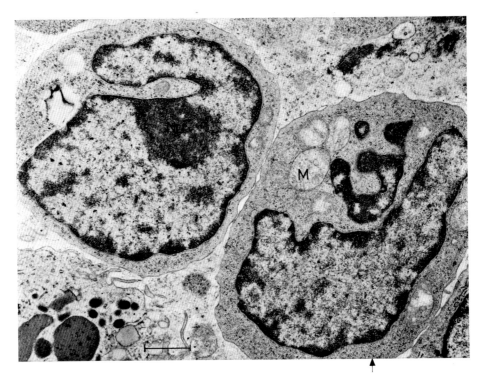

Fig. 384. *Burkitt tumor* (Burkitt, 1958). *Malignant lymphoma* (similar to lymphosarcoma). Figure 384 shows the distinct pleomorphism of the tumor cells and the irregular, clump-like divisions of heterochromatin and the large nucleolus (Nu). The cytoplasm is rich in free ribosomes and polysomes (e. g., →) but poor in mitochondria (M). Probably of viral origin (Stewart, 1966; Soustek, 1965). 10,000 × (Dr. Bernhard).

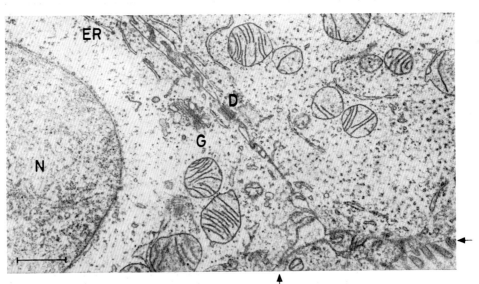

Fig. 385. Section of two cells of *a gastric carcinoma* (human). Both cells have a loose nuclear structure. The cytoplasm is "dedifferentiated," with only isolated profiles of rough ER. Diffusely distributed free-lying ribosomes and polysomes. The mitochondria are of different sizes with anomalies of the cristae. G = Golgi complex, → margin of an adjacent cell with microvilli, D = desmosome = attachment between the cells (normal). 13,000 × (Dr. Gusek).

1 See the reviews of the electron microscopy of tumors by Bernhard, 1960, 1961; Parry *et al.*, 1965.

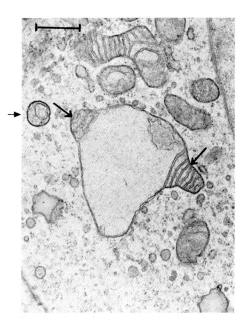

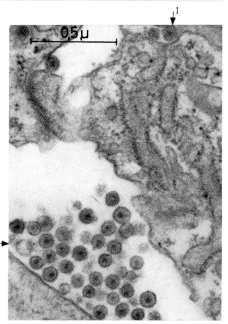

Fig. 386. Anomalous mitochondria in a hamster tumor cell. Large, deformed mitochondrion with dilatation of the mid-portion of the mitochondrial body. To the right and the left of this, the cristae are still regular (→ in the picture). → = autolysosome. 20,000 × (Dr. BERNHARD).

Fig. 387. Rous sarcoma virus (chicken). Intracellular (→ 1) and extracellular (→ 2) virus particles with dense internal bodies. 60,000 × (BERNHARD, 1960).

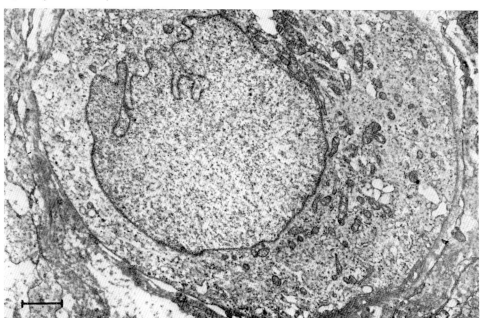

Fig. 388. *Hodgkin cell* (see Fig. 279). Loosely structured nucleus with imperfect membrane. In the cytoplasm, there are a few mitochondria of various sizes distributed in a focal fashion. The rough ER is increased. There are many free ribosomes. 9,000 × (Dr. GUSEK).

Fibroepithelioma

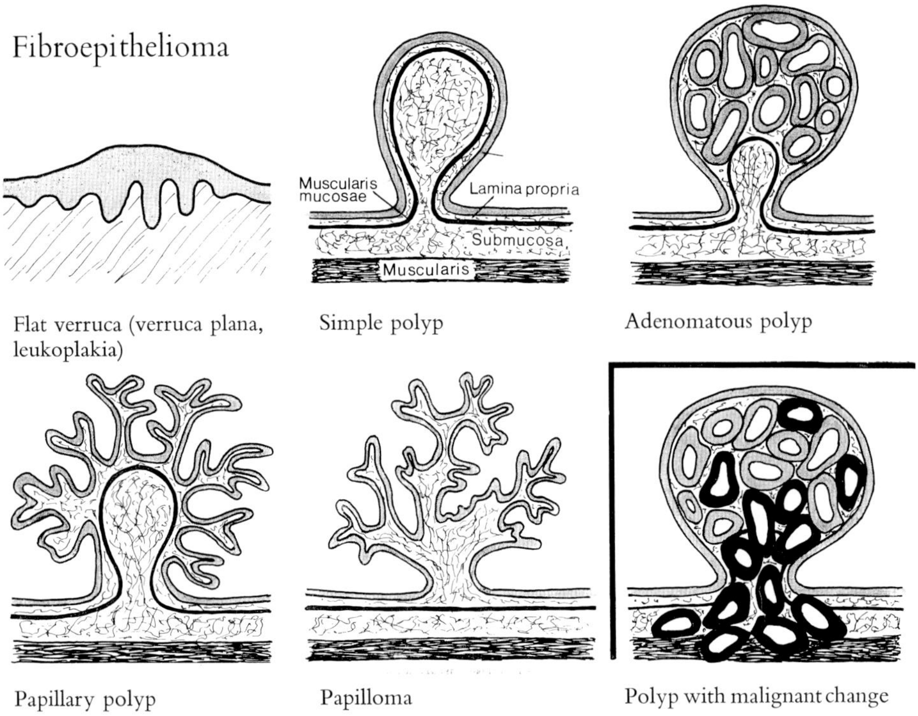

Flat verruca (verruca plana, leukoplakia)

Simple polyp

Muscularis mucosae
Lamina propria
Submucosa
Muscularis

Adenomatous polyp

Papillary polyp

Papilloma

Polyp with malignant change

Fig. 389. Microscopic features of fibroepitheliomas.

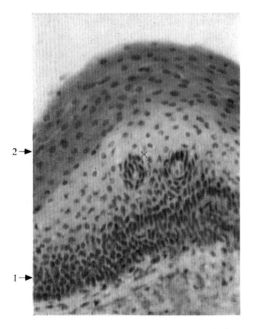

Fig. 390. Leukoplakia of the uterine cervical mucosa; H & E, 320 ×.

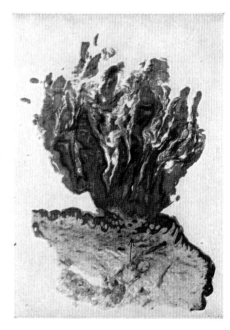

Fig. 391. Papillary wart (verruca vulgaris); H & E, 10 ×.

Benign Epithelial Tumors

Two growth patterns are recognized: 1. *Fibroepithelial arising from the epidermis or mucous membranes and producing an exophytic tumor* (**polyp, papilloma**). 2. **Adenoma,** *an endophytic tumor of parenchymatous organs with an organoid structure and showing expansile growth.* Both patterns of growth have in common the primary proliferation of epithelium into which vascularized nutrient connective tissue grows from adjacent tissues.

The various kinds of exophytic, fibroepithelial tumors are illustrated in Figure 389. **Leukoplakia,** or **verruca plana,** consists principally of *thickening of the epithelium.* **Polyps:** nodular structures with a connective tissue stalk: formed of cylindrical epithelium resting on a stalk which arises from the submucosa (varieties: simple polyp, adenomatous polyp, papillary polyp, see p.237). **Papilloma:** branching, arborescent epithelial growth arising from squamous or transitional epithelium. The connective tissue stalk originates from the lamina propria.

In leukoplakia of the cervical mucous membrane (Fig. 390), there is an increase in thickness of both the basal cell layer (→ 1) and the cornified layer which, in addition, shows pyknotic nuclei (parakeratosis → 2). The two round nodules in the epithelium (×) are pegs of connective tissue cut in cross section.

Verruca vulgaris, or papillary wart (Fig. 391), shows papillary overgrowth of the epidermis which rests on a delicate base of vascularized connective tissue. The rete pegs are elongated and extend into the verruca like spokes radiating from the axle of a wheel (→). The epithelium is covered by a thick horny layer (hyperkeratosis with slight parakeratosis).

Papillomas of the mucous membranes such as, for example, those arising from epithelium of the urinary bladder (Figs. 392, 393), show tree-like branching of the connective tissue stalk (matrix). It must be remembered, when such a pattern is discovered in histological sections, that only a two-dimensional plane surface is seen and, therefore, the branches and twigs may be revealed only by examining many sections. Figure 392 is of a portion of a urinary bladder papilloma in which the connective tissue stalk shows extensive branching. The upper portion appears separated from the lower due to the fact that the base of the branch is not in the plane of the section. Higher magnification (Fig. 393) shows multilayered transitional epithelium with a superficial layer of surface epithelium. The nuclei are uniform. If cellular and nuclear atypia were present, they would suggest the possibility of malignant change.

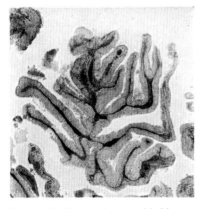

Fig. 392. Papilloma of urinary bladder; H & E, 27×.

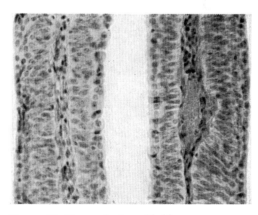

Fig. 393. Papilloma of urinary bladder; H & E, 155×.

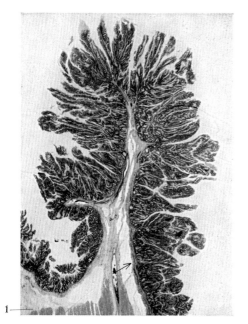

Fig. 394. Papillary polyp of colonic mucosa;
H & E, 3×.

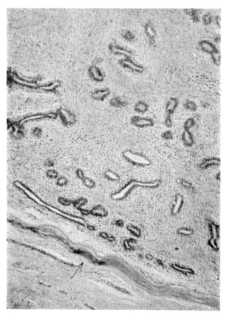

Fig. 395. Extracanalicular fibroadenoma of
breast;
van Gieson stain, 70×.

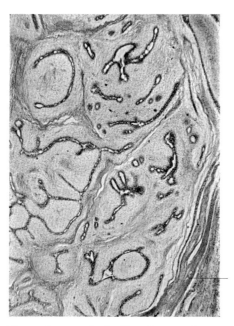

Fig. 396. Intracanalicular fibroadenoma of
breast;
van Gieson stain, 33×.

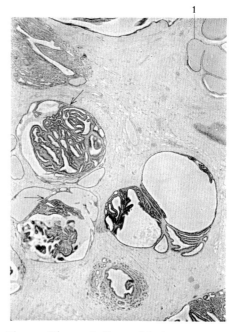

Fig. 397. Fibrocystic disease of the breast;
H & E, 23×.

Polyps

Papillary or adenomatous growths of mucous membranes covered with cylindrical epithelium are called *polyps* (see Fig. 389, p. 234 and Fig. 394). They originate as a focal area of *evaginated mucous membrane* and eventually show *accompanying glandular proliferation* (adenomatous polyp). In polyps of the colon, the stalk is formed by the submucosa and mucosa muscularis. Accordingly, in histological preparations, it is possible to trace the mucosa muscularis from the normal colon into the connective tissue stalk of the polyp. The glands are arranged in papillary fashion *(papillary polyp)*. If such *papillary polyps* are broad based they show malignant change in about 50% of cases. *Adenomatous polyps* – with or without a connective tissue stalk – can be solitary (malignant change is rare) or multiple *(intestinal polyposis,* see p. 249; a familial disease; eventually 50% show malignant change). If *malignant change* occurs, first the stalk and then the intestinal wall is invaded (see Fig. 389, p. 234, and Fig. 417, p. 248).

Figure 394 shows a **papillary polyp of the mucosa of the large bowel** with the colonic muscularis (→ 1) and the submucosa and mucosa muscularis (→), which can be clearly seen to lead into the stalk. Small branches and twigs covered with cylindrical epithelium arise from the central stalk as though from the trunk of a tree.

Macroscopic: Stalked or broad-based tumors situated on mucous membranes.

Adenoma

Adenomas or **fibroadenomas,** which show *endophytic growth,* are comparable to the fibro-epitheliomas which show an *exophytic growth* pattern, because, in both, glandular proliferation is accompanied by new growth of connective tissue.

Fibroadenoma of the breast (Figs. 395, 396). Histologically, there is a well-circumscribed nodule with a capsule formed by compressed surrounding connective tissue (red tissue → in Figs. 395, 396). There is primarily an outgrowth of the ductal epithelium (double-layered cuboidal epithelium) accompanied by overgrowth of connective tissue which either grows around the proliferated tubular-glandular structures like a mantle (**extracanalicular fibroadenoma,** Fig. 395), or focally compresses the glandular lumens so that the glands and ducts appear to branch (**intracanalicular fibroadenoma,** Fig. 396). In either case, the ducts are lined with a double layer of cuboidal epithelium, and the surrounding connective tissue is loose and moderately cellular.

The **intracanalicular fibroadenoma** in Figure 396 shows the connective tissue capsule as well as the elongated, drawn-out ducts, which have a branching pattern. The young connective tissue lying alongside the tubule-like glands contains fewer mature fibers (stained bright red in van Gieson preparations) than the connective tissue septa that lie between.

Macroscopic: Sharply circumscribed, firm, grayish white nodules.

Fibrocystic disease of the breast (Fig. 397). *This is not a true tumor at all, but an endocrine-induced, nodular overgrowth of ductal and glandular epithelium with cyst formation and increase in connective tissue.* In contrast to a fibroadenoma, there is no sharply defined nodule, but a diffuse, poorly defined overgrowth of connective tissue and newly formed milk ducts, which, for the most part, are widely dilated and cystic. Even with low magnification, the numerous cysts can be recognized. The lining epithelium is flat and atrophic (→ 1). Some areas also show pseudopapillary (without connective tissue stalks) or papillary growths with many-layered epithelium (→). This proliferative type of chronic cystic disease is regarded by some authors as precancerous.

Macroscopic: Firm, grayish white breast tissue containing numerous cysts.

237

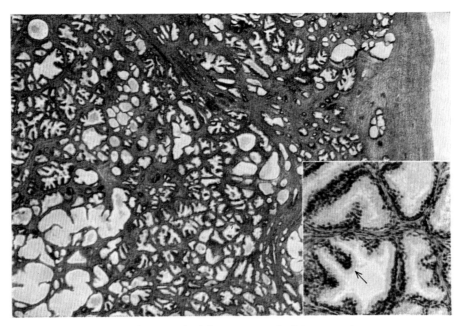

Fig. 398. So-called prostatic hypertrophy (adenomyomatosis of the prostate);
H & E, 17× (inset magnified 120×).

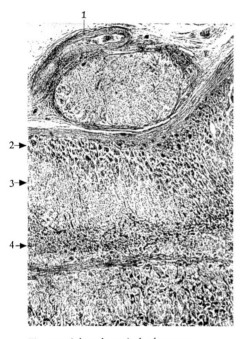

Fig. 399. Adrenal cortical adenoma;
H & E, 35×.

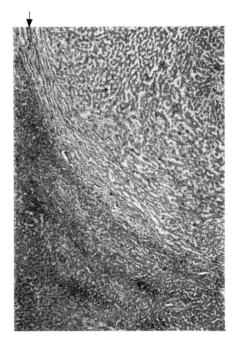

Fig. 400. Liver cell adenoma;
H & E, 36×.

238

So-called **prostatic hypertrophy (adenomyomatosis of the prostate,** Fig. 398). *This is a hormonally conditioned tumor-like enlargement consisting of nodular hyperplasia of the portion of the prostate surrounding the urethra (so-called internal gland) which may be predominantly of glandular (adenomatous), glandulomuscular (adenomyomatous) or even purely myomatous character. This results in compression of the remaining portion of the prostate and the formation of a so-called surgical capsule.* Under low magnification, many nodular areas of glandular hyperplasia can be seen with closely approx- imated and sometimes cystically dilated glands that are lined with flattened epithelium. Here and there are pseudopapillary growths (→ in the inset for Fig. 398), so that the glands appear to have various shapes when seen in cross sections. In other portions, the glands are separated by an excess of stromal tissue which, with van Gieson stain, is seen to be smooth muscle. High magni- fication (inset in Fig. 398) reveals cylindrical lining cells with pale cytoplasm and basally placed nuclei. Homogeneous protein masses and laminated concrements are found in the lumens of many of the cystically dilated glands.

Macroscopic: Nodular enlargement of the prostate, with the nodules either projecting into the urinary bladder or outside it ("lateral nodular hypertrophy"). Concrements appear as black stippling on the cut surfaces.

Typical examples of benign **glandular new growths** with a preponderant parenchymatous component can be found in the glands of internal secretion and in the liver and kidney. *The classification of adenomas of the glands of internal secretion as true tumors is by no means undisputed;* many authors regard them as examples of *hyperplastic adaptation.* Thus, nodular hyperplasia of the adrenal cortex (see p. 187) frequently can be distinguished from a capsular adenoma only with difficulty. Figure 399 **(adenoma of the adrenal cortex)** shows an adenoma situated in the capsule of the adrenal gland and arising from detached adrenal cortical tissue. The capsule of connective tissue is easily recognized (→ 1 shows an overlying artery), as are the cortical cells which are arranged in cords resembling the architecture of the zona fasciculata (columns of cells with capillaries between) (→ 2: zona glomerulosa of the adrenal cortex, → 3: zona fasciculata, → 4: zona reticularis).

Macroscopic: Yellow, sharply circumscribed nodules. Adenomas can actively secrete hormone, in which case *Cushing's disease* may develop (see p. 187).

A liver cell adenoma (Fig. 400) has been chosen as an example of an adenoma developing in a large parenchymatous organ. The normal parenchyma is compressed by the tumor and forms a thin capsule of atrophic liver cells (→). The cells of the adenoma are arranged in the typical cord pattern found in the liver, but are not as well organized as in normal liver lobules and show no radiation from a central vein. The surrounding normal liver tissue shows hyperemia which, however, is not present in the adenoma.

Macroscopic: Grayish red nodules, mostly only 2–3 cm. in diameter.

These adenomas are of dysontogenetic origin and, for the most part, are *not* a precursor of liver cell car- cinoma. Primary carcinoma of the liver arises usually in a cirrhotic liver (hepatocellular carcinoma, bile duct or cholangiocellular carcinoma).

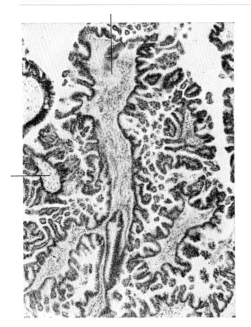

Fig. 401. Serous cystadenoma;
H & E, 58×.

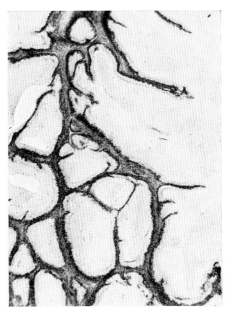

Fig. 402. Pseudomucinous cystadenoma of the ovary;
H & E, 50×.

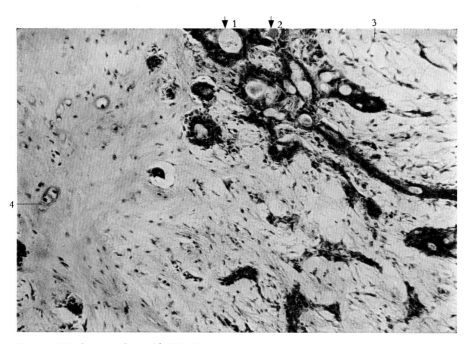

Fig. 403. Mixed tumor of parotid; H & E, 130×.

Cystadenoma of the Ovary

This is a cystic ovarian adenoma that is derived in some cases from peritoneal epithelium (mesothelium) or medullary cords (rete ovarii) forming a serous cystadenoma and, in other cases, from the epithelium of the Müllerian ducts (pseudomucinous cystadenoma).

Serous cystadenomas (papillary serous cystadenoma) (Fig. 401) occur, for the most part, as bilateral, multilocular growths having a connective tissue capsule and cystic spaces divided by fibrous septa. The inner surfaces of the cysts are covered either with a single layer of epithelium or with extensively branching papillary processes showing stalks of vascularized fibrous tissue (→). There is a single layer of covering cylindrical epithelium having centrally placed nuclei. The cysts contain serous fluid. Not infrequently, these cysts become malignant (25%). The morphological indications of such a malignant change are heaping up of the epithelium, cellular pleomorphism, invasion of the fibrous septa and penetration of the capsule.

Pseudomucinous cystadenoma, or mucinous cystadenoma (Fig. 402), usually arises as a unilateral growth with a smooth capsule and multiple mucus-containing cysts of various sizes. Histologically, the cysts are lined with mucus-secreting epithelium. **High magnification** (Fig. 404) shows the goblet-like structure of the cells and the basally situated nuclei. Malignant change is much less common (5%) than in serous cystadenomas.

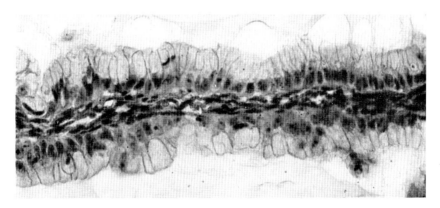

Fig. 404. Pseudomucinous cystadenoma; H & E, 260 ×.

Mixed tumor of parotid gland (Fig. 403).

Mixed tumors may arise in any of the salivary glands in the neck or oral cavity. Current opinion is that they are true adenomas with pseudomesenchymal differentiation (mesenchymal metaplasia); that is, they are pleomorphic adenomas. The constituent ground substances, such as mucus, hyalin and cartilage are interpreted as excretory products of the cells of the glands.

Examination under low power shows areas composed of many different tissues. There are solid columns of cuboidal or cylindrical epithelial cells, which may also form gland-like structures (→ 1) that contain homogeneous hyalin masses (→ 2). The solid columns of epithelium are embedded in homogeneous tissue rich in blue-staining ground substance and containing ramifying cells with stellate-shaped processes (mucoid portion: → 3). These latter may also appear as isolated cartilage-like cells with halos (→ 4).

Macroscopic: Well-circumscribed, grayish white tumors often with mucinous cut surfaces.

Malignant Epithelial Tumors

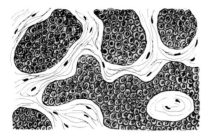

Carcinoma simplex

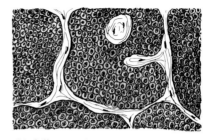

Medullary carcinoma

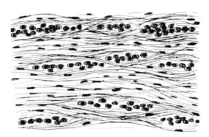

Scirrhous carcinoma

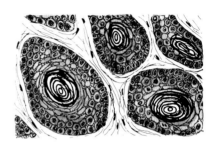

Squamous cell carcinoma

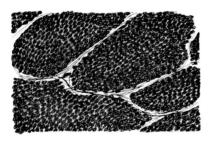

Small cell bronchial carcinoma

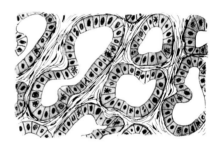

Adenocarcinoma

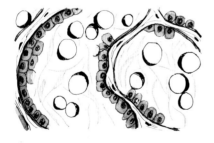

Mucinous carcinoma

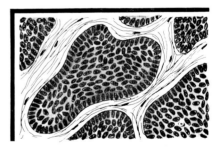

Basal cell carcinoma (basalioma)

Fig. 405. Diagram of the histological appearances of malignant epithelial tumors, including basal cell carcinoma (basalioma).

Malignant Epithelial Tumors

The different histological appearances of the malignant epithelial tumors can be grouped as follows according to their fibrous stroma content (Fig. 405):

1. **Carcinoma simplex** (see Fig. 406). Epithelium and fibrous stroma are present in about equal amounts (ratio 1:1).
2. **Medullary carcinoma** (see Fig. 407). Epithelial tissue predominates over fibrous stroma (ratio 9:1).
3. **Scirrhous carcinoma** (see Figs. 408, 409). The fibrous stroma predominates, and the cancer cells are present in small nests or masses.

This grouping is based solely upon the quantitative relation between stroma and parenchyma and not upon the degree of differentiation of the epithelial cells.

From the viewpoint of their *histogenesis*, the following kinds of tumors can be recognized: **keratinized** and **non-keratinized squamous cell carcinomas** (Figs. 410, 411 on pages 244, 245), **transitional cell carcinoma and columnar cell carcinoma.** Finally, tumors can be divided according to the degree of differentiation as undifferentiated **solid carcinoma** simplex Figs. 406, 407), **adenocarcinoma** (Figs. 417, 418, p. 248), **mucinous carcinoma** (Fig. 419, p. 248) and **papillary carcinoma** (Fig. 433, p. 255). **Small cell carcinoma** is regarded as an undifferentiated medullary carcinoma (Figs. 412, 416). For basal cell carcinoma, see Figs. 413, 414, p. 246.

Solid carcinoma simplex (Fig. 406) consists of large epithelial masses without differentiation. It arises chiefly from glands (in this case, breast) and can be conceived as a solid growth of epithelium which has not differentiated further into glandular structures. In Figure 406 can be seen the thickly layered cells, most of which are round with palely stained cytoplasm and large pleomorphic nuclei. They are grouped into large clusters or masses and have invaded the mammary fat tissue.

Medullary carcinoma (Fig. 407), which has a soft, fungus-like gross appearance, shows expanding columns of undifferentiated epithelial cells supported by delicate, vascularized, fibrous tissue septa (→ 1). Figure 407 shows the pleomorphic character of the tumor cells with their large nucleoli and numerous atypical mitoses (→ 2: metaphase with chromosome separation, × : anaphase, → 3: prophase).

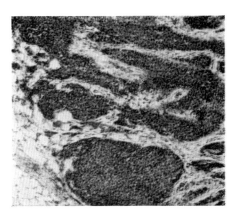

Fig. 406. Solid carcinoma simplex;
H & E, 76×.

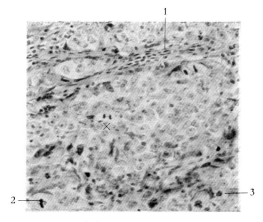

Fig. 407. Medullary carcinoma;
H & E, 215×.

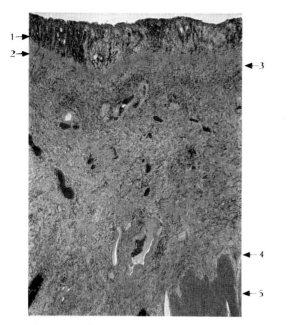

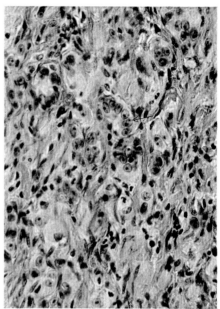

Fig. 408. Scirrhous carcinoma of the stomach; H & E, 24×.

Fig. 409. Scirrhous carcinoma of the stomach; van Gieson stain, 320×.

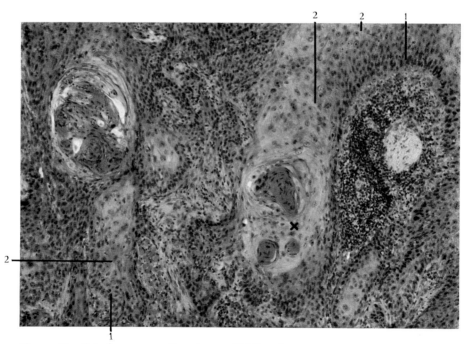

Fig. 410. Keratinized squamous cell carcinoma; H & E, 116×.

In the stomach, **scirrhous carcinoma** (Figs. 408, 409) predominantly invades the submucosa. With very low magnification, the extensive proliferation of fibrous tissue can be easily recognized, as well as the diffuse invasion of the submucosa by the cancer cells (between → 3 and 4; → 1 is mucosa, → 2 is muscularis mucosa and → 5 is muscularis). Higher magnification (Fig. 409) shows nests of cuboidal or round tumor cells lying between bundles of collagen fibers and fibroblasts. Most of the tumor cells have large nuclei and distinct nucleoli and are arranged in the shape of quotation marks (→ in the picture). Solitary tumor cells are often difficult to differentiate from large fibroblasts.

Macroscopic: Diffuse, firm, grayish white infiltration of the stomach wall. In the metastases (for example, those in the perigastric lymph nodes), scirrhous carcinoma may grow like an adenocarcinoma and have well-differentiated glands and little fibrous tissue.

Squamous cell carcinoma (Figs. 410, 411) arises from surface epithelium and sends irregular, peg-shaped extensions into the underlying supporting tissues. Figure 411 shows a **slightly keratinized squamous cell carcinoma** of the skin. In contrast to epidermal acanthosis (→ 1), the carcinoma cells are growing in plump cords and have extended widely into the depths of the corium. The surface of the tumor is ulcerated. Occasional epithelial pearls can be seen in the middle of the cords of cancer cells (→ 2). At the margins of the tumor, there is a chronic inflammatory infiltrate (→ 3, Fig. 411).

Under **high magnification** (Fig. 410), the imitation of the histological structure of normal epidermis becomes clear and the three cell layers of the epidermis can be recognized in the cancerous tissue (basal cell, prickle cell and cornified layers). The outermost layer of the columns of cells consists of relatively small cells (→ 1) with nuclei that are round to ovoid shaped or large and polymorphic with greatly increased chromatin content (corresponding to the basal cell layer of the epidermis). Next comes a layer of big cells with elongated, eosinophilic cytoplasm and large, round, pleomorphic nuclei and distinct nucleoli, corresponding to the prickle cell layer (→ 2). In the center are large cornified or keratinized masses, the epithelial pearls (×). With higher magnification, intracellular bridges can be seen in the cells in the prickle cell layer (carcinoma spinocellulare, prickle cell carcinoma). The *diagnosis of carcinoma* is made solely on finding *invasion* by the epithelial cells. The characterization of the type of epithelium (i. e., squamous epithelium) is made by finding intercellular bridges.

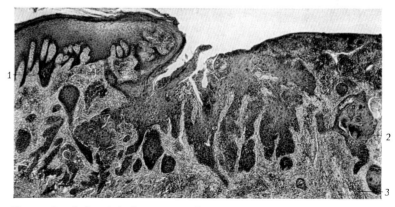

Fig. 411. Poorly keratinized squamous cell carcinoma of the skin; H & E, 31×.

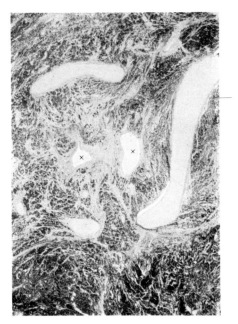

Fig. 412. Small cell carcinoma of the bronchus;
H & E, 13×.

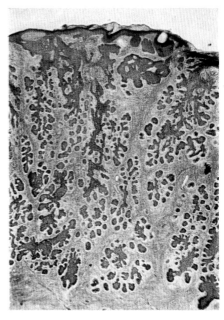

Fig. 413. Basal cell carcinoma (basalioma);
H & E, 23×.

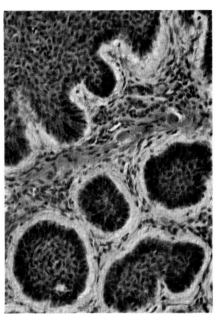

Fig. 414. Basal cell carcinoma (basalioma);
H & E, 295×.

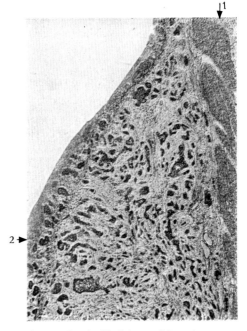

Fig. 415. Carcinoid of the small intestine;
H & E, 48×.

Small cell carcinoma of the bronchus (Figs. 412, 416) is an undifferentiated medullary carcinoma (very scanty stroma) which arises from a large or small bronchus and consists of large accumulations of small, round or oval cells (in Fig. 412 →: bronchial cartilage, ×: remaining bronchial lumen). The epithelial nature of the tumor is often so little apparent that the uninitiated observer can easily mistake it for a sarcoma. High magnification (Fig. 416) discloses the cells to be somewhat larger than lymphocytes and to have scanty, often scarcely detectable, cytoplasm and round or spindle-shaped hyperchromatic nuclei (oat cell carcinoma).

These tumors are highly malignant (the time interval between clinical diagnosis and death is often only 6 months, whereas for squamous cell carcinoma of the bronchus the clinical course is 1–2 years).

Basal cell carcinoma, or basalioma (Figs. 413, 414). *This is an epithelial tumor of the corium which develops principally in the skin about the face of older men, grows by infiltration and ulcerates (rodent ulcer) but practically never metastasizes. It can be differentiated from squamous cell carcinoma morphologically and also biologically, since the latter may metastasize. The term "basal cell carcinoma"* (KROMPECHER, *1900*) *is not entirely correct, since the tumor has only a semimalignant behavior. Rarely, a malignant basalioma with metastasis is observed* (Dr. TEN SELDAM, University of Perth, Australia, personal communication. ASSOR, 1967).

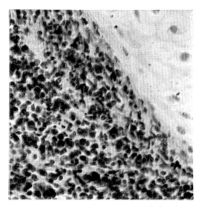

Fig. 416. Small cell carcinoma of the bronchus; H & E, 290×.

Histologically (Fig. 413), basal cell carcinomas consist of solid columns of epithelial cells growing in staghorn-like fashion. They arise in the corium and frequently connect directly with the epidermis or the skin appendages. Just as in squamous cell carcinoma, there is clear invasive growth, but metastases do not develop, except very rarely. If the cellular masses are examined under **high magnification** (Fig. 414), the differences from squamous cell carcinoma become clear: the cells in the margins of the tumor cords have a palisade arrangement; the cells in the interior of the cords are arranged haphazardly – *but in both places the cells are of the same type*, i. e., the small, undifferentiated cells of the basal layer of the epidermis or skin appendages (ALBERTINI, 1955). Certain kinds of basal cell carcinomas may show considerable maturation (keratinization, etc.), but in comparison with squamous cell carcinomas, they lack the anaplasia of the cancer cells.

Carcinoids (Fig. 415) of the small intestine (also appendix and bronchus) arise from enterochromic cells (serotonin-producing) and, like basal cell carcinomas, occupy an *intermediate position* between benign and malignant tumors. Figure 415 shows the solid, partly alveolar epithelial structure of the tumors and the infiltrative type of growth which extends to the muscularis (→ 1; → 2: mucosa). Carcinoids are composed of uniform, small, polygonal cells with faintly eosinophilic or clear (argentophilic) cytoplasm and round-to-oval nuclei. There is a rich fibrous stroma.

These tumors produce serotonin and kallikrein and may be manifested clinically by the carcinoid syndrome. Malignant forms with metastases are also encountered.

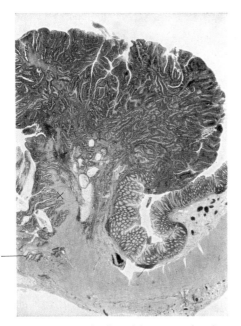

Fig. 417. Mucosal polyp of the rectum showing malignant change (adenocarcinoma); H & E, 6.5×.

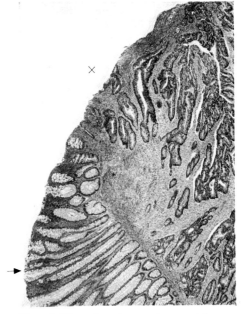

Fig. 418. Ulcerating adenocarcinoma of the rectum; H & E, 26×.

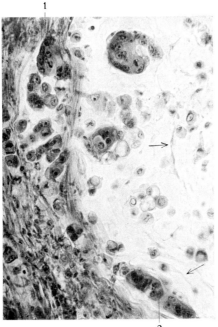

Fig. 419. Mucinous adenocarcinoma; H & E, 216×.

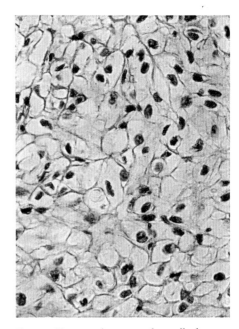

Fig. 420. Hypernephroma or clear cell adeno-carcinoma of the kidney; H & E, 312×.

Mucosal polyp of the rectum with malignant change (Fig. 417). *Adenomatous polyps of the colon* (see Fig. 389) *may become malignant (up to 50% in intestinal polyposis).* The initial stage is invasion of the stalk of the polyp by cells transformed from the normal clear, mucus-producing columnar epithelium into cells with basophilic cytoplasm. The glands are more plentiful and have become irregular in shape. Figure 417 shows a polyp that is already nearly completely permeated with atypical, ramifying glands. The stalk is infiltrated in several places (×) and the tumor is already invading the muscularis (→).

Ulcerating adenocarcinoma of the rectum (Fig. 418). This carcinoma shows superficial ulceration (×) and a normal marginal mucosa (→). The adenoid structure of the carcinoma mimics normal glands, but the tumorous glands grow by ramification and have slit-like lumens. High magnification shows multi-layered columnar epithelial cells with oval, often only slightly atypical, nuclei. Mitoses are frequent. The carcinoma has undermined the normal mucosa.

Macroscopic: Bulky tumors of the large bowel causing stenosis of the lumen. In the terminal stages, the tumor may encircle the gut and show secondary ulceration. *Clinical:* Bright red blood in the stools. Palpable on rectal examination!

Mucinous adenocarcinoma (Fig. 419). Mucinous carcinoma (gelatinous carcinoma) has a very typical histological appearance. Low-power examination discloses numerous large, faintly stained, pale areas scattered throughout the tissue. Medium magnification shows pale blue-stained, delicately fibrillar deposits of mucin (→), in which solitary cells or groups of cells can be seen. At the margins, the tumor is solid (→ 1, → 2), infiltrates the connective tissue, and shows multiple layers of large, round cells with abundant cytoplasm and pleomorphic nuclei. **High magnification** (Fig. 421) shows that mucus vacuoles have appeared in the cytoplasm and pressed the nuclei toward the periphery of the cell (*signet ring cells*; a cytoplasmic ring → 1 frames a vacuole of mucin; nucleus →).

Macroscopic: The cut surface of the tumors is gray, mucinous, and transparent.

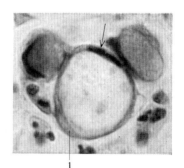

Fig. 421. Signet ring cells in mucinous carcinoma; H & E, 900×.

Hypernephroma (Fig. 420) is a tumor made up of tissues of varying degrees of maturity and has a malignant potential. The typical tumor possesses a connective tissue capsule and consists of cords of cells bearing a resemblance to plant cells. The optically empty cytoplasm contains glycogen. The cell boundaries are distinct (actually a narrow rim of cytoplasm). The nuclei are round or oval. Although these tumors often show the histological characteristics of a benign tumor, nevertheless, they may metastasize (compare metastasizing thyroid adenomas). *As a general rule, hypernephromas under 3 cm. do not usually metastasize.* **Hypernephroid carcinomas or clear cell adenocarcinomas** are frankly invasive tumors that histologically closely resemble hypernephromas. They grow into the renal vessels, especially veins, and produce pulmonary metastases. The tumors may have a strong resemblance to adrenal adenomas, but have nothing to do with adrenal rests.

Macroscopic: Mostly round, sharply demarcated tumors with yellow or reddish yellow, speckled cut surfaces.

249

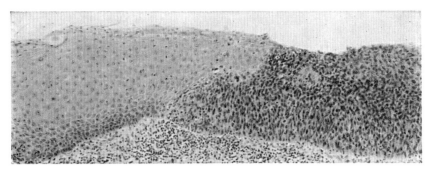

Fig. 422. Carcinoma in situ of the uterine cervix (simple replacement); H & E, 111×.

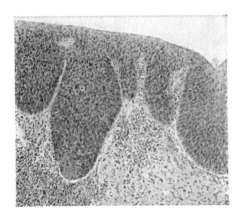

Fig. 423. Carcinoma in situ of the uterine cervix (proliferative downgrowth); H & E, 78×.

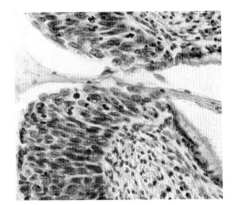

Fig. 424. Carcinoma in situ of the uterine cervix (growth in the cervical glands); H & E, 255×.

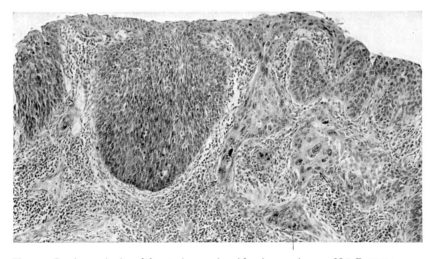

Fig. 425. Carcinoma in situ of the uterine cervix with microcarcinoma; H & E, 120×.

Precancerous Lesions of the Uterine Cervix

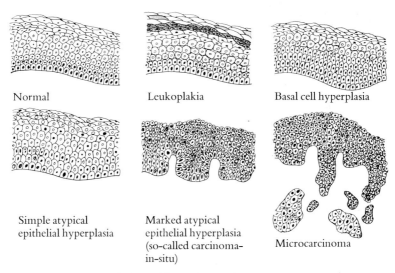

Normal   Leukoplakia   Basal cell hyperplasia

Simple atypical
epithelial hyperplasia

Marked atypical
epithelial hyperplasia
(so-called carcinoma-
in-situ)

Microcarcinoma

Fig. 426. Precancerous lesions of the uterine cervix.

Precancerous lesions will be briefly mentioned and illustrated here because of their fundamental importance in the study of tumors. *Precancerous lesions, in the strict sense of the term, are conceived of as those tissue changes which, in a definite percentage of cases (more than 20–30%), are precursors of malignancy.* They can be especially well studied in the **squamous epithelium of the uterine cervix** (Fig. 426) or of the skin. **Leukoplakia** is usually a harmless epithelial change in which the basal cell layer is thickened by simple numerical increase of the epithelial cells (see Fig. 390 on p. 234). There is a thick layer of keratinization with pyknotic nuclei (parakeratosis, see Fig. 390). No atypical cells are present in the thickened basal cell layer. In **simple atypical hyperplasia,** the normal stratification of the epithelium is preserved, but individual atypical epithelial cells appear, showing hyperchromasia and slight pleomorphism. The normal progressive maturation of the cells is preserved. In **markedly atypical epithelium,** this progressive cellular maturation is lost *(carcinoma in situ).*

Figure 422 **(carcinoma-in-situ of the uterine cervix)** shows, on the left, normal epithelium onto which abuts markedly atypical epithelium. The cells are elongated and multi-layered in fish-scale fashion. The cytoplasm is scanty and the nuclei are ovoid, hyperchromatic and somewhat pleomorphic. Mitoses are present in all layers of the richly cellular epithelium. The underlying connective tissue shows chronic inflammation. Such markedly atypical epithelium is designated as *carcinoma-in-situ,* since many clinical, histochemical and biochemical facts support the idea that a carcinoma is growing within the epithelium (intraepithelial) and in many cases will ultimately show a stepwise progression to invasive carcinoma. Figure 423 shows one of the steps in the malignant conversion of a growth which is *advancing in the form of broad pegs.* The atypical epithelium may also extend into *cervical glands* and displace the columnar epithelium (Fig. 424). At a later stage, delicate cords of the carcinoma-in-situ may invade the connective tissue, so that a **true invasive carcinoma (microcarcinoma)** develops. Figure 425 shows the crowded arrangement of the cells in a carcinoma-in-situ and beneath it the cords of pleomorphic cells forming an invasive squamous cell carcinoma (→). The cells in the invasive carcinoma are larger than those in the carcinoma-in-situ, their cytoplasm is eosinophilic and the nuclei large, pleomorphic and hyperchromatic. Invasive carcinoma is observed in about 30% of cases of carcinoma-in-situ.

251

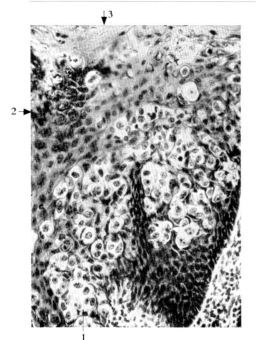

Fig. 427. Paget's disease;
H & E, 395×.

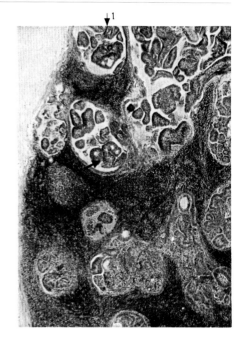

Fig. 428. Lymph node metastasis from a
carcinoma of the ovary;
H & E, 48×.

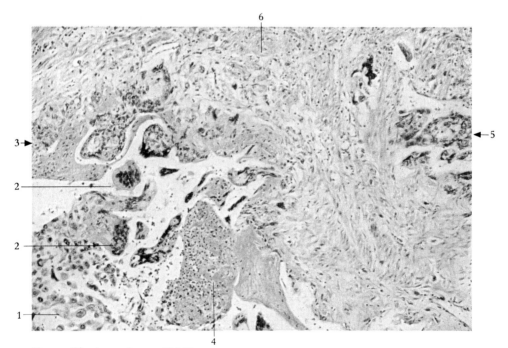

Fig. 429. Chorioncarcinoma; H & E, 109×.

Paget's disease (Fig. 427). This condition usually develops unilaterally in the breasts of women and is thought by some to be *carcinoma-in-situ of the epidermis*. In most cases, however, there is at the same time an underlaying intraductal carcinoma of the breast, so that most observers believe the lesion is an unusual intraepithelial metastasis from the ductal carcinoma. Histologically (Fig. 427), the epidermis is infiltrated by large ballooned cells, Paget cells, with optically empty cytoplasm containing glycogen (→ 1). The nuclei are hyperchromatic, pleomorphic and often contain large nucleoli. The epidermis is thickened by marked acanthosis (lower right-hand side of the picture). The stratum granulosum (→ 2) is frequently increased, as is also the keratin layer (→ 3). The atypical Paget cells are confined to the epidermis and do not invade the corium.

Macroscopic: A dark red, sharply circumscribed lesion of the nipple or areola with superficial crusting and spread into surrounding structures.
Extramammary Paget's disease usually is seen in the genital region and in the axilla. In these places, also, the characteristic balloon cells appear, frequently in clumps. The changes are very similar to those of *Bowen's disease* (precancer or cancer-in-situ of the skin).

Lymph node metastasis from an ovarian carcinoma (Fig. 428). Spread of malignant epithelial tumors customarily takes place by way of the lymphatics (carcinomatous lymphangiosis, not lymphangitis, since there is no inflammation), with involvement of regional lymph nodes. Nests of cancer cells are found first in the sinuses of the cortex and medulla. Later, the entire lymph node may be infiltrated. Figure 428 shows the metastasis of a papillary carcinoma of the ovary. Nests of cancer cells lie in widely dilated lymphatic sinuses (→ 1 and → in the picture) and show papillae with stalks of connective tissue covered with atypical columnar cells.

Macroscopic: The lymph nodes are enlarged, with grayish white cut surfaces.

Chorioncarcinoma (Fig. 429). *This is a malignant tumor of the epithelium of the placental chorionic villi but not of the accompanying stroma. Thus, it is a malignant transformation of both the (basal) Langhans layer and the superficial syncytial cell layer of the chorionic villi (see Figs. 307, 309).* Low magnification shows, for the most part, swollen, necrotic and hemorrhagic masses of tissue, at the edges of which there is still viable tumor tissue. Medium magnification shows large syncytial sheets of cells (→ 1) with pleomorphic nuclei and without recognizable cell boundaries. Next to these there are syncytial giant cells (→ 2). The Langhans cell layer is represented by regularly arranged cuboidal cells with pale cytoplasm and round or oval nuclei (→ 3). In one place can be seen a mixture of necrotic tissue and fibrin (→ 4). Sheets of pleomorphic tumor cells have invaded veins (→ 5) and these give rise to secondary deposits in the lungs. The myometrium is seen at → 6.

Macroscopic: Hemorrhagic (dark reddish brown) and necrotic tumors which metastasize by way of the blood (to lung).

Clinically, the patients show increased chorio-gonadotropin excretion. Chorioncarcinoma arises frequently in a hydatid mole (30–60%). The incidence is about 0.05–3.7% of births.

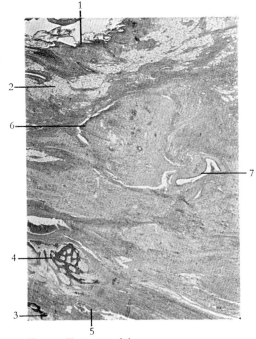

Fig. 430. Teratoma of the ovary;
H & E, 16×.

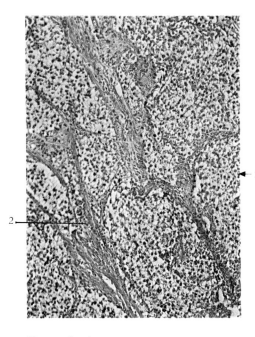

Fig. 431. Seminoma;
H & E, 80×.

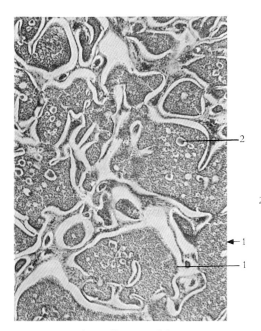

Fig. 432. Granulosa cell tumor of the ovary:
H & E, 70×.

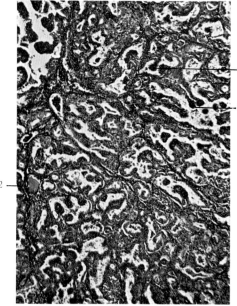

Fig. 433. Papillary adenocarcinoma of the
thyroid; H & E, 70×.

Teratoma of the ovary (Fig. 430). *Teratomas are mixed tumors composed of different tissue elements. They are malformations and may arise in different parts of the body, but show a preference for regions with germinal glands. They make up 35–50% of testicular and 15% of ovarian tumors. The testicular teratomas are mostly malignant, the ovarian preponderantly benign. The simplest ovarian teratomas are dermoid cysts, which are lined with squamous epithelium and contain sebaceous and sweat glands and hair follicles in the wall. There is commonly an area of extra thickness in the wall which often contains bone tissue or teeth. In complex teratomas, a variety of many other sorts of tissues may be found.*

Figure 430 shows an ovarian teratoma at very low magnification. There is a variety of different tissues which can best be discovered and identified with higher magnification. Cornified squamous epithelium containing numerous hair follicles (→ 1) is easily recognized, as well as attached fat tissue (→ 2), cartilage (→ 3) and bone (→ 4). Nearby is a tubule with a narrow lumen that is lined with ciliated epithelium of the kind seen in a bronchus (→ 5). In addition, there is nerve tissue containing many ganglion cells (→ 6) and a neural canal lined with ependyma (→ 7). Thyroid tissue is also commonly found (struma ovarii), or salivary gland, lung and liver tissue.

The preponderantly malignant testicular teratomas lack this rich variety of mature tissues. They are composed of rapidly growing, highly pleomorphic tissue which, in some places, resembles carcinoma and in others sarcoma.

Macroscopic: Dermoid cysts with a simple structure are identified by the presence of sebaceous and scaly cornified material and the presence of hair in the contents of the cyst. Dermoid cysts with a complex structure are mostly solid, often with alternating clefts and cysts and have an irregular and variegated appearance, depending upon the kinds of tissues that make them up. Malignant teratomas have a partly medullary, partly fish-flesh appearance and usually show focal necrosis and hemorrhage.

Seminoma (Fig. 431). *This is a malignant tumor arising from testicular tissue and presenting as undifferentiated germinal tissue cells.* The histological picture is characterized by large areas of organoid tissue composed of large, clear, polygonal cells having a central, round nucleus. In addition, groups of small, round, lymphocyte-like cells are seen.

Figure 431 shows the large, alternating fields of proliferating pale tumor cells (→ 1). Between the tumor areas run broad bands of eosinophilic collagen fibers and vascularized connective tissue (→ 2). In many places, there are nests of small round cells.

Macroscopic: Grayish white medullary tumors spreading within the tunica albuginea and markedly displacing the testis. Large tumors have yellow, map-like areas of necrosis. Many cases metastasize widely.

Granulosa cell tumor of the ovary (Fig. 432). *This ovarian tumor frequently shows hormonal activity. It can produce estrogen and cause atypical cystic hyperplasia of the uterine mucosa. Most are benign, but nevertheless have a marked tendency to recurrence, and about 10–20% of patients develop metastases (semi-malignant).*

The histological structure may show considerable variation: solid, follicular, tubulo-adenoid, cylindromatous and sarcomatous forms are seen in different tumors. Correspondingly, the individual cells of these tumors also can be of many shapes and, in occasional cases, can store fat. Figure 432 illustrates the solid (→ 1) and the follicular (→ 2) forms of this tumor. The uniform, medium-size, polygonal cells with deeply stained, oval nuclei resemble the granulosa cells of the graafian follicle morphologically.

Papillary adenocarcinoma of the thyroid (Fig. 433). *Thyroid papillary carcinoma will serve as an example of the various kinds of malignant epithelial thyroid tumors (malignant adenoma: regular pattern resembling normal thyroid tissue. Follicular carcinoma: follicular pattern and of intermediate malignancy. Undifferentiated carcinoma).*

Histologically, thyroid papillary carcinoma shows irregular islands of papillary and adenoid tissue with an irregular vascularized matrix of connective tissue supporting the pleomorphic, strongly basophilic cylindrical or cuboidal epithelial cells. The hyperchromatic nuclei are round. Frequently, there are proliferating buds of deeply basophilic epithelial cells at the tips of the papillae (→ 1). In some places, the colloid structure of the thyroid is still present (→ 2).

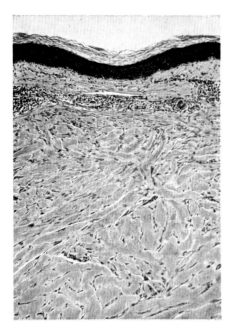

Fig. 434. Keloid;
H & E, 62×.

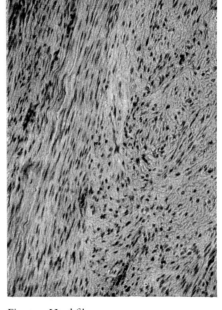

Fig. 435. Hard fibroma;
H & E, 103×.

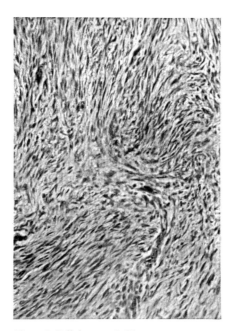

Fig. 436. Cellular or soft fibroma;
H & E, 165×.

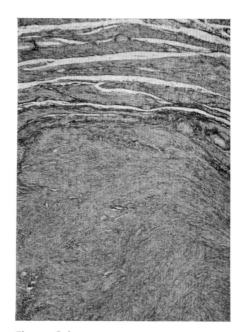

Fig. 437. Leiomyoma;
van Gieson stain, 90×.

Mesenchymal Tumors

Both benign and malignant mesenchymal tumors are encountered:

1. *Benign mesenchymal tumors.* These are composed of well-matured tissues and resemble closely the tissue of their origin (homologous). They grow by expansion. The following tumors belong to this group: fibroma (soft-hard, fibromas, keloid), myxoma, lipoma, chondroma, osteoma, myoma (leiomyoma, rhabdomyoma), hemangioma.

2. *Malignant mesenchymal tumors.* These tumors show less resemblance to the tissue of their origin (heterologous). They grow by invasion and metastasize by way of the blood stream. Some show no differentiation of the intercellular substance, such as fibers or other products (immature type), some do show such differentiation (mature type). a) *immature or undifferentiated types:* round cell sarcoma, spindle cell sarcoma, polymorphocellular sarcoma. b) *mature or differentiated types:* these tumors produce definite intercellular products: fibrosarcoma (collagen fibers), myxosarcoma (mucopolysaccharide ground substance) chondrosarcoma (cartilage), osteosarcoma (bone), myosarcoma (muscle fibers), reticulum cell sarcoma (often produce agyrophilic fibers).

Keloid (Fig. 434). Keloids usually do not appear as spontaneous tumors *(keloid fibroma)* but rather as an excessive overgrowth of hyalinized connective tissue *(scar keloid of the skin)*. Histologically, they show in the corium broad bundles of hyalinized, homogeneous, eosinophilic connective tissue with a few spindle-shaped fibroblasts. In Figure 434 there is a narrow rim of lymphocytes beneath the atrophic epidermis.

Macroscopic: Either firm nodules or cord-like elevations (scar keloids).

Fibroma (Figs. 435, 436). True fibromas differ from keloids in the richness of their cellularity and in the absence of hyalinized connective tissue. **Hard fibromas** (Fig. 435) consist of bundles of collagenous fibers which interlace with one another so that some are seen in cross section and others in longitudinal or oblique section. The fibroblasts have spindle-shaped nuclei. Transitions are seen between this richly fibrous and poorly cellular type and the richly cellular and poorly fibrous type of fibroma (Fig. 436 **cellular fibroma**). Macroscopically, because of their slight fibrous content, cellular fibromas are soft. The elongated nuclei (spindle-shaped fibroblasts) are completely uniform, showing neither pleomorphism nor hyperchromasia (compare this to spindle cell sarcoma, Figs. 447, 448).

Macroscopic: Most fibromas do not possess a capsule, but merge imperceptibly into the surrounding normal tissue. Nonetheless, their benign character is attested by the high degree of tissue differentiation. In cellular fibromas, the differential diagnosis from spindle cell carcinoma can be very difficult.

Leiomyoma (Fig. 437). This is a benign tumor of smooth muscle and is particularly common in the myometrium. Leiomyomas, too, show an interlacing arrangement, but of bundles of smooth muscle fibers. The cytoplasm of the muscle fibers is colored yellow with van Gieson's stain, whereas the connective tissue between the muscle fibers stains red. The nuclei are also elongated but, in contrast to those in a fibroma, have blunted ends (cylindrical shape). The expansile type of growth is clearly shown in the illustration, for the surrounding myometrium is atrophic and compressed into a sort of capsule (in upper part of illustration).

Macroscopic: Myomas appear sharply circumscribed, and most of them are firm. The central portion is frequently hyalinized and the muscle necrotic because of interference with the circulation.

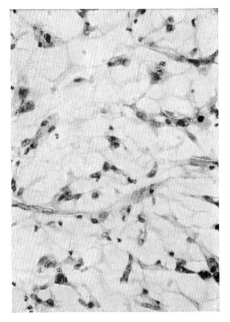

Fig. 438. Myxoma;
H & E, 296×.

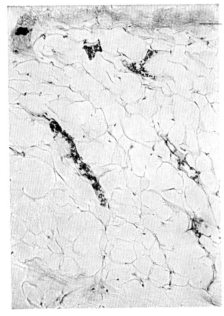

Fig. 439. Lipoma;
H & E, 105×.

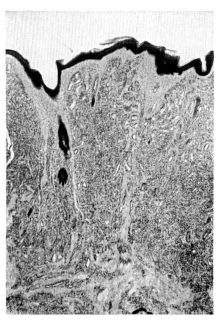

Fig. 440. Capillary hemangioma of skin;
H & E, 30×.

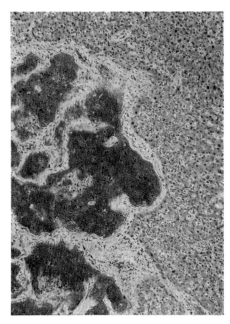

Fig. 441. Cavernous hemangioma of the liver;
H & E, 56×.

Myxoma (Fig. 438). These are infrequent tumors which arise from mucoid connective tissue. They consist of stellate-shaped cells with interlacing cytoplasmic processes. Between the cells there is a pale blue-staining ground substance that gives a positive reaction for mucin. Collagen fibers may also be present (myxofibroma). Figure 438 shows the stellate cells, which resemble the cells of embryonal mucoid tissue (e. g., umbilical cord). Frequently, foci of myxomatous tissue are found in other mesenchymal tumors (chondromyxoma, myxofibroma, etc.), the myxomatous portion either arising from immature portions of the tumor (matrix of the tumor) or being secondary to interstitial edema.

Macroscopic: The tumors are soft, with glassy cut surfaces covered with tenacious mucin.

Lipoma (Fig. 439). These tumors of the fat tissue have a lobulated structure and are sharply circumscribed by a fibrous tissue capsule (→). Histologically, they are composed of typical fat cells that appear little different from normal fat tissue.

Hemangiomas *are benign new formations of blood vessels that are due, for the most part, to congenital malformations (hamartomas, dysontogenetic tumors).* The hemangiomas may have a *capillary, cavernous* (sinusoidal) or, rarely, an *arterial* pattern. *Glomus tumor,* which is a neuro-myo-epithelial tumor, is a special variant.

The most frequent variety is the **capillary hemangioma** (Fig. 440). *It occurs particularly in the skin of children, either as a flat lesion (port wine stain) or as a small, round, slightly raised nodule.* Histologically, under low magnification, the lower part of the tumor consists of poorly defined cellular lobules. The tumor is situated in the corium, lacks clear demarcation and frequently extends into the subcutaneous fat tissue.

Medium magnification (Figure 442) shows clefts and ovoid spaces, lined with elongated endothelial cells, that are either empty (→ 2) or filled with erythrocytes (typical capillaries → 1). In addition, there are solid sprouts of endothelial-like cells without canalization. Between them there is reticular connective tissue (→ 3). The poorly defined boundaries of the lesion are noteworthy and

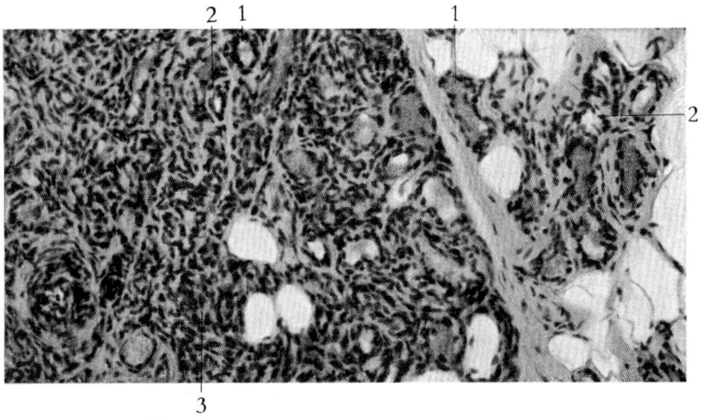

Fig. 442. Capillary hemangioma; H & E, 150×.

can be observed in the photograph as "infiltrative growth" into the subcutaneous fat tissue. In spite of this, the tumor is benign and should not be mistaken for a sarcoma.

A **cavernous hemangioma** (Fig. 441) has essentially the same simple structure. It occurs mostly in the subcapsular region of the liver (hamartoma) and macroscopically is sharply delineated and has a dark red cut surface. Low magnification shows large, blood-filled spaces separated by thin septa of connective tissue covered with endothelial cells. The surrounding liver cells show pressure atrophy.

The malignant form of the tumor is called a *malignant hemangioendothelioma* (see Fig. 450) and has a special tendency to spread to the thyroid.

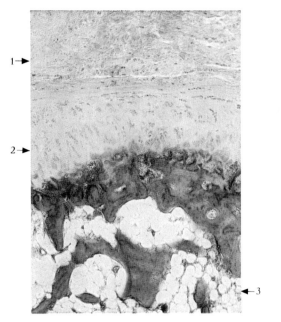

Fig. 443. Cartilaginous exostosis;
H & E, 36×.

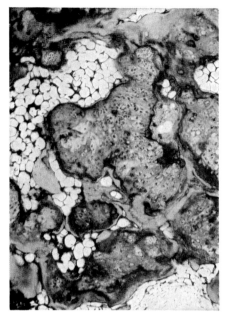

Fig. 444. Enchondroma;
H & E, 41×.

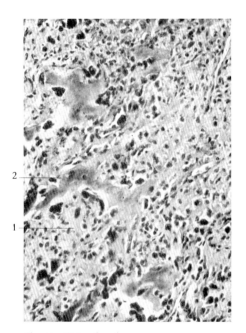

Fig. 445. Osteochondrosarcoma;
H & E, 102×.

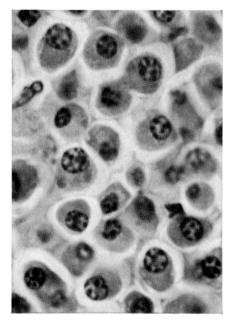

Fig. 446. Plasmacytoma;
H & E, 1,200×.

260

Cartilaginous exostosis (Fig. 443). *Cartilaginous exostoses are considered to be developmental abnormalities and not true tumors. They are hereditary and usually multiple.* Their structure is reminiscent of normal cartilaginous bone growth (enchondral ossification). At the top of the picture, there is periosteal connective tissue (→ 1). Next to this, there is a layer of cartilage which shows distinct columnar organization (→ 2) and a tendency to form irregular cancellous trabeculae. In the uppermost layers, these have lined up as in compact bone. The cancellous bone contains fat tissue and a single focus of hematopoiesis (→ 3).

Enchondroma (Fig. 444). *Chondromas, confined chiefly to the hands and feet, occur as either ecchondromas (periosteal chondroma) or enchondromas of the epiphyseal region, from where they grow into the bone.* Histologically, masses of hyalin cartilage of varying shapes can be seen, which, in this particular instance, have developed in the fatty marrow *(enchondroma)*. Most of the cartilaginous ground substance appears blue (calcification, *ossified chondroma*). It is only in the marginal areas that small reddish blue areas of unmineralized cartilage are seen. Typical cartilage cells may be seen in the lacunae of the ground substance. There is a dense and more irregular arrangement of these cells than would be expected normally.

Osteochondrosarcoma (Fig. 445). The osteogenic sarcomas have a very varied morphological appearance. They destroy the normal bone tissue but, at the same time, promote development of pathologic bone from connective tissue and cartilage (ALBERTINI, 1955). Aside from the true osteoblastic sarcomas with or without giant cells, osteochondrosarcomas exist consisting of cartilaginous portions and areas of bone formation (osteoid bone trabeculae). Osteoblastic sarcomas containing numerous giant cells may very well resemble giant cell tumors of bone (compare Fig. 353, p. 214). Figure 445 reveals polymorphocellular tumor tissue containing cartilage-like structures with a homogeneous ground substance (hyalin cartilage). Atypical cartilage cells can be seen embedded in lacunae (→ 1). In some places (→ 2), structures are found that are reminiscent of uncalcified bony trabeculae (osteoid). The tumor cells are capable, just like osteoblasts, of lining the trabeculae. There are, however, some totally undifferentiated portions which have the appearance of polymorphocellular sarcoma.

Clinical: Although osteochondrosarcomas are seen particularly in children, they also occur in somewhat older age groups (peak incidence at 16–20 years). Sites of predilection are the epiphyses and metaphyses of the femur (distal) and tibia (proximal). The remainder of the skeleton is more rarely affected. Radiologically, these tumors may give the impression of either an osteolytic or osteoblastic tumor. In order to make a histological diagnosis of bone tumors, it is essential to know the clinical and x-ray findings.

Plasmacytoma or Multiple Myeloma (Fig. 446) *is a circumscribed or diffusely growing tumor of bone marrow which destroys the bone. There is an accompanying increase of globulins in the blood plasma* (β-, or γ-globulin producing plasmacytoma, according to the newest nomenclature, γG and γA). The kidneys frequently excrete a pathological protein (Bence Jones protein, light chain protein), which is reabsorbed and produces hyalin droplet degeneration in the tubular epithelium (compare Fig. 225, p. 140). The disease is also frequently associated with amyloidosis. A smear or section of the bone marrow reveals the characteristic atypical plasma cells with eccentrically placed nuclei and pronounced wheel-spoke arrangement of the chromatin. The cytoplasm is strongly basophilic (increased RNA).

Macroscopic: Focal lesions in the cranial tables (x-ray!) and focal or diffuse lesions in the spinal column, sternum, pelvis, etc., with concomitant osteolysis. Red or grayish red, gelatinous nodular lesions.

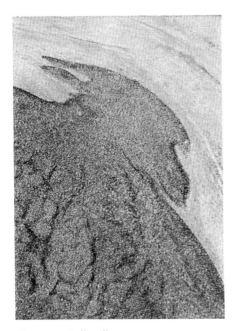

Fig. 447. Spindle cell sarcoma;
H & E, 20×.

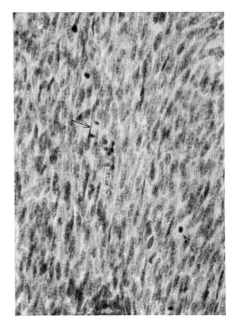

Fig. 448. Spindle cell sarcoma;
H & E, 320×.

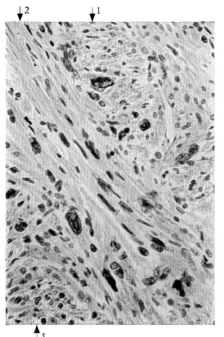

Fig. 449. Polymorphocellular leiomyosarcoma;
H & E, 190×.

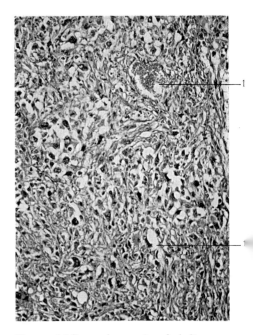

Fig. 450. Malignant hemangioendothelioma.

Sarcomas

The malignant tumors of the connective and supporting tissues may have the appearance of markedly immature or *undifferentiated sarcomas* consisting of cells with little or no differentiation (round cell sarcoma, spindle cell sarcoma, polymorphocellular sarcoma). *The mature types* are characterized by formation of fibers (fibrosarcoma, myosarcoma), intercellular substance (chondrosarcoma, osteosarcoma) or other products of differentiation (myxosarcoma, liposarcoma).

Spindle cell sarcoma (Figs. 447, 448). Spindle cell sarcoma may be considered to be the malignant form of cellular fibroma. Histologically, the tumor tissue shows a very cellular, uniform structure. It grows into the surrounding connective tissue partly by expansion and partly by infiltration (Fig. 447). Medium power reveals a rough organization into individual broad bundles of fibers sectioned at all angles. Under high power (Fig. 448), the densely packed ovoid or spindle-shaped cells may be seen. They are arranged in broad bands and thus give the impression of a certain order. The cytoplasm is elongated and mitoses are frequent (→). The nuclei are slightly pleomorphic and hyperchromatic.

Such slightly differentiated *spindle cell sarcomas*, in which only sparse collagen fibers develop between the cells, *recur* (75%) and *metastasize more frequently* (24%) than the so-called *semimalignant* fibrosarcomas which do not metastasize, but do evidence *destructive local growth* and *recur* in about 40% of cases (STOUT, 1953).

Polymorphocellular leiomyosarcoma (Fig. 449). These tumors arise in smooth muscle (uterus, gastrointestinal tract, retroperitoneal vessels) and metastasize relatively early via the vascular system (metastases to the lungs). Microscopically, there are elongated spindle-shaped cells with eosinophilic cytoplasm, which often are arranged in clumps (in this picture, the cells are cut partly in cross section [→ 1] and partly longitudinally [→ 2]). The nuclei have rounded ends; bizarre giant cell nuclei also occur. In some areas, the nuclei are lined up in palisade fashion. At times, myofibrils may be demonstrable in the cytoplasm of the cells. The cytoplasm is yellow with van Gieson stain.

Malignant hemangioendothelioma (Fig. 450). *This relatively uncommon tumor is composed of vascular endothelium.* Histologically, the tumor has a sarcomatous structure, with many atypical cells which, in part, line irregular clefts and, in part, form solid pegs. There is a connective tissue stroma containing numerous collagen fibers. The tumor cells have a variety of shapes. Spindle cells, polygonal cells and giant cells give rise to a variegated picture. The nuclei also are extremely pleomorphic. Phagocytosed erythrocytes or leukocytes can often be seen in the cytoplasm. Frequently, cytoplasmic processes seem to join individual cells, giving the impression of a reticular tissue (ALBERTINI, 1955), which has led to the interruption of these tumors as an angioblastic reticulum cell sarcoma. Figure 450 is from a section of a malignant hemangioendothelioma of the thyroid and shows marked cellular and nuclear pleomorphism. At → 1 there are blood-filled lumina.

Macroscopic: Most of these tumors arise in the thyroid (colloid goiters) or in the liver. The cut surface is dark red and friable. They have a marked tendency to metastasize.

263

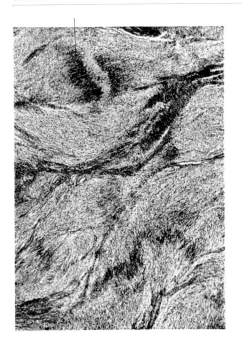

Fig. 451. Neurinoma;
van Gieson, 47×.

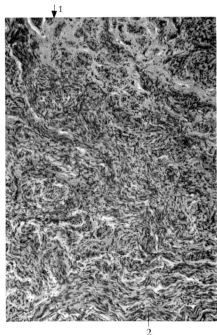

Fig. 452. Neurofibroma (amputation
neuroma);
H & E, 90×.

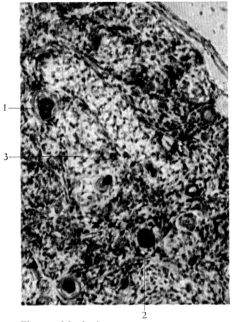

Fig. 453. Meningioma;
van Gieson, 180×.

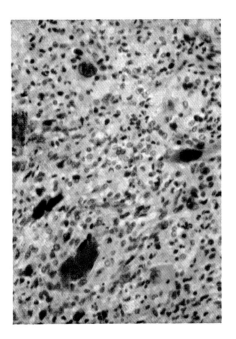

Fig. 454. Glioblastoma multiforme;
H & E, 190×.

Tumors of Nerve Tissues

The neuromas are tumors of nerves, and they may be subdivided into tumors of true nerve tissue (e. g., ganglioneuroma derived from ganglion cells and nerve cells) and tumors derived from nerve sheaths (neurinoma, neurofibroma). The latter consist of proliferated Schwann cells and connective tissue.

The **neurinomas** (Fig. 451) present a typical histological picture, even when examined only with a scanning lens. There are densely packed spindle-shaped cells and fibers arranged in wide bands. The nuclei are pointed and have an orderly, rhythmic arrangement (so-called palisading of the nuclei: →). Medium magnification of a van Gieson preparation reveals the yellow, drawn-out cytoplasm of the cells which form a syncytium. These cells are derived from the Schwann cells of the nerve sheath ("schwannoma").

Macroscopic: Round, discrete tumors, e. g., in the pontine-cerebellar angle.

Neurofibroma (Fig. 452) may be solitary or multiple and frequently are generalized (as part of *von Recklinghausen's neurofibromatosis*). It is only the large amount of collagenous fibrous tissue that distinguishes them from the neurinomas. The tumors are essentially fibromas, infiltrated by nerve fibers and proliferated Schwann cells. The bundles of nerve fibers (van Gieson yellow) are divided and pressed apart by the proliferating connective tissue (→ 1: van Gieson: red). Figure 452 shows a so-called *amputation neuroma*, i.e., a club-shaped proliferation of nerve fibers (→ 2) and connective tissue following injury or severance of a nerve. Such a lesion is probably not a true neoplastic condition; rather, it appears to be compensatory regeneration.

Meningioma (Fig. 453). *Grossly, most meningiomas are spherical tumors situated on the dura and compressing the brain. They derive from the arachnoid fibroblast.* The typical structures can be best located under low magnification. There are spindle-shaped cells in an onion-skin arrangement (→ 1), in the center of which there are hyalin or calcified nodules (necrotic cells) arranged concentrically – the so-called *dural psammoma body* (→ 2). In Figure 453, even the cellular peripheral portions of the onion-skin-like formations have become hyalinized (van Gieson: red). Scattered between these foci, there are solid portions containing great numbers of ovoid cells (→ 3) surrounded by collagenous fibrous tissue. Should proliferation of connective tissue predominate, the tumor will resemble a fibroma histologically. The displaced brain tissue is seen in the upper right-hand corner of the picture.

Glioblastoma multiforme (Fig. 454). The glioblastoma multiforme is the most common malignant brain tumor of adults. Histologically, the tumor is highly cellular with focal areas of necrosis and hemorrhage. A prominent feature is the marked variation of the cells, which have pleomorphic cytoplasm and bizarre, hyperchromatic and pleomorphic nuclei, and frequently are arranged in perivascular fashion. Scattered throughout the tissue there are small round cells. It is not possible to identify any of these cells specifically as either glial cells or astrocytes.

Macroscopic: Variegated cut surface with a mixture of red hemorrhagic portions, yellow areas of necrosis and gray tumor tissue. Frequently, the surrounding brain tissue is edematous (yellowish gray, gelatinous).

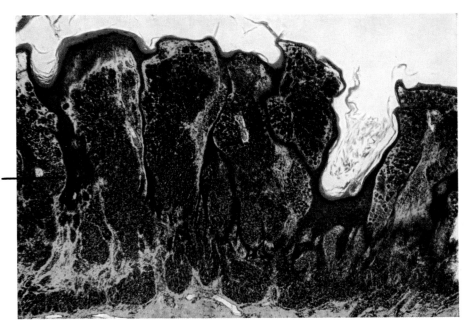

Fig. 455. Pigmented nevus; H & E, 58 ×.

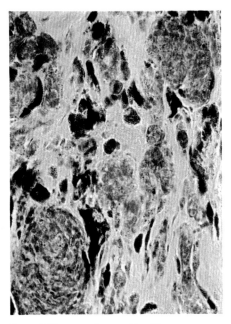

Fig. 456. Pigmented nevus (detail);
H & E, 270 ×.

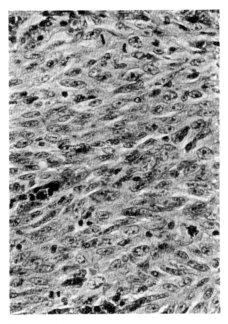

Fig. 457. Malignant melanoma;
H & E, 350 ×.

Melanomas

Melanomas are tumors of the skin or, less frequently, of mucous membranes that originate from the pigment-forming cells. Benign melanomas constitute one category, being derived histogenetically from the *pigment cells in the epidermis (epidermal nevus)*, or from similar cells in the dermis, the latter also called *intradermal nevus*. The malignant tumors are called *malignant melanomas*. The term *nevus* is only a very general descriptive name for a congenital malformation of the skin (also called a mole or birthmark), including various unrelated dysontogenetic tumors or hamartomas (e.g., a vascular nevus = a hemangioma; a sebaceous nevus = focal sebaceous gland hyperplasia, etc.). The correct designation of a nevus should therefore always indicate the particular attributes of the lesion. The term nevus, when used without other qualification, refers to a pigmented cellular nevus, although there are actually both pigmented and non-pigmented types.

An *intradermal nevus* (blue nevus, normal Mongolian spots) is a collection of pigment-producing cells in the *dermis* without involvement of the epidermis. It is composed of pigmented spindle-shaped cells (notice the elongated cellular elements in Fig. 456). Malignant transformation occurs relatively seldom.

The **epidermal pigmented nevus** (Figs. 455, 456) develops in the *epidermal papillae* of the skin. The nevus cells are derived from the melanoblasts of the epidermis (neuroectodermal origin, Masson, 1932). These tumors may be *flat* or have epidermal *papillary excrescences (papillomatous or verrucous nevus)*. Histologically (Fig. 455), the tumor is cellular and involves the entire corium. The epidermal papillae are markedly elongated and acanthotic (→: rete pegs). The nevus cells are clustered in nodules in the upper portion of the corium. Subsequently, long, solid cellular columns may be seen in which the cells are arranged like epithelial tissue. At a deeper level, the columns are broken up into small groups of cells between which there is collagenous fibrous tissue. The indefinite margin of the lesion is noteworthy but is not an indication of malignancy. **Higher magnification** (Fig. 456) shows the nest-like conglomerations of cells. For the most part, they have round nuclei and poorly demarcated, pale cytoplasm. Pigment is commonly found in the cytoplasm or the nucleus. Some individual cells contain only small amounts of pigment, whereas in others both the nucleus and the cytoplasm are densely packed with it.

From these "quiescent" nevi without atypical cells, transitions may occur to "active" nevi, with varying degrees of cellular *atypia* and *mitoses*, and infiltration of the epidermis. Especially liable to malignant transformation are so-called *junctional nevi*, in which nests of nevus cells occupy the upper corium and much of the epidermis.

A *precancerous lesion* occurs with intraepidermal proliferation of nevus cells (precancerous melanosis circumscripta of Dubreuilh), which appears grossly as a brown or black spotty discoloration of the skin. This change always leads to the development of malignant melanoma after a variable latent period.

Malignant melanoma (Fig. 457). A malignant melanoma is characterized by greater pleomorphism and hyperchromasia of the nuclei than is the case in a quiescent nevus. The cells are arranged partly in epithelial-like formations, partly in sarcoma-like structures. The metastases may or may not contain pigment.

A sharp differentiation must be made between the adult type of malignant melanoma and the so-called juvenile melanoma seen in children and youths. In the latter case, there is an "active" cellular nevus, which, although showing slight cellular pleomorphism, occasional mitotic figures and giant cells, never metastasizes.

Macroscopically, the malignant melanoma shows partly "white", partly black metastases in almost all organs.

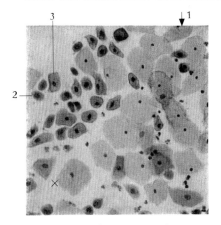

Fig. 458. Vaginal smear, normal;
Papanicolaou stain, 340×.

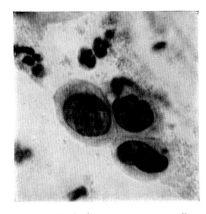

Fig. 459. Vaginal smear, squamous cell
carcinoma; H & E, 800×.

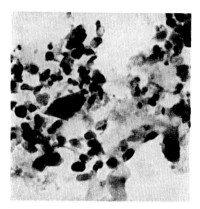

Fig. 460. Cells of a squamous cell carcinoma
in sputum; H & E. 350×.

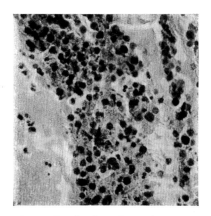

Fig. 461. Small cell carcinoma in sputum;
H & E, 350×.

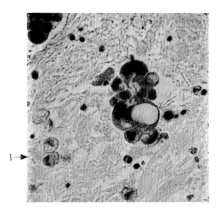

Fig. 462. Sputum with clumps of cells from
an adenocarcinoma;
H & E, 350×.

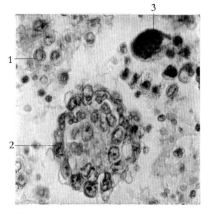

Fig. 463. Malignant tumor cells in pleural
exudate;
H & E, 350×.

Cytodiagnosis

Cytodiagnosis, first used extensively by G. PAPANICOLAOU, should be mentioned at this time, since it is being used ever more widely as a tool to *detect cancer*. The method has proved very useful in the early detection of carcinoma of the cervix and its precursor; in the diagnosis of bronchial carcinoma, cytodiagnosis has an accuracy of 70%. The degree of error is 20%, and occurs largely in patients with chronic bronchitis and tuberculosis (according to the most recent statistics, the accuracy is 85–90% and mistaken diagnoses 5%). Nowadays, stomach, colon, pleura and joint smears are being routinely examined for cancer cells.

Cytological diagnosis can give only a provisional diagnosis, since invasion and metastasis are required to make a firm diagnosis of a malignant tumor. Cellular anaplasia, as described on page 231, can only be regarded as suggestive evidence for the presence of malignant cells.

The pictures on page 268 show the most essential cellular characteristics upon which cytological diagnosis rests: *hyperchromatism* and *irregularity of size* of nuclei, increase in *nuclear cytoplasmic ratio*, *prominent nucleoli* and *marked basophilia of the cytoplasm*. The difficulties of cytological diagnosis stem from the fact that even normal cells, e. g., in chronic cervicitis or bronchitis with some squamous metaplasia, may show similar atypical cells and thereby lead to the making of a false positive diagnosis. *An unequivocal diagnosis of a malignant tumor should be made only from an excised biopsy specimen.*

From what has just been said, it should be clear that a great deal of experience is needed correctly to diagnose cytological preparations. The reader should therefore be warned not to use these pages as a basis for cytological diagnosis. They should serve only to point out the importance of the technique and how it may be used clinically. Cytodiagnosis belongs in the hands of the expert.

Figure 458 shows **normal cells in a vaginal smear** stained by Papanicolaou's method. There are acidophilic (red → 1) and basophilic (blue ×) superficial surface cells with pyknotic nuclei (estrogen effect), basophilic parabasal cells (→ 2) and intermediate cells (→ 3).

Figure 459 is from a vaginal smear and shows the **atypical epithelial cells of a squamous cell carcinoma** under high magnification. There is marked nuclear hyperchromatism and irregularity of size, and the nuclear cytoplasmic ratio is increased.

Various types of cells from malignant tumors may occur in **sputum.** Figure 460 shows a group of cells from a **squamous cell carcinoma** with very marked cellular and nuclear pleomorphism and rather characteristic eosinophilic cytoplasm. In **small cell carcinoma** (Fig. 461), groups of only slightly pleomorphic cells with scanty cytoplasm and strongly hyperchromatic nuclei may be found. The nuclei are larger than those of lymphocytes and have denser chromatin.

Infrequently, sputum may reveal clumps of cells from a metastatic tumor in the lungs. Figure 462 shows such a clump from an **adenocarcinoma** containing a signet ring cell (→). At the margin of the picture, there is normal alveolar epithelium (→ 1). The appearance in the sputum of atypical columnar cells (particularly in women) should lead to suspicion of an underlying *adenomatosis* of the lung.

In pleural effusions (Fig. 463), clusters of tumor cells (→ 2) may be found intermingled with normal epithelial cells (→ 1). In this preparation, there is also a markedly pleomorphic cell with a hyperchromatic nucleus (→ 3).

Fungi – Parasites

This chapter has been added in order to facilitate a basic knowledge of these important and frequent diseases. Professor SALFELDER[1]) has kindly provided the following pages, which are written from the viewpoint of a pathologist working in a subtropical or tropical region. Nonetheless, this addition to the book is not without importance for physicians in temperate zones for two chief reasons: On the one hand, we are confronted today with an increasing international commerce, and on the other hand, modern therapeutic agents (cortisone, antibiotics, cytotoxic drugs, etc.) have changed the pattern of infectious diseases, with the result that overwhelming fungal infections are common.

The following introduction gives some suggestions for the identification of fungi and parasites (Table 10). For ameba, which are easily confused with large tissue cells, the PAS-reaction is recommended. If parasites of small size are found in routine hematoxylin and eosin slides, or Chagas disease, kala-azar or leishmaniasis is suspected, it is helpful to remember that they are negative with the Gram stain for fibrin. For the identification of fungi in tissue, the Grocott stain is superior to all other methods. In tissues, dead fungi retain their structural integrity and staining properties for a long time. The mucicarmine stain is recommended for staining the capsule of Crytococcus in sections. India ink demonstrates the thick capsule of the Cryptococcus very well in smears. The capsule remains colorless, bright and shining. In unstained smears, undesired cell and tissue constituents, especially keratin, can be dissolved with 10% potassium hydroxide (10 min.), which makes the search for infecting organisms easier. Several species are easily identified with the fluorescent antibody technique (COONS and KAPLAN).

Table 10. Methods Used for Identification of the Fungi.

Method	Result	Remarks
Hematoxylin-eosin (H+E)	Blue	Not all fungal elements stain
Fibrin (Weigert)-Gram	Blue	Only partially stained
PAS[2])	Red	Cells of small fungi can be overlooked
Gridley[2])	Reddish blue	Stains nearly all fungi
Grocott[2])	Black	Ideal stain, good contrast against light background. Also useful for smears. Note: Coal pigment also stains black, as do erythrocytes and elastic fibers
Mucicarmine[2])	Red	Cryptococcus positive. Excludes other fungi
Polarized light	Shining yellowish blue	Shows double refraction and Maltese crosses of yeast-like fungi in tissue
Fluorescent antibody	Variable	Fungi of many types positive. Specificity destroyed through cross reactions
Unstained smear	—	Round forms with doubly contoured capsule-suspect fungi
Smear treated for 10 min. with KOH 10%	—	Fungi detected easier because of destruction of other cells and tissues
India ink smear	Black	Wide wall of cryptococcus shines forth against dark background
Giemsa, Wright, May-Grünwald Giemsa (smear)	Blue	Stains yeasts and cysts of Pneumocystis carinii

1 Director of the Institute of Anatomic Pathology, University of the Andes, Merida, Venezuela.
2 Staining of control preparation recommended.

Fig. 464. Outline of Various Mycoses

Morphology	Mycosis	Fungus	Tissue Reaction	Fungus in Tissue	Size
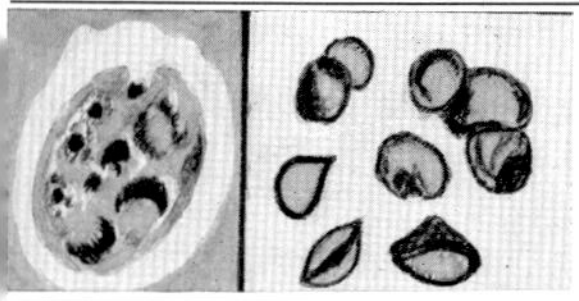	Pneumo-cystosis[1]) Fig. 465	Pneumocystis carinii (Pn. car.)	Interstitial plasma cell infiltrate; lung	Grocott: Round, small; Giemsa: cysts (C) with internal bodies (I)	3–4 µ C 5–12 µ I 0.1–2 µ
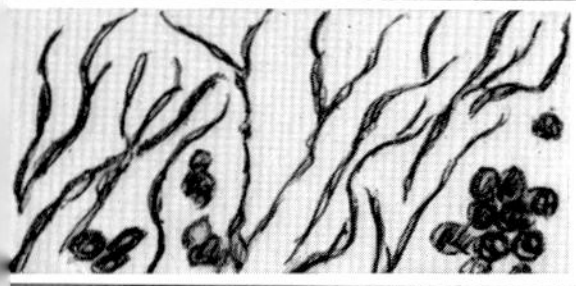	Candidiasis Fig. 466	Candida albicans, tropic, etc. (Cand. albic.)	Non-specific granulation tissue	Hyphae and small yeast cells	2–4 µ
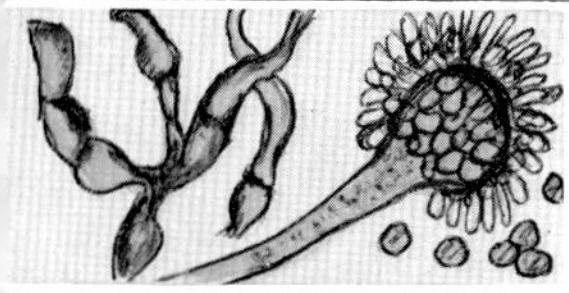	Aspergillosis Fig. 469	Aspergillus fumigatus	Non-specific; usually granulomas with eosinophils and giant cells	Septated hyphae, conidia "Fruiting bodies"	Variable
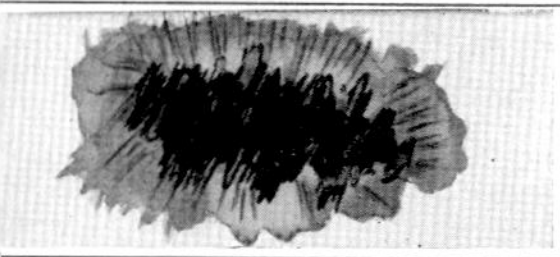	Actino-mycosis Fig. 471	Actino-mycosis israeli or bovis (Actin. isr.)	Abscesses with foam cells. Yellow color. Fistulae	Thick mycellial masses; peripherally radiating process	Variable
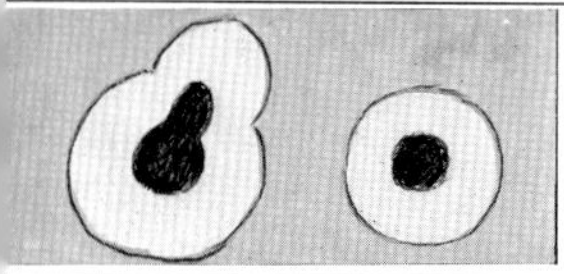	Crypto-coccosis Fig. 473	Cryptococcus neoformans (Cr. neof.)	Increase in histio-cytes, granulomas	Thick-walled buds	4–20 µ
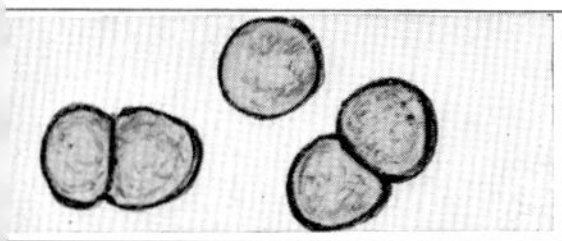	Chromo-blastomycosis Figs. 444–447	Hormo-dendrum and Phialophora	Microabscesses and granulomas of the skin	Brown round sep-tated fungal cells	5–12 µ
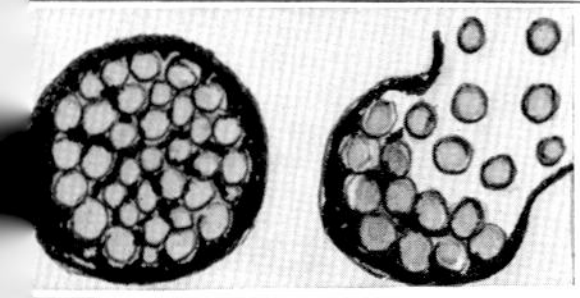	Coccidioido-mycosis Figs. 475, 476	Coccidioides immitis (Cocc. imm.)	Abscesses, granulomas	Large cysts, Endospores	30–60 µ
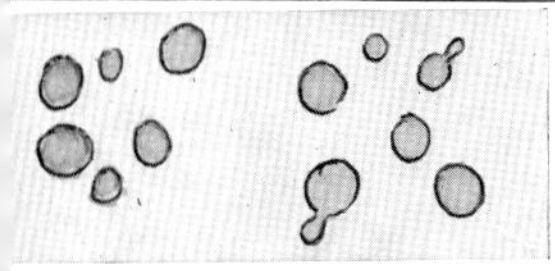	Histo-plasmosis Figs. 478–480	Histoplasma capsulatum (H. caps.)	Proliferation of histiocytic tuber-culoid granulomas, calcification	Small round yeast-like fungal cells; intracellular	2–5 µ
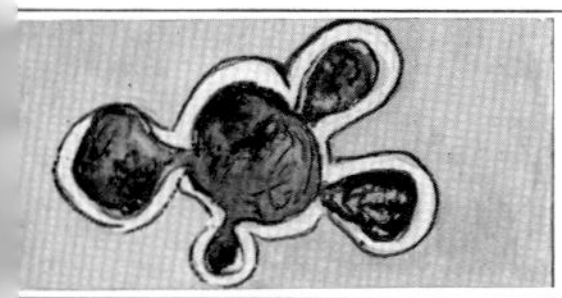	Paracoccidio-idomycosis (South Ame-ric. blastomy-cosis) Fig. 481	Para-coccidioides brasiliensis (Parac. bras.)	Abscesses, granulomas	Yeast-like multiple budding (steering wheel)	5–30 µ
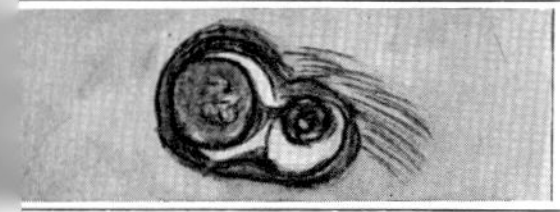	Blastomycosis (N. American) Fig. 482	Blastomyces dermatitidis (Blas. derm.)	Abscesses, granulomas	Large yeast-like cells, solitary budding; figure 8 shape	8–15 µ

Fungal nature not proved.

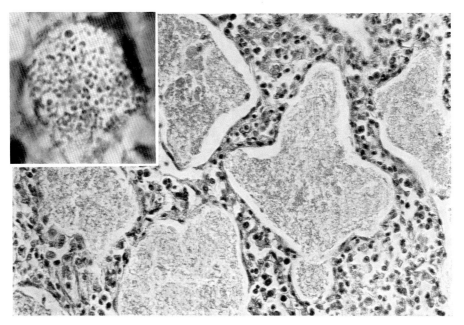

Fig. 465. Pneumocystosis with interstitial pneumonia; H & E, 396×.
Inset: Pneumocystis carinii in smear; Giemsa, 1,500×.

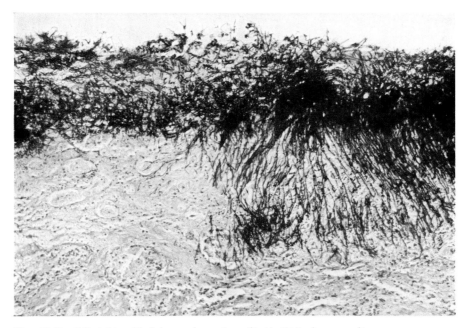

Fig. 466. Candidiasis (thrush) of the esophagus (moniliasis); PAS – hematoxylin, 77×.

Pneumocystosis with interstitial pneumonia (Figs. 465, 467). *Pneumocystosis with interstitial pneumonia occurs frequently in prematurely born infants in the 3rd–6th month of life, but also may occur in older children. When it occurs in adults it is mostly in the end stages of malignant disease (leukemia, sarcoma, carcinoma), particularly after treatment with cytotoxic agents.* **Pneumocystis carinii** is the etiological agent but whether this is a protozoa or a fungus is still debated. Pneumocystis carinii was first seen in Brazil in the lungs of animals (CARINI, 1910). VANEK and JIROVEC (1952) and GIESE (1952) proved the etiological agent in man about 15 years ago. The disease is frequently characterized by an interstitial pneumonia with plasma cell infiltration. H & E sections show finely honeycombed granular material in the alveoli (Fig. 465). The alveolar lumens are reduced by a thick exudate of alveolar septal cells, lymphocytes, histiocytes and plasma cells. The appearance, indeed, may lead to confusing this form of interstitial pneumonia with atelectasis. The increased cell content of the alveoli and the type of cells should, however, lead to a correct diagnosis. The organisms may be seen in smear preparations stained with Giemsa in which they appear as cystic forms with internal bodies originating from the honeycombed alveolar contents (see inset in Fig. 465). With the Grocott stain, numerous yeast-like bodies 3-4 μ in diameter are seen which are often indented and wrinkled (Fig. 467).

Macroscopic: The cut surface resembles liver and is grayish red, homogeneous and firm.

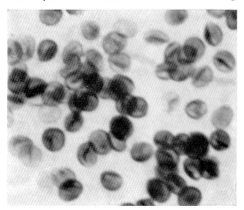

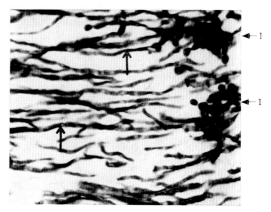

Fig. 467. Pneumocystis in a smear; Grocott stain, 1,140×.

Fig. 468. Hyphae and yeast forms of Candida albicans; Grocott stain, 800×.

Candidiasis *(thrush) of the esophagus* **(candidiasis, moniliasis)** (Figs. 466, 468). *Various species of Candida, but chiefly Candida albicans, cause a mycosis that is localized predominantly in the mucous membranes. Spread to the internal organs occurs infrequently (sepsis), mostly in patients with weakened resistance. Macroscopically,* white plaques or membranes are seen on the mucosa of all the upper alimentary and respiratory tracts. *Microscopically,* numerous fungal filaments forming a mycelium are seen with H & E, but better with PAS staining (Fig. 466). The mycelial filaments penetrate between and into the epithelial cells of the mucous membrane, localizing particularly in the zone between the epithelium and tunica propria (see Fig. 466). They penetrate like the roots of a plant into the upper layers of the connective tissue. The tunica propria is infiltrated by lymphocytes. Fig. 468 shows the fungal filaments under higher magnification (hyphae, → in the picture). Yeast forms 2-4μ in diameter are also present (blastospores, → 1) which show budding and pseudohyphae formation. If only yeast forms of Candida are present, it may be confused with similar forms of Histoplasma capsulatum or Blastomyces.

273

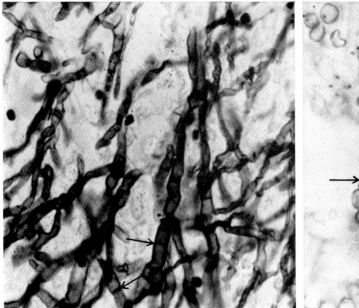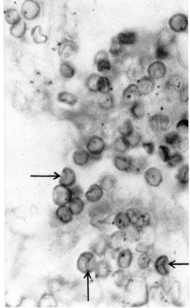

Fig. 469. Aspergillus mycelium with hyphae; Grocott stain, 800×.

Fig. 470. Conidia of aspergillus; Grocott stain, 800×.

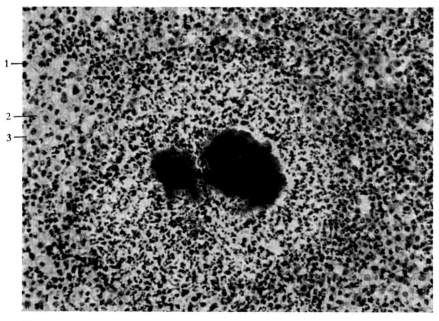

Fig. 471. Actinomycosis; H & E, 300×.

Aspergillosis (Figs. 469, 470, 472). *Aspergillus is a fungus of world-wide distribution. The various species produce changes in the lungs and mucous membranes. Less frequently, there is hematogenous spread to other organs. The fungus is a saprophyte like Candida and the Phycomytes. Aspergillosis occurs frequently in animals, especially birds. The infection is established mostly by inhalation of spores. The mycosis often is seen secondarily in patients whose power of resistance has become greatly reduced (malignant tumors, steroid-antibiotic-cytotoxic treatment or x-irradiation).*

The diagnosis is based upon the demonstration of septate forms (→ in Fig. 469) and dichotomous branching of hyphae (Fig. 469), which form a network (mycelium). They can penetrate the walls of vessels and other hindrances. In addition, conidia are found (Fig. 470). If only conidia are observed in tissues stained with Grocott stain, they can easily be confused with the yeast forms of Candida or Pneumocystis. The conidia are indented and wrinkled (→ in the illustration) similarly to Pneumocystis carinii (see Fig. 467). So-called fruiting bodies (Fig. 472) occur in infections with Aspergillus fumigatus, particularly in areas of the body that produce acid (lungs, mucous membranes). The fruiting bodies develop on the end of the hyphae, bear sterigmata and also are known as conidiophores. From the sterigmata, conidia are formed, which then fall from them and lie free in the tissue.

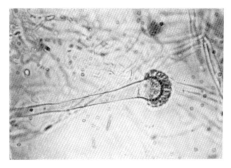

Fig. 472. Fruiting body of Aspergillus fumigatus;
H & E, 675×.

The tissue reaction is predominantly a non-specific granuloma showing eosinophilic leukocytes and giant cells. Not uncommonly, a tuberculous or bronchiectatic cavity becomes secondarily infected and filled with a so-called fungus ball which may resemble a tumorous mass and for this reason is called an "aspergilloma". Hematogenous spread can lead to involvement of practically all organs (brain, meninges, kidney, spleen, heart, etc.).

Actinomycosis (ray fungus disease) (Fig. 471). *In man, the disease is caused chiefly by Actinomyces israeli, and in cattle by Actinomyces bovis. The portal of entry is usually a break in a mucous membrane (e. g., in the oral cavity, a tooth extraction), the lungs or the gut (appendix). Further spread results from either blood stream invasion (e. g., liver, bone marrow) or lymphatic invasion.*

The fungi occur in conglomerations and form so-called nodules with characteristic ray-like runners to the periphery. Figure 471 shows several nodules in the center of an abscess (polymorphonuclear leukocytes and tissue destruction). Granulation tissue containing numerous foam cells (→ 1, → 2, 3) with cytoplasmic fat droplets (foam cells) forms a wall around the abscess. In this way, the abscesses become confluent and form fistulous tracts (especially common, for example, in infections of the mandible). Yellow granules, which contain the nodules, may be demonstrated in the secretion of the fistulas.

Macroscopic: Hard, brawny induration of the skin with numerous fistulas. Sulfur yellow abscess wall (granulation tissue with foam cells).

In the tropics, a **mycetoma** (Madura foot) in the extremities is most frequently due to actinomycosis. The nodules and the tissue reaction in mycetoma have similarities to those in actinomycosis.

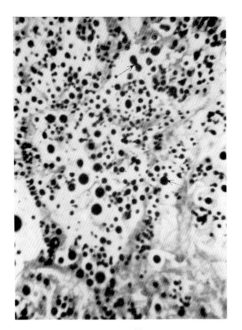

Fig. 473. Cryptococcosis of lung;
Grocott stain, 185×.

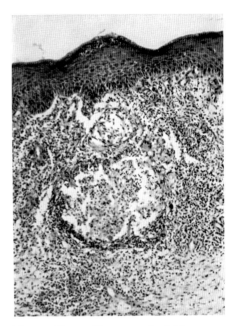

Fig. 474. Chromoblastomycosis of skin;
H & E, 104×.

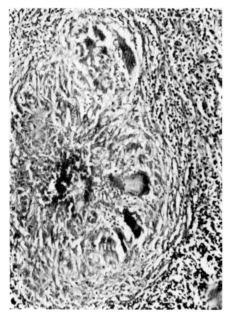

Fig. 475. Coccidioidomycosis granuloma
of lung;
H & E, 54×.

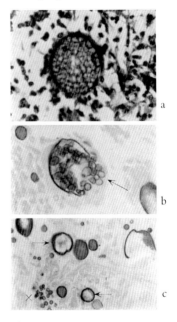

Fig. 476a. Intact spherule of Coccidioides
immitis in tissue; H & E, 138×.
b. Endospores released from a spherule;
Grocott stain, 92×.
c. Empty fungus spherule and small endospores;
Grocott stain, 102×.

Cryptococcosis of the lung (*torulosis, European blastomycosis*, Fig. 473). *Cryptococcus neo-formans* (Sanfelice, Busse-Buschke) *has a world-wide distribution. A prime source of infection is the excrement in the nesting places of pigeons. The central nervous system and, above all, the leptomeninges are favored sites for localization of the lesions, although they may occur in any organ. The portal of entry is probably the lungs, where healing results in the development of nodules.*

Figure 473 shows several yeast cells lying free in alveoli. The infecting organisms appear as round bodies 4–20 μ in diameter and show buds (→ in the picture). In massive infections, the fungi elicit only a marked histiocytic reaction. Chronic granulomatous foci contain only a few fungi. They are usually embedded in dense granulation tissue and, for this reason, often are difficult to discover and easy to confuse with foreign bodies.

Macroscopic: Gelatinous foci which look like a myxomatous tumor. Often the lesions resemble caseating tuberculosis macroscopically.

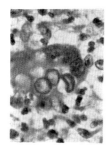

Chromoblastomycosis (Chromomycosis) (Figs. 474, 477). *This fungus has an intrinsic dark brown color, hence the designation. There are five species of Hormodendrum and Phialophora which may produce this mycosis. Local-ization occurs in the skin, particularly of the lower extremities. Seldom does lymphatic spread occur and only exceptionally hematogenous dissemination, usually to the brain and meninges. Chronic verrucous, ulcerated and crusted lesions of the skin may result in considerable deformity of the extremities and invalidism. The mycosis is found in many tropical and subtropical countries, primarily in farm workers.*

Histologically, the corium shows microabscesses composed of numerous granulocytes and marginal granulation tissue containing giant cells (Fig. 474). Tuberculoid granuloma may also be produced. As in American blastomycosis, the overlying epidermis is hyperplastic. The brown, round fungus cells (Fig. 477) frequently are septate, have a diameter of 5–12 μ and often lie within giant cells.

Fig. 477. Chromo-blastomycosis. Giant cell containing three fungus bodies; H & E, 480 ×.

The macroscopic diagnosis is not easy and may be confused with epithelioma.

Coccidioidomycosis (*San Joaquin Valley fever*) (Figs. 475, 476a, b, c). *The disease occurs most frequently in California and Arizona and certain parts of Central and South America, particularly where deserts exist. A large part of the population in an area may be infected. Coccidioides immitis occurs in dusty soil, attacks the lungs and mostly produces a benign disease. Much less frequently, spread occurs to internal organs, which is often fatal.*

Histologically, there are abscesses with a thick wall of tuberculoid granulation tissue showing Langhans giant cells and epithelioid cells (Fig. 475). So-called coccidioidoma has been described, which shows extensive necrosis and, in contrast to histoplasmosis, only a slight tendency to calci-fication. Macroscopically, the lesions are similar to tuberculosis, which is true also of many other "deep" mycoses.

The fungus shows so-called dimorphism (as do Histoplasma capsulatum, Blastomyces dermatitidis, etc.), that is, it can grow in saprophytic form both in its natural habitat and in cultures grown at room temperature. The fungus also grows in parasitic form (as a mold with hyphae and arthro-spores) in animals and humans (large spherules or sporocysts with numerous endospores which are expelled from the spherule or mother cell). The spherules (Fig. 476a) measure 30–60 μ in size and are round. The endospores are extravasated from the spherule (in Fig. 476b) and can attain the size of a white blood cell. Empty spherules (Fig. 476a →, × endospores) can be confused with Blasto-myces dermatitidis, and endospores (Fig. 476b and c) with Histoplasma capsulatum and Crypto-coccus neoformans.

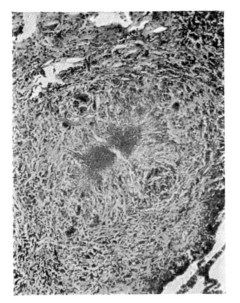

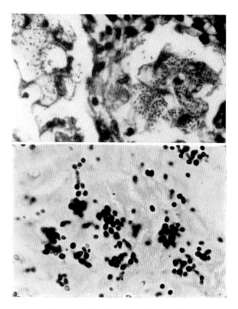

Fig. 478. Fresh histoplasma granuloma in the lung; H & E, 105×.

Fig. 479. (Upper) alveolar epithelium with histoplasmas; H & E, 160×.
Fig. 480. (Lower) yeast form of Histoplasma capsulatum; Grocott stain, 320×.

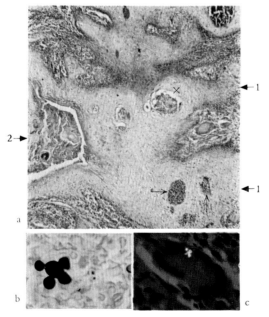

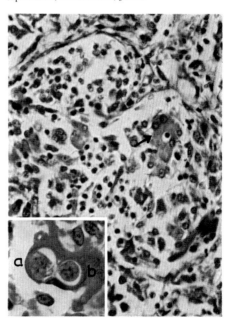

Fig. 481 a. Paracoccidioidomycosis (South American blastomycosis) of the skin; H & E, 55×. b. Multiple budding of Paracoccidioides brasiliensis in tissue; Grocott stain, 500×. c. Fungal cell (Parac. bras.) in a giant cell, polarized light (so-called Maltese cross); H & E, 550×.

Fig. 482. North American blastomycosis of the lung; H & E, 525×. Inset: Solitary bud of Blasto. derm.; a) mother cell; b) daughter cell; H & E, 1,050×.

Histoplasmosis (Figs. 478, 479, 480). *Histoplasmosis is one of the most widely distributed mycoses. In the United States, it is estimated that more than 30 million persons have been infected. The clinical and pathological similarities to tuberculosis and the predominantly benign course prevented its recognition for a long time, with the result that most of the significant features of this mycosis have been recognized only in the past 20 years. Spontaneous cases are rare in Europe. The disease also occurs spontaneously in animals.*
Histoplasma capsulatum (DARLING) *grows best in the soil of chicken houses, is spread apparently through the air and causes a primary lung infection. Most cases heal with a residue of focal calcification in the lung and hilar lymph nodes, where fungi can be demonstrated for a long time. Seldom, and only under special conditions, does the disease in the lung become generalized and have a fatal outcome. In addition to the calcified residual foci in the lungs, cases are encountered with multiple scattered nodules, cavitation or histoplasmomas. Extrapulmonary histoplasmosis may involve any organ, the adrenals being affected frequently.*

Histologically, the lungs show histiocytic granulomas with central necrosis, an epithelioid cell type of granulation tissue and giant cells (Fig. 478). The tissue picture can be very similar to that of a tuberculous granuloma. Higher magnification shows that the fungi are almost exclusively in the cytoplasm of histiocytes or alveolar epithelial cells (Fig. 479, small black granules). With hematoxylin and eosin stains, the fungi are not often recognized, but with the Grocott stain (Fig. 480), the organisms can be seen distinctly. There are also yeast-like forms 2–5 μ in diameter. A larger fungus *(Histoplasma duboisii)* produces African histoplasmosis.

Paracoccidioidomycosis *(South American blastomycosis)*, Figs. 481 a, b, c. *As the name indicates, this disease occurs in South America, although not in Chile. In Brazil, it is a major sanitary problem. Paracoccidioidomycosis is not encountered spontaneously in animals. In man, minor tissue changes attributed to the fungus have been seen in almost all organs. Chiefly attacked are the lungs, skin, mucous membranes and adrenals.*

Histologically, there is a combination of abscesses and granulation tissue. Calcification is rare. Figure 481 shows pseudoepitheliomatous hyperplasia of the epidermis with broad, deeply penetrating epidermal pegs (→ 1, → 2 surface of the epidermis with keratin scales). Within the epidermis, there are numerous microabscesses (→ in the picture) as well as granulomas (×). The diagnosis rests on demonstration of large yeast-like fungi showing multiple budding (Fig. 481 b). Frequently, the granulomas contain giant cells with enclosed fungi appearing as Maltese crosses in polarized light (Fig. 481 c).

North American blastomycosis (Fig. 482) *occurs practically only in North America. Frequently, secondary skin lesions appear first. The lungs are the portal of entry for the fungus and from there hematogenous dissemination occurs. Spontaneous animal infections occur (dogs).* The microscopic changes are similar to those seen in South American blastomycosis. Figure 482 shows granulocytes in a lung alveolus as well as a giant cell which has phagocytized a fungus cell (→). In tissues, the round, yeast-like fungi produce single daughter cells only (solitary budding). Figure 482: mother cell (a), daughter cell (b).

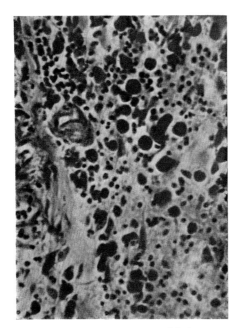

Fig. 483. Amebae in the submucosa of the large intestine (amebic dysentery); PAS-hematoxylin stains, 420 ×.

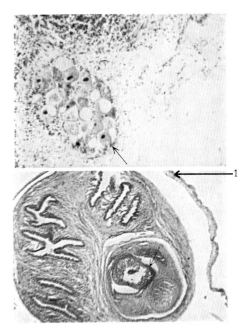

Fig. 484 (above). Balantidium dysentery; H & E, 168 ×.
Fig. 485 (below). Cysticercus; H & E, 105 ×.

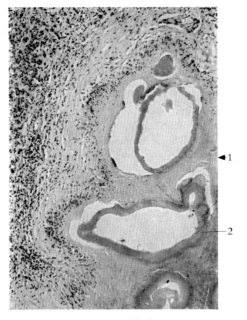

Fig. 486. Echinococcus cyst of the liver; H & E, 80 ×.

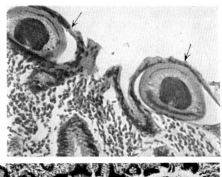

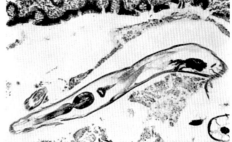

Fig. 487 (above). Trichuris larvae in the mucosa of the appendix; H & E, 310 ×.
Fig. 488 (below). Appendix with Enterobius vermicularis (oxyuris); H & E, 53 ×.

Amebic dysentery (Fig. 483). *Amebic dysentery occurs chiefly in warm climates. Of the various types occurring in man, only the vegetative form of Entamoeba histolytica is seen in tissues. The existence of a non-pathogenic small type of Entamoeba histolytica that can change into the pathogenic large form which penetrates the wall of the intestine is still unsettled. It is also disputed whether E. histolytica always is pathogenic.* The intestinal lesions are usually confined to the colon. Ameba actively penetrate the intestinal wall and have both cytological and histolytical effects. At first, there is extensive necrosis of tissue, with formation of crater-like ulcers with undermined margins (see Fig. 165). **Histologically,** the base of the ulcers shows fibrin, necrotic tissue and many granulocytes. Careful inspection is necessary to discover the amebae in the submucosa of the large intestine. They appear as round cells with an eccentrically placed nucleus (Fig. 483). The cytoplasm is distinctly red with PAS-stain; with H & E, the protozoans can be easily overlooked or confused with reticulum cells, macrophages or ganglion cells. Fig. 483 shows, in addition, infiltration of tissues with round cells and granulocytes.

Peritonitis from perforation is a frequent complication, along with dissemination of the ameba through the portal vein to the liver and other organs, where abscesses may form.

Balantidium dysentery (Fig. 484). *Balantidium coli occurs in man and animals independently of climatic influence.* The pathological changes in the tissues are similar to those of amebic dysentery. The living etiological agent has no histolytic effect. Inflammation is produced primarily by the presence of a large number of dead Balantidia as is perhaps also true in amebic dysentery. The disease is commonly accompanied by bacterial infection. Extra-intestinal dissemination of the protozoans has been observed. Figure 484 shows Balantidia (→) in a lymph vessel in the periphery of a lymph node.

Cysticercosis (Fig. 485). *This implies the seeding of larva (Cysticercus cellulosae) of the swine tapeworm (Taenia solium) in the various organs of man or swine. Generalized and localized forms occur. Cysticercus is found in eastern Europe, Asia, South America and Central America. The larva are found predominantly in the central nervous system, eyes and skeletal muscles.* **Histologically,** the larvae are found enclosed in a vesicle (→ 1 vesicle wall) arising from invagination. Often, the head end is visible (→). The diameter of a Cysticercus seldom is larger than 1.5 cm. The shape is variable. After the worm dies, a foreign body reaction occurs. Secondary calcification (χ-ray) and the development of epilepsy, if the central nervous system is involved, provide clues for clinical diagnosis.

Echinococcosis (Fig. 486). *The larvae of Taenia echinococcus (dog tapeworm) pass through the portal vein into the liver, where they form cysts (hydatid cysts).* Figure 486 shows cysts the wall of which consists of a ring of collagenous fibrous tissue (→ 1) on which rests a homogeneous, lamellar red chitinous layer (cuticle → 2). Scolices are often seen near the cuticle. The adjacent liver shows atrophy and lymphocytic infiltration.

Macroscopic: Either a large unilocular cyst or several cysts filled with daughter cysts. They are especially common in the right lobe of the liver. Echinococcus alveolaris (2% in humans): multiple small cysts bounded by a capsule of connective tissue.

Intestinal worms (Figs. 487, 488). In tropical countries, *Ascaris* and *Trichuris trichiura* frequently are found in the lumen of the intestine. Hookworm *(Ancylostoma duodenale* and *Necator americanus)* causes severe anemia and wasting, which often leads to death in children. Larvae of *Trichuris trichiura* (Fig. 487) occasionally penetrate into the mucous membrane of the intestine. In Fig. 487, two larvae are seen covered by a layer of intestinal mucosal epithelium (→). *Enterobius vermicularis*, commonly called pinworm (Fig. 488), is seen commonly in the lumen of the appendix or less seldom in the mucosa. Abscesses with eosinophils may develop as a reaction to the worms or their eggs.

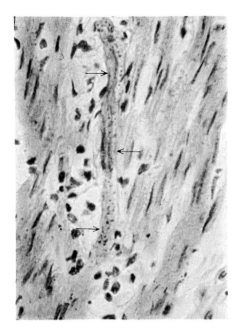

Fig. 489. Larva migrans in the intestinal
musculature;
H & E, 630×.

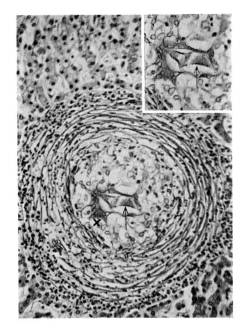

Fig. 490. Schistosoma granuloma in the liver;
H & E, 300×.
Inset at upper right, egg from the center of the
granuloma;
H & E, 490×.

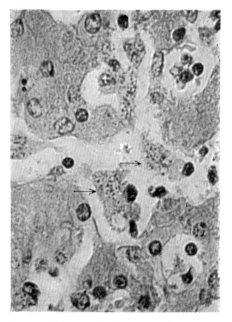

Fig. 491. Kala-azar (liver);
H & E, 1,550×.

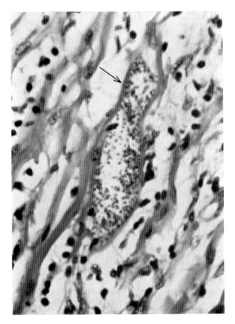

Fig. 492. Chagas myocarditis (mouse);
H & E, 840×.

Larva migrans (Fig. 489). *This includes all conditions in which larvae and microfilaria invade the body tissues. The disease occurs mostly in children and causes symptoms of a general infection with fever and, in addition, shows blood eosinophilia. The larvae are found most particularly in infections with* **Strongyloides, Ancylostoma, Ascaris lumbricoides suum** as well as **Toxocara canis and cati.** In the last-named disease, man is a secondary host and the disease is known as visceral larva migrans. The larvae elicit a tissue reaction consisting of eosinophils and granulomas. The parasites are not ordinarily detected in the tissue (→). In most cases, exact classification is difficult.

Schistosomiasis (*Bilharziasis,* Fig. 490). *Schistosoma belong to the* **trematodes.** *Three types are found in man.* **Schistosoma haematobium** *occurs in Africa and bordering countries,* **Schistosoma mansoni** *in Africa and South America and* **Schistosoma japonicum** *in Asia. The worm spends its youth in the outside world. Snails act as the intermediate host. Infection is the result of contact with infected water. Adult Schistosoma are found in the paravesicular tissues (Schistosoma haematobium) and mesenteric veins (Schistosoma haematobium and japonicum). The tissue changes and symptoms of the disease are caused by the eggs of the Schistosoma, which have characteristic structures that allow diagnosis of the type of parasite causing the infection. In Schistosoma hematobium, the eggs are found in the liver, ureter and genital organs (occasionally rectum and lungs). Schistosoma mansoni and japonicum eggs occur particularly in the walls of the intestines and liver, less commonly in abdominal lymph nodes and lungs. Even less frequently, eggs localize in the central nervous system and spleen.* The eggs of trematodes cause a granulocytic or eosinophilic reaction in the earliest stages. Later, a typical granuloma forms which heals with calcification and connective tissue scarring. Complications are carcinoma of the urinary bladder, hepatic cirrhosis, cor pulmonale and, in the central nervous system, focal symptoms, depending upon the site. Figure 490 shows a Schistosoma granuloma in the liver. In the center, there is a trematode egg, shown enlarged in the upper right inset. The egg shows a tapering pointed process (Schistosoma mansoni). A giant cell granuloma has formed as a reaction (giant cell ×) with histiocytes on the inside and on the outside a capsule of loose collagen fibers infiltrated by lymphocytes.

Kala-azar (**visceral leishmaniasis,** Fig. 491). *The name comes from India and means "black disease". It occurs also in Asia, Africa, southern Europe and South America. The protozoan Leishmania donovani produces visceral changes, as opposed to Leishmania tropica and brasiliensis, which produce only skin and mucous membrane lesions (mucocutaneous Leishmaniasis). Natural infection occurs in dogs, foxes and jackals, and the etiological agent is transmitted by Phlebotomus (sand fly).* Clinically, there is hepatosplenomegaly with fever, pancytopenia and increase of plasma globulins. After a subacute to chronic course, death generally results unless treatment is given. The causative agent measures 2–5 μ and is distinguished by a kinetoplast. It is found in the cytoplasm of reticuloendothelial cells. Figure 491 shows small corpuscular elements in Kupffer cells (→).

Chagas' disease (*American trypanosomiasis,* Fig. 492). **Trypanosoma cruzi** *is found only in blood. The carriers are reduviid bugs (Triatomiae). The disease, occurs only in Central and South America, where millions of persons are infested. A specific treatment is not known.*
Trypanosomiasis may cause chronic myocarditis producing symptoms only after decades but eventually leads to death. The agent is found in tissues in early stages only. Fig. 492 shows cystic nests of Trypanosomes (→) in heart muscle and accompanying interstitial lymphohistiocytic myocarditis. In late stages of the disease, the diagnosis is difficult, for then there is merely cardiac hypertrophy with mural thrombosis and a lymphocytic, histiocytic interstitial myocarditis with occasional eosinophils and giant cells. Morphologically, in this later stage it cannot be differentiated from Fiedler's idiopathic myocarditis (see p. 45).

Selected References

The following references are either review articles (indicated by ★) which contain additional references or original papers of historical interest or special significance for the subject under discussion.
Many of the references in German or other foreign languages have been omitted from the English edition, since many English-speaking readers would find difficulty in reading them. The complete bibliography is, of course, contained in the 2nd German edition of *Histopathologie* which is available in many libraries. Where serious omissions occurred because of deletion of German papers, comparable papers written in English have been substituted. – Ed.

Staining

DAVENPORT, H. A.: Histological and Histochemical Technics (Philadelphia: W. B. Saunders Company, 1960).★

HUMASON, G. L.: Animal Tissue Techniques (San Francisco: W. H. Freeman Company, 1962).★

LILLIE, R. D.: Histopathologic Technic and Practical Histochemistry (3d ed.; New York: McGraw-Hill Book Company, 1965).★

PEARSE, A. G. E.: Histochemistry (London: J. & A. Churchill, Ltd., 1960).★

General and Special Pathology

ANDERSON, W. A. D.: Pathology (5th ed.; St. Louis: C. V. Mosby Company, 1961).★

BOYD, W.: Pathology for the Physician (Philadelphia: Lea & Febiger, 1965).★

CAPPELL, D. F.: Muir's Textbook of Pathology (8th ed.; Baltimore: The Williams & Wilkins Company, 1965).★

DE DUVE, C.: Lysosomes (New York: Ronald Press Co., 1959), p. 128.★

DUMONT, A.: Lab. Invest. *14:* 2034 (1965).

FLOREY, H. W.: General Pathology (3d ed.; Philadelphia: W. B. Saunders Company, 1962).★

GIESEKING, R.: Mesenchymale Gewebe und ihre Reaktionsformen im elektronenoptischen Bild (Stuttgart: G. Fischer, 1966).★

GUSEK, W.: Submikroskopische Untersuchungen zur Feinstruktur aktiver Bindegewebszellen. Veröffentl. aus der morphologischen Pathologie (Stuttgart: G. Fischer, 1962).★

HENKE, F., O. LUBARSCH: Handbuch der speziellen pathologischen Anatomie und Histologie (Berlin: Springer-Verlag, 1931).★

KING, D. W., ed.: Ultrastructural Aspects of Disease (New York: Hoeber, 1966).

MAJNO, G., G. E. PALADE: J. Biophys. Biochem. Cytol. *11:* 571 (1961).

MONTGOMERY, G. L.: Textbook of Pathology (Baltimore: The Williams & Wilkins Company, 1965).★

PEREZ-TAMAYO, R.: Mechanisms of Disease (Philadelphia: W. B. Saunders Company, 1961).★

ROBBINS, S. L.: Textbook of Pathology (3rd ed.; Philadelphia: W. B. Saunders Company, 1967).★

SCHÄFER, A., R. BÄSSLER: Frankfurt. Ztschr. Path. *75:* 37 (1966).

SMITH, D. E., ed.: Survey of Pathology in Medicine and Surgery. Baltimore: Williams and Wilkins (Bimonthly review).

TRUMP, B. F., J. L. ERICSSON: In ZWEIFACH, B. W., GRANT, L., and McCLUSKEY, R. T.: The Inflammatory Process (New York: Academic Press, Inc., 1965).

WARTMAN, W. B.: Evaluation of Biopsy Diagnosis, Am. J. Clin. Path. *32:* 207 (1959).

WARTMAN, W. B., ed.: Year Book of Pathology and Clinical Pathology. Chicago; Year Book Medical Publishers (annual review).

WEISSMANN, G.: New England J. Med. *273:* 1084 (1965).

WESSEL, W., P. GEDIGK: Virchows Arch. path. Anat. *332:* 508 (1959).

Histology

BLOOM, W., D. W. FAWCETT: A Textbook of Histology (8th ed.; Philadelphia: W. B. Saunders Company. 1962).★

KARLSON, P.: Introduction to Modern Biochemistry (2d ed.; New York and London: Academic Press, Inc., 1965). (Good correlation of biochemistry and morphology.)

PORTER, K. R.: An Introduction to the Fine Structure of Cells and Tissues, K. R PORTER and M. A. BONNE-VILLE (eds.) (2d ed.; Philadelphia: Lea & Febiger, 1964).★

Heart

General
GOULD, S. E.: Pathology of the Heart (2d ed.; Springfield, Ill.: Charles C. Thomas, Publisher, 1960).★
HUDSON, R. E.: Cardiovascular Pathology (Baltimore: The Williams & Wilkins Company, 1965).

Hypertrophy
SANDRITTER, W., G. SCOMMAZONI, G.: Nature *202*: 100 (1964).
WARTMANN, W. B. and HILL, W. T.: In GOULD, S. E.: Pathology of the Heart, 2nd ed.; Springfield, Ill.: C. C. Thomas, 1960.

Atrophy
HELLERSTEIN, D., SANTIAGO-STEVENSON: Circulation *1:* 93 (1950).

Myocardial Infarct – Coronary Insufficiency
BÜCHNER, F.: Die Coronarinsuffizienz (Dresden, Leipzig: Steinkopff, 1939).★
CUSHING, E. H., H. S. FEIL, E. S. STANTON, W. B. WARTMAN: Infarction of the Cardiac Auricles. Brit. Heart J. *6:* 115 (1944).
JENNINGS, R. B., J. H. BAUM, P. B. HERDSON: Arch. Path. *79:* 135 (1965).
MALLORY, G. K., P. D. WHITE, J. SALCEDO-SALGAR: Am. Heart J. *18:* 647 (1939).
MITCHELL, J. R. A., C. J. SCHWARTZ: Arterial Disease (Oxford: Blackwell Scientific Publications, 1965).★
SOMMERS, H. M., R. B. JENNINGS: Lab. Invest. *13:* 1491 (1964).
WARTMAN, W. B.: Definition of Myocardial Infarction, in: The Etiology of Myocardial Infarction, T. N. JAMES and J. W. KEYES (eds.) (Boston: Little, Brown & Company, 1961).
WARTMAN, W. B., H. K. HELLERSTEIN: Incidence of Heart Disease. Ann. Int. Med. *28:* 41 (1948).

Myocarditis
BLANKENHORN, M. A., E. A. GALL: Circulation *13:* 217 (1956).★
SAPHIR, O.: Arch. Path. *32:* 1000 (1941).
SAPHIR, O.: Bull. Soc. int. Chir. *19:* 463 (1960).

Endocarditis
WARTMAN, W. B.: Research in Burns. *9:* 6 (1962).

Rheumatic Fever
ASCHOFF, L.: Verhandl. deutsch. Gesellsch. Path. *8:* 46 (1904).

Pericarditis
SCHORN, J.: In: Das Herz des Menschen (Stuttgart: Georg Thieme, 1956).★

Blood Vessels
ROKITANSKY, C.: Über einige der wichtigsten Krankheiten der Arterien (Wien: Hof- u. Staatsdruckerei, 1852).
WARTMAN, W. B.: Hemorrhage into the Arterial Wall. Am. Heart J. *39:* 79 (1950).

Coronary Arteriosclerosis
ENOS, F., R. H. HOLMES, J. BEYER: J. A. M. A. *152:* 1090 (1953).
FULTON, W. F. M.: The Coronary Arteries (Springfield, Ill.: Charles C. Thomas Publisher, 1965).★
KLEMPERER, P.: Am. J. Cardiol. *5:* 94 (1960).

Inflammation
BUERGER, L.: Am. J. M. Sc. *136:* 567 (1908).
LEWIS, T.: Clin. Sc. *3:* 287 (1938). (Raynaud's disease.)

Thrombosis
RODMAN, N. F., Jr., R. G. MASON, K. M. BRINKHOUS: Fed. Proc. *22:* 1356 (1963).
RODMAN, N. F., Jr., J. C. PAINTER, N. B. McDEVITT: J. Cell Biol. *16:* 225 (1963).
SANDRITTER, W.: Behringwerk-Mitteilungen *41:* 37 (1962).
SANDRITTER, W., G. BENEKE: In E. KAUFMANN and M. STAEMMLER: Lehrbuch der speziellen pathologischen Anatomie (Berlin: W. de Gruyter, 1965).★
ZAHN, W.: Int. Beitr. wissensch. Med. *2:* 199 (1891).

Lung

General
SCHULTZ, H.: Die submikroskopische Anatomie und Pathologie der Lunge (Berlin: Springer-Verlag, 1959).★

SPENCER, H.: Pathology of the Lung (Oxford: Pergamon Press, 1962).★

Fat Embolism
SEVITT, S.: Fat Embolism (London: Butterworth & Co., 1962).★

Asthma
DUNNIL, M. S.: J. Clin. Path. *13:* 27 (1960).

Interstitial Pneumonia
HAMMAN, L., A. R. RICH: Bull. Johns Hopkins Hosp. *74:* 177 (1944).

Anthracosis
ANDERSON, R. B., F. D. GUNN: Am. J. Path. *26:* 735 (1950).

Tuberculosis
Diagnostic Standards and Classification of Tuberculosis. National Tuberculosis Association, New York, 1961.★
KOCH, R.: Berl. klin. Wchnschr. *1882:* 221.
LANGHANS, TH.: Virchows Arch. path. Anat. *42:* 382 (1868).

Alimentary Tract

General
BOCKUS, H. L.: Gastroenterology (2d ed.; Philadelphia: W. B. Saunders Company, 1963).★
SHEEHY, T. W., M. H. FLOCH: The Small Intestine (New York: Hoeber Medical Division, Harper & Row, Publishers, 1964).★

Fungal Infections
EMMONS, C. W., C. H. BINFORD, J. P. UTZ: Medical Mycology (Philadelphia: Lea & Febiger, 1963).★

Gastritis
PALMER, E. D.: Medicine *33:* 199 (1954).★

Gastric Ulcer
ILLINGWORTH, C. F. W.: Peptic Ulcer (Edinburgh: E. & S. Livingstone, Ltd., 1953).★

Typhoid Fever
HUCKSTEP, R. L.: Typhoid Fever and Other Salmonella Infections (Edinburgh: E. & S. Livingstone, Ltd., 1962).★

Appendix
ASCHOFF, L.: Appendicitis (trans.) (London: G. C. Pether, 1932).

Enterocolitis
BROBERGER, O., P. PERLMANN: J. Exper. Med. *110:* 657 (1959).
KRONEBERG, G., W. SANDRITTER: Ztschr. ges. exper. Med. *120:* 329 (1953).
MOHR, H. J.: Chemotherapia *6:* 1 (1963).
SANDRITTER, W., H. G. LASCH: Pathologic Aspects of Shock, in: Methods and Achievements in Experimental Pathology (Basel: S. Karger AG., 1966).★

Regional Ileitis
CROHN, B. B., L. GINZBURG, G. D. OPPENHEIMER: J. A. M. A. *99:* 1923 (1932).

Whipple's Disease
CHEARS, W. C., C. T. ASHWORTH: Gastroenterology *41:* 129 (1961).
WHIPPLE, G. H.: Bull. Johns Hopkins Hosp. *18:* 382 (1907).

Mucoviscidosis
ANDERSON, D. H.: Ann. New York Acad. Sc. *93:* 500 (1962).

Liver

General
POPPER, H., F. SCHAFFNER: Liver: Structure and Function (New York: McGraw-Hill Book Company, Inc., 1957).★
RAPPAPORT, A. M., Z. J. BOROWY, W. M. LOUGHEED, W. H. LOTTO: Anat. Rec. *119:* 11 (1954).

Amyloidosis
TEILUM, G.: Acta path. scandinav. *61:* 21 (1964).

Eclampsia
BLACK-SCHAFFER, B., D. S. JOHNSON, W. G. GOBBEL: Am. J. Path. *26:* 397 (1950).

DEXTER, L., S. WEISS, F. W. HAYNES, H. S. SISE: J. A. M. A. *122:* 145 (1943).

Cirrhosis
SHERLOCK, S.: Diseases of the Liver and Biliary System (3d ed.; Oxford: Blackwell Scientific Publications, 1963).*
STEINER, P. E., J. HIGGINSON: Acta Un. internat. contra cancrum *17:* 581 (1961).

Erythroblastosis
ALLEN, F. H., L. K. DIAMOND: Erythroblastosis Fetalis (Boston: Little, Brown & Company, 1957).
POTTER, E. L.: Arch. Path. *41:* 223 (1946).

Electron Microscopy
ASHWORTH, C. T., D. J. WERNER, M. D. GLASS, N. J. ARNOL: Am. J. Path. *47:* 917 (1965).
BIAVA, C.: Lab. Invest. *13:* 301 (1964).
BIAVA, C.: Lab. Invest. *13:* 1099 (1964).
BIAVA, C., M. MUKLOVA-MONTIEL: Am. J. Path. *46:* 775 (1965).
HERDSON, P. B., J. P. KALTENBACH: J. Cell Biol. *25:* 485 (1965).
MALLORY, K. G.: Lab. Invest. *9:* 132 (1960).
REYNOLDS, E. S.: J. Cell Biol. *19:* 139 (1963).

Kidney

General
ALLEN, A. C.: The Kidney (New York: Grune & Stratton, Inc., 1962).*
BELL, E. T.: Renal Diseases (Philadelphia: Lea & Febiger, 1950).*
BLACK, D. A. K.: Renal Disease (Oxford: Blackwell Scientific Publications, 1962).*
HEPTINSTALL, R. H.: Pathology of the Kidney (Boston: Little, Brown & Co., 1966).
VOLHARD, F., TH. FAHR: Die Brightsche Nierenkrankheit (Berlin: Springer–Verlag, 1914).*

Nephrosis
EARLE, D. P., R. B. JENNINGS, M. BERNIK: Prog. Cardiovas. Dis. *4:* 148 (1961).

Arterio-Arteriolosclerosis
SMITH, J. P.: J. Path. Bact. *69:* 147 (1955).

Kimmelstiel – Wilson's Glomerulosclerosis
KIMMELSTIEL, P., C. WILSON: Am. J. Path. *12:* 83 (1936).

Glomerulonephritis
ELLIS, A.: Lancet *1:* 1 (1942).
HERDSON, P. B., R. B. JENNINGS, D. P. EARLE: Arch. Path. *81:* 117 (1966).
JENNINGS, R. B., D. P. EARLE: J. Clin. Invest. *40:* 1525 (1961).
MASUGI, M., Y. SATO: Virchows Arch. path. Anat. *293:* 615 (1934).
PFEIFFER, E. F., W. SANDRITTER, K. SCHÖFFLING, G. TRESER, E. KRAUS, W. MENK, M. HERRMANN: Ztschr. ges. exper. Med. *132:* 436 (1960).
SANDRITTER, W., E. F. PFEIFFER: Verhandl. deutsch. Gesellsch. Path. *43:* 213 (1959).

Pyelonephritis
QUINN, E. L., E. H. KASS: Biology of Pyelonephritis (Boston: Little, Brown & Company, 1960).*

Cysts
OSATHANONDH, V., E. L. POTTER: Arch. Path. *77:* 459 (1964).

Electron Microscopy
DALTON, A. J., F. HAGUENAU, ed.: Ultrastructure of the Kidney, New York – London: Academic Press, 1967.
MILLER, F., G. E. PALADE: J. Cell Biol. *23:* 519 (1964).
THOENES, W.: Zwanglose Abhandlung aus dem Gebiet der normalen und pathologischen Anatomie (Stuttgart: Georg Thieme, 1964).*
TOTOVIĆ, V.: Virchows Arch. path. Anat. *340:* 251 (1966).
WACHSTEIN, M., M. BESEN: Am. J. Path. *44:* 383 (1964).

Spleen and Lymph Nodes

Spleen
BLAUSTEIN, A.: The Spleen (New York: Blakiston Division, McGraw-Hill Book Company, Inc., 1963).*

Amyloid
BENDITT, E. P., N. ERIKSEN: Proc. Nat. Acad. Sc. *55:* 308 (1966).
BOERÉ, H., L. RUINEN, J. H. SCHOLTEN: J. Lab. & Clin. Med. *66:* 943 (1965).
CAESAR, R.: Path. et microbiol. (Basel) *24:* 387 (1961).
COHEN, A. S., E. GROSS, T. SHIRAHAMA: Am. J. Path. *47:* 1079 (1965).
PUCHTLER, H., F. SWEAT, M. LEVINE: J. Histochem. *10:* 355 (1962).
PUCHTLER, H., F. SWEAT: J. Histochem. *13:* 693 (1965).
SCHNEIDER, G.: Ergebn. allg. Path. u. Path. Anat. *46:* 1 (1964).★
TEILUM, G.: Am. J. Path. *32:* 945 (1956).

Lymph Nodes
MARSHALL, A. H. E.: An Outline of the Cytology and Pathology of the Reticular Tissue (London: Oliver & Boyd, Ltd., 1956).★
MASSHOFF, W.: Deutsche med. Wchnschr. *87:* 915 (1962).
PIRINGER-KUCHINKA, A.: Verhandl. deutsch. Gesellsch. Path. *36:* 352 (1953).
PIRINGER-KUCHINKA, A., I. MARTIN, O. THALHAMMER: Arch. path. Anat. *331:* 522 (1958).
WARTMAN, W. B.: Sinus Cell Hyperplasia of Lymph Nodes. Brit. J. Cancer. *13:* 389 (1959).

Boeck's Disease
FREIMAN, D. G.: New England J. Med. *239:* 664, 709, 742 (1948).

Hodgkin's Disease
FRESEN, O.: Ann. New York Acad. Sc. 73 (1958).
HOSTER, H. A., M. B. DRATMAN, L. F. CRAVER, H. A. ROLNICK: Cancer Res. *8:* 17 (1948).★

Blood and Bone Marrow
WHITBY, L. E. H., C. J. C. BRITTON: Disorders of the Blood (9th ed.; London: J. & A. Churchill, Ltd., 1963).★
WINTROBE, M. M.: Clinical Hematology (5th ed.; London: Henry Kimpton, 1961).★

Endocrine Glands

KUPPERMANN, H. S.: Human Endocrinology (London: Blackwell Scientific Publications, 1963).★
SHERWIN, R. P., V. J. ROSEN: Am. J. Clin. Path. *43:* 200 (1965).

Genital Organs
HAINES, M., C. W. TAYLOR: Gynecological Pathology (London: J. & A. Churchill, Ltd., 1962).★
KLINEFELTER, A. F., E. C. REIFENSTEIN, F. ALBRIGHT: J. Clin. Endocrinol. *2:* 615 (1942).
NOVAK, E.: Gynecologic and Obstetric Pathology (Philadelphia: W. B. Saunders Company, 1953).★

Skin and Muscle
ADAMS, R. D., D. DENNY-BROWN, C. M. PEARSON: Disease of Muscle (2d ed.; New York: Hoeber Medical Division, Harper & Row, Publishers, 1962).★
GREENFIELD, J. G., G. M. SHY, E. C. ALVORD, L. BERG: An Atlas of Muscle Pathology in Neuromuscular Diseases (Edinburgh: E. & S. Livingstone, Ltd., 1957).★
LEVER, W. F.: Histopathology of the Skin (3d ed.; Philadelphia: J. B. Lippincott Company, 1961).★

Bones and Joints

HARRISON, C. V.: Diseases of Bone, Chapter IX in Recent Advances in Pathology (7th ed.; London: J. & A. Churchill, Ltd., 1960).
JAFFE, H. L.: Tumours and Tumorous Conditions of the Bones and Joints (London: Henry Kimpton, 1958).★
LICHTENSTEIN, L.: Bone Tumors (St. Louis: C. V. Mosby Company, 1959).★
PAGET, J.: Med. Chir. Tr., London *60:* 37 (1877).

Brain and Spinal Cord

General
BLACKWOOD, W., W. H. MCMENEMEY, A. EYER, R. M. NORMAN, D. S. RUSSEL: In Greenfield: Neuropathology (London: Edward Arnold & Co., 1963).★
WARTMAN, W. B.: Pathology of Epidemic Typhus. Arch. Path. *56:* 397, 512 (1953).

Tumors

Reviews
AMBROSE, E. J., F. J. ROE: The Biology of Cancer (London: D. van Nostrand, 1963).
Atlas of Tumor Pathology. Armed Forces Institute, Washington, D. C., 1953.★
BERNHARD, W., N. GRANBOULAN: Exper. Cell. Res., suppl. 9, 1963.
BUSCH, H.: Biochemistry of the Cancer Cell (New York: Academic Press, Inc., 1962).★
DENOIX, P.: Mechanism of Invasion in Cancer (U.I.C.C. Monograph, vol. 6. Heidelberg: Springer, 1967).
HAMPERL, H.: Atlas der Tumornomenklatur (Heidelberg: Springer, 1965).★
HOMBURGER, F.: The Physiopathology of Cancer (New York: Hoeber Medical Division, Harper & Row, Publishers, 1953).★
POTTER, V. R.: Cancer Res. *24:* 1085 (1964).★
WILLIS, R. A.: Pathology of Tumours (London: Butterworth & Co., Ltd., 1960).★

Carcinogenesis
Ciba Foundation Symposium on Carcinogenesis (London: J. & A. Churchill, Ltd., 1959).★

Electron Microscopy
BERNHARD, W.: Cancer Res. *20:* 712 (1960).★
BERNHARD, W.: Verhandl. deutsch. Gesellsch. Path. 1961, S. 8. G. Fischer, Stuttgart.★
BURKITT, D.: Brit. J. Surg. *46:* 218 (1958).
PARRY, E. W., F. N. GHADIALLY: Cancer *18:* 1026 (1965).
STEWART, S. E.: Tr. New York Acad. Sc. *28:* 290 (1966).

Tumors of Skin and Mucosae
DUKES, C. E.: J. Path. & Bact. *50:* 527 (1940).
MACKEE, G. M., A. C. CIPOLLARO: Am. J. Cancer, 1937.★
STOUT, A. P.: Tumors of the Stomach. Atlas of Tumor Pathology. Bd. VI/21. Armed Forces Institute of Pathology, Washington, D. C., 1953.★

Mammary Tumors
BONSER, G. M., I. A. DOSSE, I. W. JULL: Human and Experimental Breast Cancer (London: Pitman, 1961).★
MUIR, R.: J. Path. & Bact. *42:* 155 (1941).

Ovarian Tumors
BARZILAI, G.: Atlas of Ovarian Tumors (New York: Grune & Stratton, Inc., 1949).★
ENGE, L. A.: Am. J. Obst. & Gynec. *68:* 348 (1954).

Basalioma
ALBERTINI, A.: Schweiz. med. Wchnschr. *1941:* 992.
KROMPECHER, E.: Beitr. path. Anat. *28:* 1 (1900).
ASSOR, D.: Cancer *20:* 2125 (1967).

Hypernephroma
KING STANTON: Renal Neoplasia. (Boston: Little, Brown & Company, 1967.)

Carcinoma In Situ
HAMPERL, H.: In Cancer of the Cervix, Ciba Foundation Study Group, No. 3 (London: J. & A. Churchill, Ltd., 1959).
SANDRITTER, W.: In A. LINKE: Früherkennung des Krebses. S. 43 (Stuttgart: F. K. Schattauer, 1962).
SANDRITTER, W.: Verhandl. deutsch. Gesellsch. Path. *48:* 34 (1964).

Paget's Carcinoma
PAGET, J.: St. Bartholomew's Hosp. Rep. X (1874).

Metastasis
WALTHER, H. E.: Krebsmetastasen (Basel: B. Schwabe, 1948).★
WILLIS, R. A.: The Spread of Tumors in the Human Body (2d ed.; London: Butterworth & Co., Ltd., 1952).★

Chorionepithelioma
AHLSTRÖM, C. G.: Acta path. scandinav. *8:* 213 (1931).

Fibroma
CAPELL, D. F., G. L. MONTGOMERY: J. Path. & Bact. *44:* 517 (1937).
STOUT, A. P.: Bull. Hosp. Joint Dis. (N. Y.) *12:* 126 (1951).
STOUT, A. P.: Cancer *7:* 953 (1954).

Keloid

GARB, J., M. J. STONE: Am. J. Surg. *58:* 315 (1942).

Myxoma

STOUT, A. P.: Ann. Surg. *127:* 706 (1948).

Hemangioma

McCARTHY, W. D., G. T. PACK: Surg., Gynec. & Obst. *91:* 465 (1950).
STOUT, A. P.: Cancer *2:* 1027 (1949).

Sarcoma

STOUT, A. P.: Cancer *1:* 30 (1948).

Fibrosarcoma

STOUT, A. P.: Tumors of the Soft Tissues. Atlas of Tumor Pathology. II/5. Armed Forces Institute of
    Pathology, Washington, D. C., 1953.

Neurinoma, Neurofibroma

RECKLINGHAUSEN, F. D. VON: Festschrift für Rudolf Virchow. S. 138 (Berlin: Hirschwald, 1882).

Brain Tumors

RUSSEL, D., L. J. RUBINSTEIN: Pathology of Tumors of the Nervous System (London: Edward Arnold
    & Co., 1959).★

Pigmented Nevus, Melanoma

AFFLECK, D. H.: Am. J. Cancer *27:* 120 (1936).
KLAUDER, J. V., H. BEERMANN: Arch. Dermat. *71:* 2 (1955).
MASSON, P.: Am. J. Path. *8:* 367 (1932).

Cytodiagnosis

GRAHAM, R. M.: The Cytologic Diagnosis of Cancer (2d ed.; Philadelphia: W. B. Saunders Company,
    1963).★
KOSS, L. G., G. R. DURFEE: Diagnostic Cytology and Its Histopathologic Bases (London: Pitman, 1961).★
PAPANICOLAOU, G. N.: Atlas of Exfoliative Cytology (Cambridge, Mass.: Harvard University Press,
    1954).★

Fungi – Parasites

General

ASH, J. E., S. SPITZ: Pathology of Tropical Diseases (Philadelphia: W. B. Saunders Company, 1947).★
EMMONS, C. W., C. H. BINFORD, J. P. UTZ: Medical Mycology (Philadelphia: Lea & Febiger, 1963).★
FAUST, E. C., P. F. RUSSELL: Craig and Faust's Clinical Parasitology (6th ed.; Philadelphia: Lea & Febiger,
    1957).★
SMITH, D. T., N. F. CONANT: Zinsser Microbiology (12th ed.; New York: Appleton-Century-Crofts,
    Inc., 1960).★

Technic

COONS, A. H., M. H. KAPLAN: J. Exper. Med. *91:* 1 (1950).
GRIDLEY, M. F.: Am. J. Clin. Path. *23:* 303 (1953).
GROCOTT, R. G.: Am. J. Clin. Path. *25:* 975, 1955.

Amebic Dysentery

FAUST, E. C.: Amebiasis (Springfield, Ill.: Charles C Thomas, Publisher, 1954).★

Cystocercosis

DIXON, H. B. F., F. M. LIPSCOMB: Med. Res. Council Ser. No. 292, London, 1961.★

Kala-Azar

DONOVAN, C.: Brit. M. J. *1903:* 79.
LEISHMAN, W. B.: Brit. M. J. *1903:* 1252.

Chagas' Disease

CHAGAS, C.: Mem. Inst. Oswaldo Cruz, *2:* 159 (1909).
GOULD, S. E.: Am. J. Path. *36:* 533 (1960).

Larva Migrans
BEAVER, P. C.: Exper. Parasitol. *5:* 587 (1956).★

Pneumocystis
CARINI, A.: Com. Soc. Med. São Paulo, p. 204, August 16, 1910.
HAMPERL, H.: Maandschr. kinderheilk. *108:* 132 (1960).

Candidiasis
LODDER, J., N. J. W. KREGER-VAN RIJ: The Yeasts (Amsterdam: North-Holland Publishing Company, 1952).★
ROBINSON, H. M.: Arch. Dermat. *70:* 640 (1954).
WINNER, H. I., R. HURLEY: Candida Albicans (London: J. & A. Churchill, Ltd., 1964).

Actinomycosis
WEED, L. A., A. H. BAGGENSTOSS: Am. J. Clin. Path. *19:* 201 (1949).

Cryptococcosis
LITTMAN, M. L., L. E. ZIMMERMANN: Cryptococcosis (New York: Grune & Stratton, Inc., 1956).★

Coccidioidomycosis
AJELLO, L.: Coccidioidomycosis (Tucson, Ariz.: Univ. Arizona Press, 1967).
FIESE, M. J.: Coccidioidomycosis (Springfield, Ill.: Charles C Thomas, Publisher, 1958).★
SMITH, L. E.: Coccidioidomycosis. H. A. Christian, Oxford Medicine, Vol. V/XIV-B. 1943.★

Histoplasmosis
BINFORD, C. H.: Am. J. Clin. Path. *25:* 25 (1955).
DARLING, S. T.: J. A. M. A. *46:* 1283 (1906).
EMMONS, C. W.: Pub. Health Rep. *64:* 892 (1949).
STRAUB, M., J. SCHWARZ: Am. J. Clin. Path. *25:* 727 (1955).
STRAUB, M., J. SCHWARZ: J. Path. et Microbiol. (Basel) *25:* 421 (1962).
SWEANY, H. C.: Histoplasmosis (Springfield, Ill.: Charles C Thomas, Publisher, 1960).★

Paracoccidioidomycosis
SALFELDER, K., M. HARTUNG: Sourcebook of Skin Diseases (New York: Hoeber Medical Division, Harper & Row, Publishers). In press.★

Blastomycosis
GILCHRIST, T. C.: Rep. Johns Hopkins Hosp. *1:* 269 (1896).
MOVAT, H. Z., N. V. P. FERNANDO: Lab. Invest. *12:* 895 (1963).
NELSON, E., K. BLINZINGER, H. HAGER: J. Neuropath. & Exper. Neurol. *21:* 155 (1962).
PROSE, P. H., L. LEE, S. D. BALK: Am. J. Path. *47:* 403 (1965).
SAMORAJSKY, T., J. M. ORDY, J. R. KEEFE: J. Cell Biol. *26:* 779 (1965).
SCHWARZ, J., G. L. BAUM: Am. J. Clin. Path. *21:* 999 (1951).
STEINER, J. W., A. JÉZÉQUEL, M. J. PHILLIPS, K. MIYAI, K. ARAKAWA: Progress in Liver Diseases (New York Grune & Stratton, Inc., 1965).★
WIENER, J., D. SPIRO, R. G. LATTES: Am. J. Path. *47:* 457 (1965).

Index